Chronic Kidney Disease

Editors

DAVID J. POLZIN
LARRY D. COWGILL

VETERINARY CLINICS
OF NORTH AMERICA:
SMALL ANIMAL PRACTICE

www.vetsmall.theclinics.com

November 2016 • Volume 46 • Number 6

ELSEVIER

1600 John F. Kennedy Boulevard • Suite 1800 • Philadelphia, Pennsylvania, 19103-2899
http://www.vetsmall.theclinics.com

VETERINARY CLINICS OF NORTH AMERICA: SMALL ANIMAL PRACTICE Volume 46, Number 6
November 2016 ISSN 0195-5616, ISBN-13: 978-0-323-47698-0

Editor: Patrick Manley
Developmental Editor: Meredith Clinton

Veterinary Clinics of North America: Small Animal Practice (ISSN 0195-5616) is published bimonthly by Elsevier Inc., 360 Park Avenue South, New York, NY 10010-1710. Months of issue are January, March, May, July, September, and November. Business and Editorial Offices: 1600 John F. Kennedy Blvd., Ste. 1800, Philadelphia, PA 19103-2899. Customer Service Office: 3251 Riverport Lane, Maryland Heights, MO 63043. Periodicals postage paid at New York, NY and additional mailing offices. Subscription prices are $310.00 per year (domestic individuals), $564.00 per year (domestic institutions), $100.00 per year (domestic students/residents), $410.00 per year (Canadian individuals), $701.00 per year (Canadian institutions), $455.00 per year (international individuals), $701.00 per year (international institutions), and $220.00 per year (international and Canadian students/residents). To receive student/resident rate, orders must be accompanied by name of affiliated institution, date of term, and the *signature* of program/residency coordinator on institution letterhead. Orders will be billed at individual rate until proof of status is received. Foreign air speed delivery is included in all *Clinics* subscription prices. All prices are subject to change without notice. **POSTMASTER:** Send address changes to *Veterinary Clinics of North America: Small Animal Practice*, Elsevier Health Sciences Division, Subscription Customer Service, 3251 Riverport Lane, Maryland Heights, MO 63043. Customer Service (orders, claims, online, change of address): Elsevier Periodicals Customer Service, Elsevier Health Sciences Division Subscription **Customer Service 3251 Riverport Lane Maryland Heights, MO 63043. Tel: 1-800-654-2452 (U.S. and Canada); 314-447-8871 (outside U.S. and Canada). Fax: 314-447-8029. E-mail: journalscustomerservice-usa@elsevier.com (for print support); journalsonlinesupport-usa@elsevier.com (for online support).**

Reprints. For copies of 100 or more of articles in this publication, please contact the Commercial Reprints Department, Elsevier Inc., 360 Park Avenue South, New York, NY 10010-1710. Tel.: 212-633-3874; Fax: 212-633-3820; E-mail: reprints@elsevier.com.

Veterinary Clinics of North America: Small Animal Practice is also published in Japanese by Inter Zoo Publishing Co., Ltd., Aoyama Crystal-Bldg 5F, 3-5-12 Kitaaoyama, Minato-ku, Tokyo 107-0061, Japan.

Veterinary Clinics of North America: Small Animal Practice is covered in *Current Contents/Agriculture, Biology and Environmental Sciences, Science Citation Index, ASCA, MEDLINE/PubMed (Index Medicus), Excerpta Medica, and BIOSIS.*

Printed in the United States of America.

Contributors

EDITORS

DAVID J. POLZIN, DVM, PhD
Diplomate, American College of Veterinary Internal Medicine; Professor and Chief of Small Animal Internal Medicine, Department of Veterinary Clinical Sciences, College of Veterinary Medicine, University of Minnesota, St Paul, Minnesota

LARRY D. COWGILL, DVM, PhD
Diplomate, American College of Veterinary Internal Medicine (Small Animal); Associate Dean, Southern California Clinical Programs; Director, University of California Veterinary Medical Center – San Diego, San Diego, California; Professor, Department of Medicine and Epidemiology, School of Veterinary Medicine, University of California, Davis, Davis, California

AUTHORS

LILLIAN R. ARONSON, VMD
Diplomate, American College of Veterinary Surgery; Professor of Surgery, Department of Clinical Studies, School of Veterinary Medicine, University of Pennsylvania, Philadelphia, Pennsylvania

SCOTT BROWN, VMD, PhD
Diplomate, American College of Veterinary Internal Medicine (Small Animal); Edward H. Gunst Professor of Small Animal Medicine; Associate Dean for Academic Affairs, Department of Physiology and Pharmacology, College of Veterinary Medicine, The University of Georgia, Athens, Georgia

JULIE A. CHURCHILL, DVM, PhD
Diplomate, American College of Veterinary Nutrition; Associate Professor and Chief of Clinical Nutrition, Department of Veterinary Clinical Sciences, College of Veterinary Medicine, University of Minnesota, St Paul, Minnesota

CELESTE CLEMENTS, DVM
Diplomate, American College of Veterinary Internal Medicine; Medical Content Specialist, Companion Animal Group Medical Organization, IDEXX, Westbrook, Maine

LARRY D. COWGILL, DVM, PhD
Diplomate, American College of Veterinary Internal Medicine (Small Animal); Associate Dean, Southern California Clinical Programs; Director, University of California Veterinary Medical Center – San Diego, San Diego, California; Professor, Department of Medicine and Epidemiology, School of Veterinary Medicine, University of California, Davis, Davis, California

WILLIAM T.N. CULP, VMD
Diplomate, American College of Veterinary Surgeons; Assistant Professor, Department of Surgical and Radiological Sciences, School of Veterinary Medicine, University of California, Davis, Davis, California

JONATHAN ELLIOTT, MA, Vet MB, PhD, Cert SAC, MRCVS
Diplomate, European College of Veterinary Pharmacology and Toxicology; Vice Principal, Research and Innovation, Professor of Veterinary Clinical Pharmacology, Department of Comparative Biomedical Sciences, Royal Veterinary College, University of London, London, United Kingdom

GIOSI FARACE, MSc, PhD
Staff Scientist, IDEXX Laboratories, Research & Development, Westbrook, Maine

JONATHAN D. FOSTER, VMD
Diplomate, American College of Veterinary Internal Medicine (Small Animal Internal Medicine); Department of Clinical Studies, University of Pennsylvania School of Veterinary Medicine, Philadelphia, Pennsylvania

GREGORY F. GRAUER, DVM, MS
Diplomate, American College of Veterinary Internal Medicine (Small Animal); Professor and Jarvis Chair of Medicine, Department of Clinical Sciences, College of Veterinary Medicine, Kansas State University, Manhattan, Kansas

ROSANNE E. JEPSON, BVSc, MVetMed, PhD, FHEA, MRCVS
Diplomate, American College of Veterinary Internal Medicine; Diplomate, European College of Veterinary Internal Medicine - Companion Animals; Department of Clinical Science and Services, Royal Veterinary College, Hertfordshire, United Kingdom

DOTTIE P. LAFLAMME, DVM, PhD
Diplomate, American College of Veterinary Nutrition; Consultant, Scientific Communications, Floyd, Virginia

CATHY LANGSTON, DVM
Diplomate, American College of Veterinary Internal Medicine (Small Animal); Associate Professor, Department of Veterinary Clinical Sciences, The Ohio State University College of Veterinary Medicine, Columbus, Ohio

JENNIFER A. LARSEN, DVM, PhD
Diplomate, American College of Veterinary Nutrition; Associate Professor of Clinical Nutrition, Molecular Biosciences, School of Veterinary Medicine, University of California, Davis, Davis, California

HAGAR MELTZER, DVM
Koret School of Veterinary Medicine, The Hebrew University of Jerusalem, Rehovot, Israel

MARY B. NABITY, DVM, PhD
Diplomate, American College of Veterinary Pathology (Clinical Pathology); Assistant Professor, Department of Veterinary Pathobiology, College of Veterinary Medicine & Biomedical Sciences, Texas A&M University, College Station, Texas

CARRIE A. PALM, DVM
Diplomate, American College of Veterinary Internal Medicine; Assistant Professor, Department of Medicine and Epidemiology, School of Veterinary Medicine, University of California, Davis, Davis, California

DAVID J. POLZIN, DVM, PhD
Diplomate, American College of Veterinary Internal Medicine; Professor and Chief of Small Animal Internal Medicine, Department of Veterinary Clinical Sciences, College of Veterinary Medicine, University of Minnesota, St Paul, Minnesota

JESSICA M. QUIMBY, DVM, PhD
Diplomate, American College of Veterinary Internal Medicine; Assistant Professor, Department of Clinical Sciences, Colorado State University, Fort Collins, Colorado

JOHN QUINN, MS
Senior Staff Scientist, IDEXX Laboratories, Research & Development, Westbrook, Maine

ROBERTA RELFORD, DVM, MS, PhD
Diplomate, American College of Veterinary Internal Medicine; Diplomate, American College of Veterinary Pathologists; Vice President; Chief Medical Officer, Companion Animal Group Medical Organization, IDEXX, Westbrook, Maine

JANE ROBERTSON, DVM
Diplomate, American College of Veterinary Internal Medicine; Director of Medical Affairs, Companion Animal Group Medical Organization, IDEXX, Westbrook, Maine

SHERI ROSS, DVM, PhD
Diplomate, American College of Veterinary Internal Medicine; Coordinator, Department of Hemodialysis/Nephrology/Urology, University of California Veterinary Medical Center – San Diego, San Diego, California

MARGIE A. SCHERK, DVM
Diplomate, American Board of Veterinary Practitioners (Feline Practice); Private Consultant, CatsINK, Vancouver, British Columbia, Canada

GILAD SEGEV, DVM
Diplomate, European College of Veterinary Internal Medicine - Companion Animals; Senior Lecturer of Veterinary Medicine; Department Head, Small Animal Internal Medicine, Koret School of Veterinary Medicine, The Hebrew University of Jerusalem, Rehovot, Israel

ANNA SHIPOV, DVM
Diplomate, European College of Veterinary Surgeons; Koret School of Veterinary Medicine, The Hebrew University of Jerusalem, Rehovot, Israel

SHELLY L. VADEN, DVM, PhD
Diplomate, American College of Veterinary Medicine; Professor of Internal Medicine, Department of Clinical Sciences, College of Veterinary Medicine, North Carolina State University, Raleigh, North Carolina

ASTRID M. VAN DONGEN, DVM
Department of Clinical Sciences of Companion Animals, Utrecht, The Netherlands

MAHA YERRAMILLI, MS, PhD
Staff Scientist, IDEXX Laboratories, Research & Development, Westbrook, Maine

MURTHY YERRAMILLI, PhD
Vice President, R&D, IDEXX Laboratories, Research & Development, Westbrook, Maine

Contents

Chronic kidney disease (CKD) is a common condition in cats and dogs,
traditionally diagnosed after substantial loss of kidney function when
serum creatinine concentrations increase. Symmetric dimethylarginine
(SDMA) is a sensitive circulating kidney biomarker whose concentrations
increase earlier than creatinine as glomerular filtration rate decreases.
Unlike creatinine, SDMA is unaffected by lean body mass. The IDEXX
SDMA test introduces a clinically relevant and reliable tool for the diagnosis and management of kidney disease. SDMA has been provisionally
incorporated into the International Renal Interest Society guidelines for
CKD to aid staging and targeted treatment of early and advanced
disease.

Chronic kidney disease (CKD) and acute kidney injury (AKI) are interconnected and the presence of one is a risk for the other. CKD is an important
predictor of AKI after exposure to nephrotoxic drugs or major surgery,
whereas persistent or repetitive injury could result in the progression of
CKD. This brings new perspectives to the diagnosis and monitoring of kidney diseases highlighting the need for a panel of kidney-specific biomarkers that reflect functional as well as structural damage and
recovery, predict potential risk and provide prognosis. This article discusses the kidney-specific biomarkers, symmetric dimethylarginine
(SDMA), clusterin, cystatin B, and inosine.

International Renal Interest Society chronic kidney disease Stage 1 and
acute kidney injury Grade I categorizations of kidney disease are often
confused or ignored because patients are nonazotemic and generally
asymptomatic. Recent evidence suggests these seemingly disparate conditions may be mechanistically linked and interrelated. Active kidney injury

biomarkers have the potential to establish a new understanding for traditional views of chronic kidney disease, including its early identification and
possible mediators of its progression, which, if validated, would establish
a new and sophisticated paradigm for the understanding and approach to
the diagnostic evaluation, and treatment of urinary disease in dogs and cats.

In cats with chronic kidney disease (CKD), the most common histopathologic finding is tubulointerstitial inflammation and fibrosis; however, these
changes reflect a nonspecific response of the kidney to any inciting injury.
The risk of developing CKD is likely to reflect the composite effects of genetic predisposition, aging, and environmental and individual factors that
affect renal function over the course of a cat's life. There is still little information available to determine exactly which individual risk factors predispose a cat to develop CKD. Although many cats diagnosed with CKD have
stable disease for years, some cats show overtly progressive disease.

Renal diets have been the mainstay of therapy for cats with chronic kidney
disease (CKD) for many decades. Clinical trials in cats with CKD have
shown them to be effective in improving survival, reducing uremic crises,
and improving serum urea nitrogen and phosphorous concentrations. It
has shown that, when food intake is adequate, renal diets can maintain
body weight and body condition scores for up to 2 years. Although
some have questioned whether renal diets provide adequate protein and
have advocated feeding higher-protein diets to cats with CKD, there is
currently no convincing evidence in support of this proposal.

Renal diets typically incorporate protein and phosphorus restriction, supplement with potassium and Omega-3 fatty acids, and address metabolic
acidosis. Compared to "maintenance" diets, these modifications appear
to benefit cats with chronic kidney disease (CKD); however, there is limited
data in cats justifying the specific amounts of the nutrients used in these
diets, and there is little evidence supporting protein restriction in cats
with CKD. Energy intake, maintenance of body weight, and muscle and
body condition need to be addressed, and may take precedence over special diets. Further research is needed to better define optimum diets for
cats with CKD.

> The role of diet in management of chronic kidney disease (CKD) is important. There are different interpretations of the current knowledge on this topic. Neither clinical trials involving product testing, nor prospective research investigating dietary influences on cats with induced kidney disease provide guidance on the utility of specific nutritional strategies. Likewise, data derived from other species also has limitations. More research is needed to further our understanding of this topic; however, practical guidance from current knowledge for the management of individual patients can be utilized with success.

> Esophagostomy feeding tubes are useful, and, in many cases essential, for the comprehensive management of cats with moderate to advanced chronic kidney disease (CKD). They should be considered a lifelong therapeutic appliance to facilitate the global management of cats with CKD thus providing improved therapeutic efficacy and quality of life. Esophagostomy tubes facilitate the maintenance of adequate hydration and increase owner compliance by facilitating the administration of medications. Finally, feeding tubes provide a means to deliver a stage-appropriate dietary prescription for cats with CKD and maintain an adequate nutritional plane in a patient that otherwise would be subject to chronic wasting.

> Proteinuria is a negative prognostic indicator for dogs and cats with chronic kidney disease. A normal dog or cat should excrete very little protein and have a urine protein:creatinine ratio that is less than 0.4, or less than 0.2, respectively; persistent proteinuria above this magnitude warrants attention. Administration of angiotensin converting enzyme inhibitors and/or angiotensin receptor blockers, blood pressure control and nutritional modification are considered a standard of care for renal proteinuria. Renal biopsy and administration of immunosuppressive agents should be considered in animals with glomerular proteinuria that have not responded to standard therapy. Targeted patient monitoring is essential when instituting management of proteinuria.

> The inappropriate phosphorus retention observed in chronic kidney disease is central to the pathophysiology of mineral and bone disorders observed in these patients. Subsequent derangements in serum fibroblast growth

factor 23, parathyroid hormone, and calcitriol concentrations play contributory roles. Therapeutic intervention involves dietary phosphorus restriction and intestinal phosphate binders in order to correct phosphorus retention and maintain normocalcemia. Additional therapies may be considered to normalize serum fibroblast growth factor 23 and parathyroid hormone.

Secondary renal hyperparathyroidism is an inevitable consequence of chronic kidney disease. In human patients, the disease is associated with decreased bone quality and increased fracture risk. Recent evidence suggests that bone quality is also decreased in companion animals, more pronouncedly in cats compared with dogs, likely because of a longer disease course. The clinical significance of these findings is yet to be determined. Clinicians should keep in mind that animals with chronic kidney disease have decreased bone quality and increased fracture risk.

Dysregulation of normal kidney functions in chronic kidney disease (CKD) leads to several pathophysiologic abnormalities that have the potential to significantly clinically affect the CKD patient. This article discusses the clinical impact of hypertension, hypokalemia, anemia, dysrexia, nausea/vomiting, and constipation in the CKD patient and therapies for these conditions. These clinical manifestations of disease may not occur in every patient and may also develop later during the progression of disease. Therefore, monitoring for, identifying, and addressing these factors is considered an important part of the medical management of CKD.

Canine and feline nephroureteral obstruction is a complex disease process that can be challenging to treat. Although the availability of various imaging modalities allows for a straightforward diagnosis to be made in most cases, the decision-making process for when a case should be taken to surgery and the optimal treatment modality that should be used for renal decompression remains controversial. In the following discussion, an overview of the perioperative management of cases with nephroureterolithiasis and nephroureteral obstruction is reviewed, with particular focus on the use of renal decompressive procedures, such as ureteral stenting and subcutaneous ureteral bypass system placement.

Kidney transplantation is a novel treatment option for cats suffering from chronic renal failure or acute irreversible renal injury. Improvement in quality of life as well as survival times of cats that have undergone transplantation has helped the technique to gain acceptance as a viable treatment option for this fatal disease. This article reviews information regarding the optimal time for intervention, congenital and acquired conditions that have been successfully treated with transplantation, recipient and donor screening, immunosuppressive therapy, recent advances in anesthetic and surgical management, postoperative monitoring and long-term management, and troubleshooting perioperative and long-term complications.

VETERINARY CLINICS OF NORTH AMERICA: SMALL ANIMAL PRACTICE

THE CLINICS ARE NOW AVAILABLE ONLINE!
Access your subscription at:
www.theclinics.com

Preface

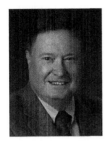
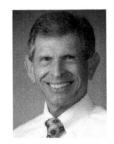

David J. Polzin, DVM, PhD, DACVIM   Larry D. Cowgill, DVM, PhD, DACVIM
Editors

Chronic kidney disease (CKD) remains an important and significant cause of morbidity and mortality in dogs and cats. The understanding, assessment, and management of CKD in veterinary practice is evolving rapidly from its foundations in serum creatinine and therapeutic diets to sophisticated diagnostic testing, novel therapies, and changing clinical paradigms. Yet, in some cases, the new advances represent merely a reunderstanding of established concepts: "old tricks for new dogs." In other cases, there are directional shifts and emerging technologies redirecting our previous understanding: "new tricks for old dogs."

In the area of evolving diagnostic assessments for CKD, novel biomarkers exemplified by symmetric dimethylarginine now provide diagnostic extension and increased sensitivity to the time-honored value of serum creatinine for the detection and monitoring of CKD. Equally exciting is the development of diagnostic markers of active kidney injury with the potential and sensitivity to detect the presence and persistence of kidney injury before it is suspected clinically or detectable by conventional diagnostics.

Deeper probing into cellular function and regulatory processes defining kidney health and kidney disease suggests the same molecular processes that control and regulate normal kidney function also may participate in the responses to kidney injury. These cellular pathways can become dysregulated by even subtle pathologic "stresses" and promote maladaptive responses that signal progressive erosion of kidney mass and function that remains subclinical in the early and evolving stages of progression. These new insights provide potential for strategic therapeutic targets to prevent progressive kidney disease. The detection and characterization of early and asymptomatic kidney disease must become a higher diagnostic priority. Logically, advanced CKD recognized at a point when it is clinically evident must have extended from a milder, less evident, and less advanced stage of CKD. Going forward, clinical practice patterns must be modified to incorporate emerging diagnostics to detect and characterize asymptomatic kidney disease (IRIS CKD stage 1). When detected early, therapeutic strategies will be more effective to slow or halt progression of CKD to more advanced stages associated with progressive morbidity and less therapeutic potential.

Vet Clin Small Anim 46 (2016) xiii–xv
http://dx.doi.org/10.1016/j.cvsm.2016.07.011
0195-5616/16/© 2016 Published by Elsevier Inc.

vetsmall.theclinics.com

The concept of spontaneous progression of CKD has been recognized for many decades, and current evidence supports that this concept is applicable to dogs and cats with CKD. Extensive research has led to a more sophisticated understanding of some of the mechanisms underlying progression of CKD, particularly in cats. The combination of improved diagnostics for recognizing early kidney disease as well as ongoing kidney injuries is potentially synergistic with the expanding understanding of progression of CKD. These exciting findings provide opportunities for intervening earlier in the course of CKD, thereby allowing us to provide a period of extending high quality of life, possibly even stopping progression of CKD before clinical signs develop.

An important controversy in Veterinary Nephrology has developed in recent years: what should be fed to cats with CKD. Although renal diets have been recommended for decades with the expectation that they will be effective in mitigating clinical signs of uremia and slowing progression of CKD, their clinical effectiveness and nutritional impact recently have been challenged. Some veterinarians have even suggested that cats with CKD should be fed high-protein diets. Three views of the current status of recommending renal diet therapy for cats are presented in this issue: the evidence supporting current feline therapeutic renal diets, the evidence questioning the current formulations of renal diets, and an overview of the disagreements concerning limiting protein content in renal diets. In addition to the impact of diet formulation, assuring adequate food ingestion is an important component of maintaining adequate nutrition in cats with CKD. The role of feeding tubes in preventing nutritional deficiencies in cats with CKD also is presented.

Two critical therapies linked to slowing progression of CKD are minimalizing proteinuria and limiting phosphorus intake. New approaches to managing proteinuria appear to enhance the effectiveness of reducing the magnitude of proteinuria, thereby potentially slowing progression of kidney disease. There are exciting new insights into the pathophysiologic events that maintain phosphorus balance in patients with CKD. Not surprising, our old construct of renal secondary hyperparathyroidism has been found lacking. Nonetheless, controlling phosphorus intake remains pivotal. An increasing variety of intestinal phosphate binders have become available for managing phosphorus balance. These have expanded our options for therapy and vary in effectiveness, side effects, and cost. In some patients, ionized hypercalcemia or ionized hypocalcemia may indicate the need for pharmacologic modification of serum calcium concentration.

Renal osteopathy is a classic and consistent feature of CKD documented and managed in human patients for decades but rarely recognized or specifically managed as a feature in dogs and cats. However, with utilization of sophisticated imaging and biomechanical techniques, reviewed in this issue, there now is compelling evidence these classic features of CKD also are pathologic features of naturally occurring CKD in dogs and cats. These new revelations require an updating of our concepts of mineral and bone disease in animal patients and reprogramming of our diagnostic approaches and holistic approach to the management of CKD. Similarly, CKD must be recognized as a polysystemic syndrome that necessitates a broad-reaching and comprehensive therapeutic approach. To be effective, the therapy must be global to ameliorate all identifiable consequences of CKD to targeted endpoints, not merely a ritualistic or uniform approach that fails to address all manifestations.

Renal transplantation, once the advanced standard for the surgical management of CKD in cats, has nearly vanished as an option for animals despite its persisting role in human nephrology. The transition in surgical interests and expertise from microvascular techniques to interventional technologies likely has contributed to this change in status. There is still opportunity and need to resurrect renal transplantation as an ongoing and future strategy for the correction of CKD in cats (and perhaps dogs) as newer advances in graph-versus-host prevention or development of genetically engineered kidneys evolves. Despite its potential impact on renal transplantation, the advent of interventional surgical expertise and devices emerged fortuitously with the emergence of ureteral obstruction as a major cause for both acute and chronic kidney disease in cats. The use of stents and subcutaneous ureteral bypass systems for the management of ureteral obstruction has provided a treatment option that is more effective and less morbid than their predecessor medical or surgical approaches.

In this issue, we have attempted to update the current and topical issues surrounding CKD in dogs and cats. We have chosen to review old issues that require conceptual updating and the conventional understanding of CKD through the lens of new technologies and insights. We hope introduction of these new concepts and therapies will catalyze future developments in the practice of veterinary nephrology.

David J. Polzin, DVM, PhD, DACVIM
Department of Veterinary Clinical Sciences
College of Veterinary Medicine
University of Minnesota
1352 Boyd Avenue, St Paul, MN 55108, USA

Larry D. Cowgill, DVM, PhD, DACVIM
Department of Medicine and Epidemiology
School of Veterinary Medicine
University of California Davis
Davis, CA 95616, USA

E-mail addresses:
polzi001@umn.edu (D.J. Polzin)
ldcowgill@ucdavis.edu (L.D. Cowgill)

Symmetric Dimethylarginine

Improving the Diagnosis and Staging of Chronic Kidney Disease in Small Animals

Roberta Relford, DVM, MS, PhD, Jane Robertson, DVM,
Celeste Clements, DVM*

KEYWORDS

- SDMA • Symmetric dimethylarginine • Renal biomarker • Chronic kidney disease
- CKD • IRIS • IDEXX SDMA test • GFR

KEY POINTS

- Symmetric dimethylarginine (SDMA) is a new kidney biomarker that accurately reflects glomerular filtration fate (GFR).
- SDMA level increases earlier in chronic kidney disease (CKD), on average with 40% reduction of GFR, compared with up to 75% reduction needed to increase creatinine level.
- Unlike creatinine, SDMA is not affected by lean body mass so it is a more sensitive indicator of kidney function in patients with muscle loss.
- The validated immunoassay for SDMA, the IDEXX SDMA test, is a clinically relevant and reliable tool for diagnosing early CKD in small animals when creatinine level is still within the reference interval.
- SDMA was added to the International Renal Interest Society CKD guidelines to complement creatinine testing in staging early and advanced disease.

INTRODUCTION

The diagnosis and management of chronic kidney disease (CKD) is a routine part of clinical small animal practice. CKD is a common problem seen throughout the lives of pets but increases in frequency as pets age. The prevalence of CKD has recently been identified to be greater than previously reported.[1] Patients diagnosed with CKD are often managed successfully for years by the partnership of a diligent veterinary staff and motivated pet owners. Use of the International Renal Interest Society

Disclosure: Drs R. Relford, J. Robertson, and C. Clements are currently employed by IDEXX.
Companion Animal Group Medical Organization, IDEXX, 1 IDEXX Drive, Westbrook, ME
04092, USA
* Corresponding author.
E-mail address: celeste-clements@idexx.com

Vet Clin Small Anim 46 (2016) 941–960
http://dx.doi.org/10.1016/j.cvsm.2016.06.010   **vetsmall.theclinics.com**
0195-5616/16/© 2016 IDEXX Laboratories Inc. Published by Elsevier Inc. This is an open access
article under the CC BY-NC-ND license (http://creativecommons.org/licenses/by-nc-nd/4.0/).

(IRIS) CKD guidelines for staging and treatment of patients with CKD encourages standardized and informed management practices to address common complications.[2] Symmetric dimethylarginine (SDMA), a novel kidney biomarker, permits earlier diagnosis of kidney disease than traditional creatinine testing, and has been included provisionally as part of the IRIS CKD guidelines, as modified in 2015, for staging of both early and advanced CKD.[2] On diagnosis of CKD, veterinarians should investigate for underlying conditions and complications that could be treated. Staging of CKD allows customized patient management for the best possible outcome.

DISCOVERY

SDMA was first identified in 1970[3] and later characterized as a molecule that is primarily cleared by the kidneys. SDMA emerged as a candidate kidney biomarker during investigations into the pathogenicity of a closely related compound, asymmetric dimethylarginine (ADMA), in people with advanced CKD.[4] Vallance and colleagues[4] found increased concentrations of both dimethylarginines, SDMA and ADMA, in a group of hemodialysis patients. They concluded that ADMA was a potent inhibitor of nitric oxide (NO) synthesis and proposed that ADMA might be contributing to the hypertension, immune dysfunction, and cardiovascular disease that complicate CKD.[4] They also recognized that significant metabolism of ADMA occurs before it reaches the kidney, whereas SDMA was primarily cleared by the kidney, which further differentiated the two molecules. SDMA's value as a kidney biomarker was not identified. Because no active role for SDMA was identified in the pathogenesis of CKD and their focus was more on hypertension and heart disease, SDMA was not the immediate target of additional research in methylated arginines.[5]

In 1997, Marescau and colleagues[6] reported a strong correlation between serum and urine concentrations of SDMA and kidney dysfunction by estimating glomerular filtration rate (GFR) with creatinine clearance (R of -0.916; $P<.0001$) in 135 people with CKD, and suggested serum SDMA as a good marker of kidney disease. Serum SDMA level increased as kidney function declined, as shown by GFR decline, in an inverse relationship, with negative correlation (R value). This work was later included as one of 18 studies in a powerful meta-analysis that showed highly significant correlations between SDMA and kidney function tests in people.[7]

In the first clinical study of SDMA in veterinary patients with spontaneous kidney disease, Jepson and colleagues[8] reported that SDMA correlated well with creatinine ($r = 0.741$; $P<.001$) in 69 cats with CKD and hypertension.

BIOCHEMISTRY
Methylarginine Synthesis

SDMA is a stable molecule that originates from intracellular proteins that play an integral role in basic cellular metabolism. SDMA and related compounds are produced in the nucleus of all cells. Their formation occurs by obligate posttranslational modification and methylation of arginine residues of various proteins and subsequent proteolysis.[7] The molecular structures of arginine, SDMA, and other methylated products of protein metabolism are shown in **Fig. 1**. The family of enzymes, arginine N-methyltransferases (PRMT), symmetrically methylate arginine residues of histones, spliceosomal Sm proteins, and receptor tyrosine kinases that generate SDMA and NG-monomethyl-L-arginine (NMMA) on their hydrolysis.[9,10] Other PRMT enzymes asymmetrically methylate histones and myelin basic protein,[11] which liberate ADMA and NMMA when degraded.[12,13] Note that although these substances are made

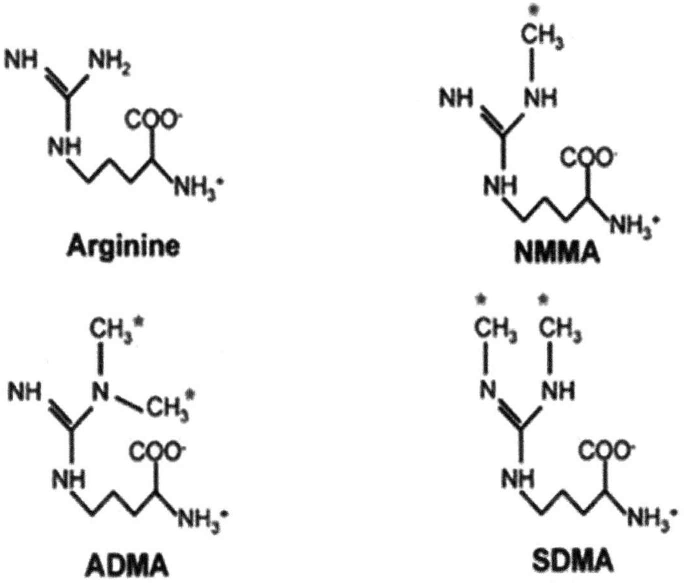

Fig. 1. Molecular structure for arginine and methylated arginines. NMMA, NG-monomethyl-L-arginine.

during a similar process, their mechanisms in the body and their clearance processes are very different.

Elimination

SDMA's small molecular size (molecular weight [MW], 202 g/mol)[14] and positive charge allow it be freely filtered by glomerular filtration. Because SDMA is largely excreted by the kidney, it is a good candidate biomarker for kidney function, whereas highly protein-bound ADMA undergoes extensive metabolism by the tissue-specific enzyme dimethylarginine dimethylaminohydrolase.[7,13] In a 2011 review, Schwedhelm and Böger[5] estimated the renal excretion of SDMA to be greater than or equal to 90%, with putative cleavage of the remainder by an unnamed enzyme. In contrast, only about 20% of ADMA is excreted into the urine.[5] The extensive renal clearance of SDMA explains its correlation with other kidney clearance markers and its potential suitability as an endogenous kidney biomarker.

CURRENT CHALLENGES WITH ASSESSING KIDNEY FUNCTION
Glomerular Filtration Rate

Direct measurement of GFR is the gold standard for quantitative assessment of kidney filtration but is not routinely performed on dogs and cats because of the need to administer a suitable filtration marker and obtain multiple timed blood samples and/or urine samples, which are both difficult for the pet and time consuming.[15] Although people might think that a gold standard is an agreed-on process, there are a variety of products, methods, and calculations to formulate GFR and there are perceived difficulties with each protocol. Renal clearance methods that measure the appearance of the marker substance in the urine were once preferred to plasma clearance methods, with inulin commonly regarded as the ideal marker substance because it is safe and inert, and is eliminated solely via glomerular filtration, without tubular reabsorption or secretion.[16] However, the complicated nature of the inulin assay and the requirement for accurate and complete urine recovery have made inulin renal clearance testing unpopular outside the research setting.[17] Alternate markers validated for GFR measurement in dogs and cats include endogenous or exogenous creatinine, cystatin C, iohexol, and radiolabeled molecules,[15] including [^{125}I] sodium iothalamate and [^{131}I] sodium iodohippurate.[17]

Plasma clearance of iohexol and exogenous creatinine offer practical and accurate methods to estimate GFR in a clinical setting. Iohexol is a commonly available iodinated contrast agent that may be given by single intravenous bolus injection. Plasma samples are collected at predetermined, accurately recorded times, usually 2, 3, and 4 hours after injection, before assay of the iodine components by mass spectroscopy or other methods, which is available only at a select few locations, without the need for urine.[18] Plasma clearance results are calculated using pharmacodynamics algorithms from marker decline on successive samples and are reported as the volume of plasma that has been cleared of the marker substance over a given interval of time, in milliliters per minute per kilogram of patient body weight,[17] ideally compared with a cohort of normal animals of the same species, breed, and size.

GFR continues to be a valuable measure of kidney function, although the complicated nature of testing and associated expense reduces the clinical utility of clearance methods. To help solve this problem in human patients, clearance methods are often replaced by calculated (rather than measured) estimates of GFR using serum creatinine (sCr) level, body weight, and various correction factors based on the patient's gender, age, and race, alone or in conjunction with a timed urine collection for a urinary creatinine clearance.[7] The muscle mass and protein intake of the individual should also be considered. However, there is no standard agreement on which formula should be used and each formula can provide a different GFR estimate, again making estimating GFR difficult. Similar algorithms for estimating GFR from sCr level in dogs and cats are inaccurate because of greater individual gender and breed variation.[19] These challenges of determining GFR continue to fuel the investigation into endogenous biomarkers of kidney function.[7]

Poor Sensitivity and Specificity of Serum Creatinine Testing

Measurement of sCr level has been the most widely used indirect estimate of GFR in veterinary medicine because its small MW[20] and neutral charge allow it to be freely filtered by the glomeruli. SCr has an inverse but nonlinear relationship to GFR; that is, sCr level increases exponentially as GFR declines. The steep curvilinear relationship between sCr and GFR poses a significant limitation to the sensitivity of sCr level for detecting early kidney disease because significant changes in GFR are reflected by modest or minimally detectable changes in sCr, and early kidney disease might be missed.[21] The converse is also true: in advanced disease, small changes in GFR make a large impact on sCr level, but this may have fewer clinical implications. SCr level has been shown to not increase beyond laboratory reference intervals until up to 75% of functional renal mass has been lost. The sensitivity of sCr level can be improved by establishing a baseline for each individual pet while in good health and then trending sCr over time using a consistent laboratory and analytical method.[21–23] Increases and degree of magnitude in sCr level cannot determine reversibility of the kidney disease or localization to renal, prerenal, or postrenal sources.[24] By the time sCr level has increased in CKD, the nephron loss is often irreversible and long-term prognosis may be poor.

A major preanalytical limitation of sCr level is dependence on muscle mass. Although regarded as a specific marker of kidney filtration, sCr level may be significantly increased in heavily muscled dogs, or significantly decreased in dogs and cats with muscle loss.[20] Comprehensive descriptions of the breed variability of sCr are lacking, but the greyhound is often cited as a breed with higher than expected sCr levels in health.[25] Evaluating kidney function in patients with increased muscle mass requires careful consideration of the patient's general health status; complete urinalysis findings, including appropriateness of the urine specific gravity; and any history, physical findings, or imaging results that suggest kidney disease. Creatinine level can significantly underestimate the degree of kidney disease present when dogs or cats lose muscle mass because of aging or any chronic disease, especially protein wasting diseases, cancer, or advanced kidney disease. In these scenarios, sCr level overestimates the degree of remaining kidney function.[26,27] These common clinical conditions create the need for a more sensitive and specific kidney biomarker.

A commonly overlooked cause of increases in sCr level is diet. A study in humans shows that sCr level can increase by 20% after eating cooked meat.[28] Studies in dogs show a similar effect following ingestion of meat. Six dogs were each fed soft moist, raw, and boiled meat in a crossover feeding trial. Following ingestion, sCr concentrations increased in all dogs; and a persistent increase was noted for several hours in the dogs fed boiled meat. The raw and soft moist diets were associated with an initial increase that was followed by a decline in sCr level.[29] These findings support the recommendation that, when measuring sCr level, the patient should be fasted for an accurate determination of kidney function.

Analytical Variability of Serum Creatinine Measurements

The fact that diagnostic reagents for measurement of sCr level are economical and widely available for reference laboratory and point-of-care testing has helped sCr to become the major predictor of kidney function. However, the commonly used Jaffe method is not specific for creatinine and, according to some estimates, noncreatinine compounds may contribute as much as 45% to 50% to reported sCr values.[18,20] The modification to the Jaffe method has addressed some of these challenges. What has remained problematic is that different laboratory reagents and methods of measurement continue to result in nonstandardized laboratory-dependent reference intervals for sCr level. Analytical variability within and between the creatinine assay is also a limitation. SDMA is a novel biomarker that can help to clarify the inaccuracies and nonkidney variables associated with sCr as a diagnostic.

Criteria for a Better Kidney Biomarker

Concentrations of soluble serum and urinary compounds that change consistently with early kidney damage have been the focus of study in people with naturally occurring kidney disease and laboratory animal models of nephrotoxicity because the current testing has limitations. As discussed previously, clinical testing for kidney disease in most species relies on sCr measurement. In addition, although sCr seems to satisfy the definition of a biomarker proposed by Puntmann,[30] namely that "A biomarker is a characteristic that can be objectively measured and evaluated as an indicator of normal biological processes, pathogenic processes or pharmacological responses to a therapeutic intervention,"[30] it has limitations and the authors suggest criteria for a better biomarker than sCr.

In the clinical setting, sCr is primarily a diagnostic and staging test. A better kidney biomarker should be more sensitive and specific than sCr, compared with the gold standard, with the clear ability to predict or exclude disease in an individual patient relative to a diverse population with many breeds, sizes, ages, and comorbidities.[30] Receiver operating curves generating R values assist with this comparison. Biomarkers for diagnosing acute conditions, like acute kidney injury, should appear early and in proportion to the magnitude of the insult, with analysis available in real time, especially at the point of care.[30]

For accurate monitoring of chronic conditions, such as CKD, a biomarker with narrow biological variability improves the assessment of longitudinal changes.[30] A good kidney biomarker should perform consistently in individual patients regardless of whether they are aged, underweight, with variable nutrition, or affected with multiple concurrent health concerns. The candidate biomarker for CKD should then be studied to show that it has a positive impact on patient outcome, with improved quality of life and survival times, compared with other methods.

Early studies of rodent and dog remnant kidney models of CKD support SDMA as an endogenous kidney biomarker. SDMA correlated well with creatinine clearance after partial nephrectomy in rats[31] and with creatinine and blood urea nitrogen (BUN) levels in rats after total nephrectomy.[32] In 10 dogs undergoing partial or complete nephrectomy, plasma SDMA concentrations increased with reductions in renal mass and correlated well with GFR by inulin clearance (r value of -0.851; $P<.0001$) and with sCr (r value of -0.749; $P = .0013$).[33]

Reviewing 18 early studies of 2136 human patients, Kielstein and colleagues[7] found that systemic SDMA concentrations correlated highly with GFR by inulin clearance ($R = 0.85$; confidence interval, 0.76–0.91; $P<.0001$), as well as with sCr ($R = 0.75$; confidence interval, 0.46–0.89; $P<.0001$), concluding that SDMA should be further investigated as a marker of renal function.[7] In recent GFR studies using continuous infusion of very-low-dose of iohexol, SDMA accurately and precisely estimated GFR in people, and was more sensitive than sCr.[34] In people with and without CKD, SDMA outperformed creatinine and creatinine-based equations in estimating kidney function compared with measured GFR.[35]

These cumulative data from animal experiments and studies in people supported the investigation of SDMA as a kidney biomarker for cats and dogs.

SYMMETRIC DIMETHYLARGININE CORRELATES WITH GLOMERULAR FILTRATION RATE
Dogs with X-linked Hereditary Nephropathy

Nabity and colleagues[22] recently published a prospective foundational study evaluating SDMA as a marker for kidney disease in a colony of dogs with progressive x-linked hereditary nephropathy (XLHN). They validated the SDMA assay for dogs using liquid chromatography–mass spectroscopy (LC-MS), then compared serial SDMA measurements with sCr and GFR by exogenous plasma iohexol clearance in a cohort of 8 affected male dogs and 4 unaffected littermate controls.

Intra-assay precision coefficient of variability (CV) of the LC-MS was 1.5% to 2.8% (mean of 2.2%) and the inter-assay precision was 2.3% to 3.7% (mean of 2.7%), both with 98% accuracy or greater, consistent with excellent analytical performance.[22] Preanalytical factors such as added hemoglobin, lipids, bilirubin, arginine, monomethylarginine, ADMA, and homocitrulline did not interfere with SDMA measurement. SDMA was highly stable in canine serum or plasma, resisting significant change at room (20°C) and refrigerator (4°C) temperatures for 14 days.[22]

The subjects were studied over 37 weeks, with 6 of 8 affected dogs reaching the targeted end point of sCr level greater than or equal to 5 mg/dL. In affected dogs, SDMA level increased during progression from preclinical disease to end-stage

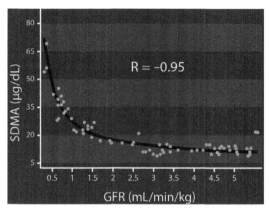

Fig. 2. Serum SDMA correlates with decreasing GFR by iohexol clearance in affected male dogs with XLHN (R = −0.95). (*From* Nabity NB, Lees GE, Boggess MM, et al. Symmetric dimethylarginine assay validation, stability, and evaluation as a marker for the detection of chronic kidney disease in dogs. J Vet Intern Med 2015;29:1040; with permission.)

kidney disease, correlating strongly with an increase in sCr level ($r = 0.95$), and with a decrease in GFR ($r = −0.95$), as shown in **Fig. 2**. An SDMA cutoff of greater than or equal to 14 μg/dL identified, on average, a less than 20% decrease in GFR, which was earlier than sCr by any comparison method, including using the sCr cutoff for azotemia at greater than or equal to 1.2 mg/dL, serial trending of sCr levels, or in comparison with sCr levels of unaffected littermates.[22] **Fig. 3** compares the rapid clinical course of an affected dog with XLHN with an unaffected littermate control.

Affected male dogs with XLHN have mutations in the genes coding for glomerular type IV collagen and develop proteinuric end-stage kidney disease between 6 and 18 months of age, creating a convenient model of rapidly progressive CKD.[36] The heterozygous carrier females develop proteinuria as juveniles, but most have sufficient normal glomerular basement membrane to maintain structural and functional integrity, with clinical normalcy, adequate urine concentrating ability, and normal sCr levels until they are about 5 years old.[37] SDMA also correlated strongly with the stable GFR of the colony's female carriers ($R^2 = 0.85$) (Mary Nabity, DVM, PhD, DACVP, College Station, TX, personal communication, 2013.).

Cats, Azotemic and Nonazotemic

In a retrospective analysis, SDMA level was measured by LC-MS on previously frozen serum samples from 10 client-owned cats and compared with their plasma creatinine concentrations and GFRs by exogenous plasma iohexol clearance from the same date. Serum SDMA levels and GFR were correlated strongly ($R^2 = 0.82$; $P<.001$) across a range of GFRs from 0.54 to 2.37 mL/min/kg (**Fig. 4**), whether cats were azotemic or not.[38]

REFERENCE INTERVAL DEVELOPMENT

Reference intervals for dogs and cats were established following Clinical Laboratory Standards Institute (CLSI) guidelines[39] to facilitate the continued development of SDMA as a clinical tool to measure kidney function.

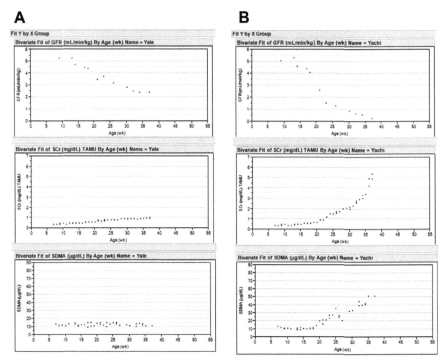

Fig. 3. Typical clinical course of progressive kidney disease over 55 weeks in a dog with XLHN compared with control litter mate, showing increasing SDMA and sCr levels as GFR declines. (A) The dog Yale represents an age-matched control from the litter. His results show an initial decline in GFR with maturation, seen in all the control pups, that plateaued after 30 weeks, with stable GFR, sCr level, and SDMA level. (B) In contrast, the affected dog Yachi's results show a progressive decline in kidney function beginning at approximately 15 weeks that reached the study end point of sCr level greater than or equal to 5 mg/dL at approximately 38 weeks of age. SDMA concentration increased as sCr level increased and GFR decreased. TAMU, Texas A&M University. (*Courtesy of* Mary Nabity, DVM, PhD, DACVP, College Station, TX, personal communication, 2013.)

Dogs

Serum samples were collected from 122 clinically healthy, adult dogs (defined as ≥1 year of age) of varying gender, age, and breed attending a heartworm clinic. The health status of each dog was based on physical examination; lack of any history of constitutional signs or illness over the last 6 months; and prescription medication limited to chemoprophylaxis for heartworm, fleas, and ticks. For each dog the following information was recorded: diet, results of comprehensive complete blood count with slide review, chemistry panel with electrolytes and total thyroxine concentrations, and when available results from a complete urinalysis, urine culture with minimum inhibitory concentration and urine protein/creatinine ratio.

There were 151 dogs examined; 28 were excluded because of age (<1 year of age) or health reasons. One dog was removed because of immeasurable sCr level. Dogs ranged in age from 1 to 15 years, with a mean age of 4.7 years. Males and females were equally represented. Body weights varied between 2.7 and 60 kg, with a wide variety of body condition scores (data courtesy of IDEXX, Westbrook, ME.)

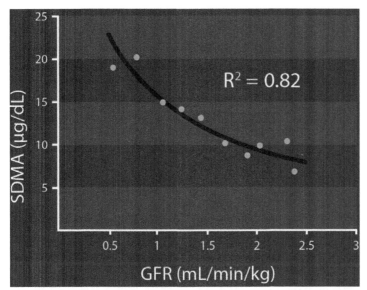

Fig. 4. The inverse relationship, with strong correlation ($R^2 = 0.82$; $P<.001$), between serum SDMA level (y axis) and GFR (x axis) in 10 client-owned cats with varied kidney function. (*Data from* Braff J, Obare E, Yerramilli M, et al. Relationship between serum symmetric dimethylarginine concentration and glomerular filtration rate in cats. J Vet Intern Med 2014;8:1699–701.)

Serum SDMA was measured by LC-MS as previously established and results analyzed with a nonparametric model, using a 2-sided 95% confidence interval. After exclusion of 2 outliers that were outside the mean, plus or minus 3 standard deviations, the reference interval for healthy adult dogs was established at less than 14 µg/dL, as shown in **Fig. 5.**[40]

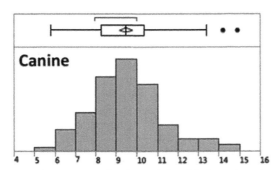

Fig. 5. Canine serum SDMA concentration (LC-MS) (µg/dL) plotted on the x axis against proportion of the reference population of healthy adult dogs (n = 122) on the y axis. The reference interval was established at less than 14 µg/dL with nonparametric analysis. The box and whiskers plot reflects the interquartile range, with outliers represented by dots. (*From* Rentko V, Nabity M, Yerramilli M, et al. Determination of serum symmetric dimethylarginine reference limit in clinically healthy dogs [ACVIM abstract P-7]. J Vet Intern Med 2013;27:750; with permission.)

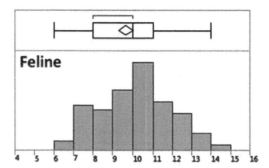

Fig. 6. Feline serum SDMA results (LC-MS) (μg/dL) plotted on the x axis against proportion of the reference population of healthy adult cats (n = 86) on the y axis. The reference interval was established at less than 14 μg/dL with nonparametric analysis. The box and whiskers plot reflects the interquartile range. (*Courtesy of* IDEXX, Westbrook, ME.)

Cats

The reference interval for serum SDMA in cats was established similarly at less than 14 μg/dL (**Fig. 6**). Data were collected from 86 clinically healthy, adult cats, aged 6 to 15 years, comprising domestic short hair (DSH), domestic longhair, Siamese, and ragdoll breeds. The cats were of both genders and weighed between 3.0 and 9.0 kg (data courtesy of IDEXX, Westbrook, ME).

SYMMETRIC DIMETHYLARGININE LEVEL INCREASES EARLIER THAN CREATININE

With normal SDMA concentrations established for healthy dogs and cats, researchers extended testing of its utility as a diagnostic tool for kidney disease.

Cats

For 21 cats with CKD living at the Hill's Pet Nutrition colony, SDMA level was measured in banked frozen serum samples and compared with available documented sCr and GFR assessments at various time points throughout the cats' lives before and after a diagnosis of CKD. In this retrospective longitudinal study, SDMA level increased to greater than the reference interval on average 17 months earlier than sCr, with a range of 1.5 to 48 months. SDMA level was found to be increased in the cats with CKD when there was on average a 40% reduction in their GFR from the median GFR of the healthy cats in the same colony. In 2 cats SDMA level was increased when there was only a 25% reduction in GFR from the designated normal for the colony. Serial results from a representative case are provided in **Fig. 7**, showing an increase in SDMA to greater than the reference interval 8 months before sCr. During this same interval, sCr level remained stable and did not trend upward as the kidney disease progressed.[41]

Dogs

A similar study performed in 19 dogs with CKD showed that SDMA increased to greater than the reference interval before sCr, in 17 of 19 dogs, on average 9.8 months earlier, with a range of 2.2 to 27 months. SDMA level was significantly correlated with GFR ($r = -0.80$; $P<.001$).[42] The longitudinal laboratory data from an 11-year-old, male, castrated Beagle in the colony are presented in **Fig. 8** to show that SDMA level increased to greater than the reference interval 19 months before sCr in this dog with CKD.[42] Postmortem renal histopathology confirmed lymphocytic/plasmacytic

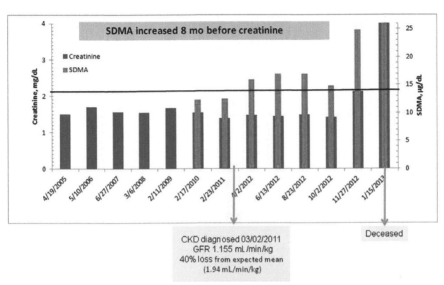

Fig. 7. Mystic, born 2001, a 12-year-old, neutered male DSH, was diagnosed with CKD in March of 2011 when GFR was 40% reduced from the expected mean of the colony. SCr level is on the left y axis and SDMA is on the right y axis. Time is on the x axis. The solid black line represents the upper end of the reference interval for both creatinine at 2.1 mg/dL and the upper end of the reference interval for SDMA at 14 μg/dL. In the bar graphs, creatinine is represented by the blue bars and SDMA is represented by the red bars. When a bar crosses over the black line, then the analyte result is increased. SDMA level increased 8 months before sCr, which was stable until a period of acute decompensation. (*From* Hall JA, Yerramilli M, Obare E, et al. Comparison of serum concentrations of symmetric dimethylarginine and creatinine as kidney function biomarkers in cats with chronic kidney disease. J Vet Intern Med 2014;28:1680; with permission.)

interstitial nephritis, with interstitial and periglomerular fibrosis, tubular ectasia, and glomerulosclerosis; changes that are consistent with CKD.[43]

SPECIFICITY OF SYMMETRIC DIMETHYLARGININE

There is considerable evidence across species supporting SDMA as a specific endogenous renal biomarker that is not influenced by extrarenal factors. In people, SDMA level did not change with acute inflammatory response,[44] hepatic disease,[45,46] cardiovascular disease,[47,48] or diabetes,[49] unless there was concurrent kidney disease. SDMA concentrations did not change in preeclampsic women receiving oral arginine supplementation.[50]

SDMA level was not significantly increased after vigorous exercise in sled dogs with normal BUN values, and was not influenced by breed or gender in a cohort of dogs, unlike ADMA and nitric oxide metabolites, which are known markers of endothelial function.[51] In a group of Cavalier King Charles spaniels, SDMA level was not affected by age or asymptomatic mitral regurgitation.[52] Internal studies at IDEXX showed no correlation between SDMA and serum arginine levels measured in dogs and cats ($R^2 = 0.002$). There was no correlation between the cardiac biomarker N-terminal pro–brain natriuretic peptide and SDMA in approximately 300 dogs over a wide range of results ($R^2 = 0.0043$). Liver enzyme concentration, as a proxy for liver disease, and SDMA level were not correlated: alkaline phosphatase ($R^2 = 0.01$), alanine transaminase ($R^2 = 0.02$), or aspartate aminotransferase ($R^2 = 0.05$) (data courtesy of IDEXX).

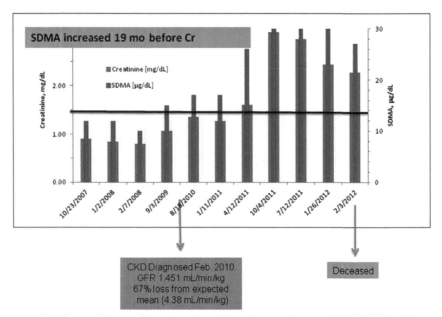

Fig. 8. Nicholas, an 11-year-old, neutered male Beagle, was diagnosed with CKD in February 2010 when his GFR was decreased by 67% of the expected mean of the healthy dogs in the same colony. Creatinine is on the left y axis and SDMA is on the right y axis. Time is on the x axis. The solid black line represents the upper end of the reference interval for both creatinine at 2.1 mg/dL and the upper end of the reference interval for SDMA at 14 μg/dL. In the bar graphs, creatinine is represented by the blue bars and SDMA is represented by the red bars. When a bar crosses over the black line, then the analyte result is increased. (*From* Hall JA, Yerramilli M, Obare E, et al. Serum concentrations of symmetric dimethylarginine and creatinine in dogs with naturally occurring chronic kidney disease. J Vet Intern Med 2016;30:799; with permission.)

Prospective veterinary studies have shown that, unlike sCr, SDMA level is independent of influences of lean body mass, so it is a more sensitive marker for kidney disease than sCr in patients with a wide variety of reasons for muscle loss. A study in older cats with age-related loss of muscle mass, as measured by dual energy x-ray absorptiometry, confirmed that creatinine level underestimates the loss of kidney function as GFR declines. In contrast, SDMA level showed no correlation with lean body mass. GFR declined with age, and serum SDMA level increased in concordance, better identifying the function loss. These results support the conclusion that SDMA is a more sensitive indicator of loss of kidney function.[26] A complementary study in healthy dogs showed comparable findings of a dependent correlation between lean body mass and creatinine level ($r = 0.54$; $P = .0003$), whereas SDMA level was not influenced by total lean body mass ($r = -0.12$; $P = .45$).[27]

INTERNATIONAL RENAL INTEREST SOCIETY CHRONIC KIDNEY DISEASE GUIDELINES INCLUSION

IRIS was created in 1998 to help veterinary practitioners better understand, diagnose, and treat renal disease in dogs and cats. The board members created standardized staging guidelines to educate and encourage the best practices for managing kidney disease after diagnosis.

In 2015, SDMA was incorporated provisionally into the updates for IRIS CKD staging guidelines, acknowledging SDMA as a renal function test to complement sCr in evaluating patients with early kidney disease, because it may be a more sensitive biomarker of renal function than fasted blood creatinine concentrations.[2] Persistent increases in SDMA greater than 14 μg/dL suggest reduced kidney function and the possibility of IRIS CKD stage 1 in patients with sCr level less than the IRIS cutoff of 1.4 mg/dL for dogs and 1.6 mg/dL for cats. Thus SDMA can help to identify dogs and cats in IRIS stage 1 and early IRIS stage 2 in which clinical signs are absent or mild and creatinine level has not increased to greater than the reference interval.

The early recognition of kidney disease provides the opportunity to investigate for an underlying cause, manage associated diseases and the CKD, and plan for monitoring the patient accordingly. Investigating when kidney disease is in the early stages increases the likelihood of finding treatable causes such as upper urinary tract infection; vector borne diseases such as Lyme disease, ehrlichiosis, or leishmaniasis; obstructive urolithiasis; or chronic toxicities. Investigating for complications such as proteinuria and hypertension that may accelerate kidney disease is an important aspect of substaging CKD.[2] Even if no underlying cause or complications are identified, earlier diagnosis and treatment may slow the rate of progression of CKD and increase the pet's life span.[53]

Monitoring SDMA in patients with CKD can help to better identify progression of disease as dogs and cats lose weight, especially if it is associated with a loss of muscle condition.[26,27] According to the IRIS guidelines, patients with low body condition scores that are in stage 2 or stage 3 based on creatinine level and that also show an increased SDMA level greater than or equal to 25 μg/dL or 45 μg/dL, respectively, may be staged inappropriately low and the degree of renal dysfunction may be underestimated. Treatment of clinical signs or laboratory findings of a more advanced stage of CKD might be appropriate; that is, CKD stage 3 and stage 4.[2] Increased practitioner awareness and use of a muscle condition scoring (MCS) system as proposed by the World Small Animal Veterinary Association Global Nutrition Committee[54] assists with proper evaluation of patients with CKD. The MCS system is helpful in targeting muscle loss because it is possible for pets to be overweight and still have muscle loss.[55]

Enhanced evaluation and recognition of kidney disease with SDMA and IRIS staging may help veterinarians to better manage CKD and assist with objective patient monitoring and communication of measurable goals. Pet owners can be engaged to participate in this important team effort to optimize their pets' renal care for improved quality and length of life. IRIS recognizes that, compared with creatinine, SDMA may be a more sensitive biomarker of excretory renal function, and that SDMA can be a useful adjunct for the early diagnosis of CKD, as well as a guide for management of more advanced CKD. SDMA testing should be run alongside sCr, BUN, and a complete urinalysis to provide a comprehensive picture of kidney function.

THE IDEXX SYMMETRIC DIMETHYLARGININE TEST
Validation

The LC-MS analysis for SDMA, although extremely accurate and considered the gold standard, can be costly and time consuming, and thus inconvenient to add to the routine laboratory minimum data base for sick and well pets. The IDEXX SDMA test is a novel, high-throughput, competitive homogeneous immunoassay using a glucose-6-phosphate dehydrogenase conjugate and anti-SDMA monoclonal antibody to quantify SDMA in serum and plasma.[56] The technique is especially useful when developing an immunoassay for a small biomarker molecule such as SDMA,[56] which is less immunogenic because of its small size.[5] The assay was validated following US Food and Drug Administration and CLSI standards for dogs and cats, using healthy and CKD populations.[57] Accuracy was confirmed by comparing the results with the LC-MS standard over a dynamic range of 5 to 100 μg/dL. In the range of 10 to 20 μg/dL, within-run precision was less than or equal to 7% CV, and total precision was less than or equal to 10% CV.[56,57]

The reference interval for the IDEXX SDMA test, established at less than or equal to 14 μg/dL, is based on transference analysis of SDMA data by LC-MS from healthy dogs and cats (data courtesy of IDEXX[40]), considering mean bias, method precision, and whole-number rounding of the original data.

Clinical Use

The SDMA test is available from IDEXX Reference Laboratories. The IDEXX SDMA test is performed along with all routine chemistries on a multichannel analyzer (Beckman Coulter, Inc, Brea, CA). SDMA results are provided at the same time as all other chemistry results without a delay in the reporting time. Serum is the preferred sample type; lithium heparin or EDTA plasma is also acceptable. The IDEXX SDMA test is not affected by mild to moderate hemolysis or any degree of lipemia or icterus. An interpretive comment is provided with all SDMA results to assist with interpretation along with creatinine results. For patient results with increased IDEXX SDMA and sCr within the reference interval, early kidney disease is likely and further investigation is indicated, as suggested in **Box 1**.

SDMA complements traditional tests for kidney disease. To diagnose kidney disease, the patient's clinical presentation, physical examination findings, and results of laboratory testing and imaging should be considered. The clinical presentation includes the signalment, consisting of age, breed, and gender; any relevant history, such as medication use, possible exposure to toxins, diet, and travel; with possible exposure to infectious diseases that may be risk factors for kidney disease, such as Lyme disease or leptospirosis.

In early CKD, clinical signs are often absent. With progression of CKD these signs are more common:

- Polyuria and polydipsia
- Decreased appetite
- Weight loss
- Lethargy

Box 1
Interpretive criteria for the IDEXX SDMA test when SDMA level is increased and creatinine level is within the reference interval

SDMA level is increased and creatinine level is within the reference interval, which indicates that early kidney disease is likely. Most animals with early kidney disease have an SDMA level between 15 and 20 μg/dL. Because SDMA level increases as kidney function decreases, SDMA levels greater than 20 μg/dL are typically seen in more advanced disease along with an increased creatinine level. SDMA is a more sensitive indicator of kidney function in poorly muscled animals. A complete urinalysis should be performed to evaluate for inappropriate specific gravity, proteinuria, and other evidence of kidney disease. SDMA results may be slightly higher (~1 μg/dL) in puppies, kittens, and greyhounds and results should be interpreted in light of other findings.

(*Courtesy of* IDEXX, Westbrook, ME.)

- Vomiting
- Bad breath

Early physical examination changes are often subtle or absent, but typically progress with advancing disease. Common physical examination findings in CKD include:

- Palpable kidney abnormalities
- Evidence of weight loss
- Dehydration
- Pallor
- Oral ulcers
- Hypertensive retinopathy

Because signs and physical examination findings are inconsistent or absent in early disease, relevant laboratory or imaging findings are necessary to assess kidney health. Urinalysis results vary in early kidney disease, with progressive loss of concentrating ability expected as the condition progresses. Inadequate concentrating ability is defined for cats as urine with specific gravity less than 1.035 and for dogs less than 1.030.[58] Making an early diagnosis of CKD commonly requires finding 1 or more of the following results:

- sCr level increasing within the reference interval
- Persistently increased SDMA level greater than 14 µg/dL
- Abnormal kidney imaging
- Persistent renal proteinuria, especially over weeks to months

With the exception of changes in kidney size, shape, or architecture that may be detected by examination or kidney imaging on the first visit (eg, finding small, irregular kidneys), these diagnostic criteria for CKD must persist over time in stable patients. Patients changing rapidly, with increasing SDMA level and the development of azotemia, should be suspected of acute kidney injury or an active primary disease and be evaluated aggressively.

With more advanced CKD, levels of both sCr and SDMA are chronically increased, and urine becomes progressively more dilute. In advanced cases of renal disease, SDMA can provide insight into the severity of disease because sCr level may be influenced by loss of muscle mass and under-represent the severity of the disease. Rarely do these patients present a diagnostic challenge to identify that kidney disease is present; instead the focus turns to managing a known problem.

PATIENT DATA AND IMPACT

SDMA data collected to date support that kidney disease is more prevalent than was previously reported, and increases with increasing pet age. In the first 750,000 or more IDEXX SDMA tests performed in the United States, dog samples outnumbered cat samples approximately 2 to 1. These samples showed that 11% of feline samples and 6% of canine samples had an increase in creatinine level to greater than the reference interval. However, there was an additional 15% of cats and 6% of dogs identified to have increased SDMA levels, whereas the creatinine level remained within the reference interval. These findings suggest that, by using SDMA, which is a more sensitive biomarker, veterinarians have the potential opportunity to diagnose kidney disease 2.4 times more often in cats and 2.0 times more often in dogs, compared with the traditional use of sCr (**Fig. 9**) (data courtesy of IDEXX).

IDEXX data gathered also highlight that the prevalence of CKD increases with increasing age and might exceed historical estimates that 1 in 3 cats[59] and 1 in 10

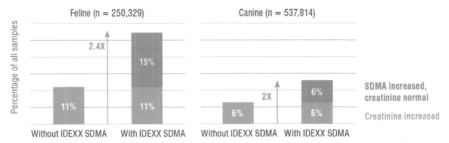

Fig. 9. Patient results for the IDEXX SDMA test and paired creatinine tests expressed as a percentage of feline and canine samples tested suggest that kidney disease may be more prevalent than estimates based on creatinine testing alone. (*Courtesy of* IDEXX, Westbrook, ME.)

dogs[60] develop CKD in their lifetimes based on creatinine alone. More than 50% of cats more than 15 years of age had increased SDMA and normal or increased Cr levels. In comparison, among dogs 15 years of age or older, 40% had increased SDMA levels and possible kidney disease (data courtesy of IDEXX). The IDEXX SDMA test data support Marino and colleagues'[1] recent report that the prevalence of CKD in cats older than 15 years was 86.2% (primarily IRIS CKD stage 1 and 2).

SUMMARY

SDMA may affect how veterinarians diagnose and manage kidney disease in dogs and cats. SDMA, a product of intranuclear protein metabolism, is freely filtered by the kidneys, and serum levels of SDMA correlate inversely with measurements of GFR in people, rats, mice, dogs, and cats. SDMA was investigated as a potential clinical renal biomarker for almost a decade, and a reference interval for SDMA has been established in healthy dogs and cats, as measured by LC-MS.

SDMA is a sensitive and specific renal biomarker. Longitudinal studies of SDMA in dogs and cats with CKD showed that SDMA level increased months earlier than sCr, when there was on average a 40% reduction in GFR, whereas sCr level increases late, when there is up to 75% reduction of GFR. Unlike sCr, SDMA is independent of lean body mass, so it is a more sensitive marker for kidney disease than sCr in patients with muscle loss. As a result of vigorous analysis and clinical review, SDMA has been included in the updated IRIS guidelines to complement sCr in the diagnostic evaluation and monitoring of CKD.

Early experience with the use of the IDEXX SDMA test, which is a new immunoassay for SDMA, in a large patient population suggests that kidney disease is more prevalent than was previously predicted by increased sCr levels alone. Kidney disease and SDMA increase more frequently as dogs and cats progress in age, supporting historical data. Earlier diagnosis of kidney disease provides an opportunity for intervention by investigation for underlying causes and complications associated with kidney disease. This, in turn, leads to more effective treatment and management.

REFERENCES

1. Marino CL, Lascelles BD, Vaden SL, et al. The prevalence and classification of chronic kidney disease in cats randomly selected from four age groups and in cats recruited for degenerative joint disease studies. J Feline Med Surg 2014; 16:465–7.

2. International Renal Interest Society guidelines. 2016. Available at: http://www.iris-kidney.com/pdf/staging-of-ckd.pdf. Accessed March 18, 2016.
3. Kakimoto Y, Akazawa S. Isolation and identification of N-G,N-G- and N-G,N'-G-dimethyl-arginine, N-epsilon-mono-, di-, and trimethyllysine, and glucosylga-lactosyl- and galactosyl-delta-hydroxylysine from human urine. J Biol Chem 1970;245:5751–8.
4. Vallance P, Leone A, Calver A, et al. Accumulation of an endogenous inhibitor of nitric oxide synthesis in chronic renal failure. Lancet 1992;339:572–5.
5. Schwedhelm E, Böger RH. The role of asymmetric and symmetric dimethylargi-nines in renal disease. Nat Rev Nephrol 2011;7:275–85.
6. Marescau B, Nagels G, Possemiers I, et al. Guanidino compounds in serum and urine of nondialyzed patients with chronic renal insufficiency. Metabolism 1997; 46:1024–31.
7. Kielstein JT, Salpeter SR, Bode-Böger SM, et al. Symmetric dimethylarginine (SDMA) as endogenous marker of renal function – a meta analysis. Nephrol Dial Transplant 2006;21:2445–51.
8. Jepson RE, Syme HM, Vallance C, et al. Plasma asymmetric dimethylarginine, symmetric dimethylarginine, l-arginine and nitrite/nitrate concentrations in cats with chronic kidney disease and hypertension. J Vet Intern Med 2008;22:317–24.
9. Sanchez SE, Petrillo E, Beckwith EJ, et al. A methyl transferase links the circadian clock to the regulation of alternative splicing. Nature 2010;468:112–6.
10. Hsu JM, Chen CT, Chou CK, et al. Crosstalk between Arg 1175 methylation and Tyr 1173 phosphorylation negatively modulates EGFR-mediated ERK activation. Nat Cell Biol 2011;13:174–81.
11. Nicholson TB, Chen T, Richard S. The physiological and pathophysiological role of PRMT1-mediated protein arginine methylation. Pharmacol Res 2009;60: 466–74.
12. Ogawa T, Kimoto M, Sasaoka K. Occurrence of a new enzyme catalysing the direct conversion of NG,NG-dimethyl-l-arginine to l-citrulline in rats. Biochem Bio-phys Res Commun 1987;148:671–7.
13. Achan V, Broadhead M, Malaki M, et al. Asymmetric dimethylarginine causes hypertension and cardiac dysfunction and is actively metabolized by dimethylar-ginine dimethylaminohydrolase. Arterioscler Thromb Vasc Biol 2003;23:1455–9.
14. Glorieux G, Neirynck N, Pletnick A, et al. Uraemic toxins: overview. In: Turner N, Lamiere N, Goldsmith DJ, et al, editors. Oxford textbook of clinical nephrology. 4th edition. Oxford (United Kingdom): Oxford University Press; 2016. p. 2161–73.
15. Pressler BM. Clinical approach to advanced renal function testing in dogs and cats. Vet Clin North Am Small Anim Pract 2013;43:1193–208.
16. Haller M, Müller W, Binder H, et al. Single-injection inulin clearance–a simple method for measuring glomerular filtration rate in dogs. Res Vet Sci 1998;64: 151–6.
17. Von Hendy-Willson VE, Pressler BM. An overview of glomerular filtration rate testing in dogs and cats. Vet J 2011;188:156–65.
18. Sanderson SL. Measuring glomerular filtration rate: practical use of clearance tests. In: Bonagura JD, Twedt DC, editors. Kirk's veterinary therapy XIV. St Louis (MO): Saunders Elsevier; 2009. p. 868–71.
19. Lefebvre HP, Craig AJ, Braun JP. GFR in the dog: breed effect. In: Proceedings of the 16th ECVIM-CA Congress. Amsterdam (Holland): European College of Veter-inary Internal Medicine–Companion Animals; 2006. p. 261.
20. Braun JP, Lefebvre HP, Watson ADJ. Creatinine in the dog: a review. Vet Clin Pathol 2003;32:162–79.

21. Grauer G. Early diagnosis of chronic kidney disease in dogs & cats: use of serum creatinine & symmetric dimethylarginine. Today's Vet Pract 2016;6:68–72. Available at: http://todaysveterinarypractice.navc.com/early-diagnosis-of-chronic-kidney-disease-in-dogs-cats-use-of-serum-creatinine-symmetric-dimethylarginine/. Accessed March 20, 2016.

22. Nabity NB, Lees GE, Boggess MM, et al. Symmetric dimethylarginine assay validation, stability, and evaluation as a marker for the detection of chronic kidney disease in dogs. J Vet Intern Med 2015;29:1036–44.

23. Nabity MB, Lees GE, Boggess M, et al. Week-to week variability of iohexal clearance, serum creatinine, and symmetric dimethylarginine in dogs with stable chronic renal disease [ACVIM abstract NU-14]. J Vet Intern Med 2013;27(3): 604–756.

24. Dibartola SP. Renal disease: clinical approach and laboratory evaluation. In: Ettinger SC, Feldman EC, editors. Textbook of veterinary internal medicine. 6th edition. St Louis (MO): Elsevier Saunders; 2005. p. 1716–30.

25. Feeman WE, Couto CG, Gray TL. Serum creatinine concentrations in retired racing greyhounds. Vet Clin Pathol 2003;32:40–2.

26. Hall JA, Yerramilli M, Obare E, et al. Comparison of serum concentrations of symmetric dimethylarginine and creatinine as kidney function biomarkers in healthy geriatric cats fed reduced protein foods enriched with fish oil, L-carnitine, and medium-chain triglycerides. Vet J 2014;202:588–96.

27. Hall JA, Yerramilli M, Obare E, et al. Relationship between lean body mass and serum renal biomarkers in healthy dogs. J Vet Intern Med 2015;3:808–14.

28. Preiss DJ, Godber IM, Lamb EJ, et al. The influence of a cooked-meat meal on estimated glomerular filtration rate. Ann Clin Biochem 2007;44:35–42.

29. Watson AD, Church DB, Fairburn AJ. Postprandial changes in plasma urea and creatinine concentrations in dogs. Am J Vet Res 1981;42:1878–80.

30. Puntmann VO. How-to guide on biomarkers: biomarker definitions, validation and applications with examples from cardiovascular disease. Postgrad Med J 2009; 85:538–45.

31. Al Banchaabouchi M, Marescau B, Possemiers I, et al. NG NG-dimethylarginine and NG, NG-dimethylarginine in renal insufficiency. Pflug Arch 2000;439:524–31.

32. Carello KA, Whitesall SE, Lloyd MC, et al. Asymmetrical dimethylarginine plasma clearance persists after acute total nephrectomy in rats. Am J Physiol Heart Circ Physiol 2006;290:H209–16.

33. Tatematsu S, Wakino S, Kanda T, et al. Role of nitric oxide-producing and -degrading pathways in coronary endothelial dysfunction in chronic kidney disease. J Am Soc Nephrol 2007;18:741–9.

34. Dixon JJ, Lane K, Dalton RN, et al. Symmetrical dimethylarginine is a more sensitive biomarker of renal dysfunction than creatinine. Crit Care 2013; 17(Suppl. 2):423.

35. Payto DA, El-Khoury JM, Bunch DR, et al. SDMA outperforms serum creatinine-based equations in estimating kidney function compared with measured GFR [AACC Annual Meeting & Clinical Lab Expo Abstract 105]. Clin Chem 2014;60:S22.

36. Lees GE, Helman G, Kashtan CE, et al. New form of X linked dominant hereditary nephritis in dogs. Am J Vet Res 1999;60:373–83.

37. Lees GE. Kidney diseases caused by glomerular basement membrane type IV collagen defects in dogs. J Vet Emerg Crit Care 2013;23:184–93.

38. Braff J, Obare E, Yerramilli M, et al. Relationship between serum symmetric dimethylarginine concentration and glomerular filtration rate in cats. J Vet Intern Med 2014;8:1699–701.

39. Clinical and Laboratory Standards Institute. Defining, establishing, and verifying reference intervals in the clinical laboratory; approved guidelines. 3rd edition. Wayne (PA): CLSI; 2010.

40. Rentko V, Nabity M, Yerramilli M, et al. Determination of serum symmetric dimethylarginine reference limit in clinically healthy dogs [ACVIM abstract P-7]. J Vet Intern Med 2013;27:750.

41. Hall JA, Yerramilli M, Obare E, et al. Comparison of serum concentrations of symmetric dimethylarginine and creatinine as kidney function biomarkers in cats with chronic kidney disease. J Vet Intern Med 2014;28:1676–83.

42. Hall JA, Yerramilli M, Obare E, et al. Serum concentrations of symmetric dimethylarginine and creatinine in dogs with naturally occurring chronic kidney disease. J Vet Intern Med 2016;30:794–802.

43. Yee J, Yu C, Kim J, et al. Histopathological study of canine renal disease in Korea, 2003-2008. J Vet Sci 2010;11:277–83.

44. Blackwell S, O'Reilly DS, Reid D, et al. Plasma dimethylarginines during the acute inflammatory response. Eur J Clin Invest 2011;4:635–41.

45. Mookerjee RP, Malaki M, Davies NA, et al. Increasing dimethylarginine levels are associated with adverse clinical outcome in severe alcoholic hepatitis. Hepatology 2007;45:62–71.

46. Lluch P, Mauricio MD, Vila JM, et al. Accumulation of symmetric dimethylarginine in hepatorenal syndrome. Exp Biol Med (Maywood) 2006;23:70–5.

47. Meinitzer A, Kielstein JT, Pilz S, et al. Symmetrical and asymmetrical dimethylarginine as predictors for mortality in patients referred for coronary angiography: the Ludwigshafen risk and cardiovascular health study. Clin Chem 2011;57: 112–21.

48. Cavalca V, Veglia F, Squellerio I, et al. Circulating levels of dimethylarginines, chronic kidney disease and long-term clinical outcome in non-ST-elevation myocardial infarction. PLoS One 2012;7:e48499.

49. Krzyzanowska K, Mittermayer F, Shnawa N, et al. Asymmetrical dimethylarginine is related to renal function, chronic inflammation and macroangiopathy in patients with type 2 diabetes and albuminuria. Diabet Med 2007;24:81–6.

50. Rytlewski K, Olszanecki R, Korbut R, et al. Effects of prolonged oral supplementation with l-arginine on blood pressure and nitric oxide synthesis in preeclampsia. Eur J Clin Invest 2005;35:32–7.

51. Moesgaard SG, Holte AV, Mogensen T, et al. Effects of breed, gender, exercise and white-coat effect on markers of endothelial function in dogs. Res Vet Sci 2007;82:409–15.

52. Pedersen LG, Tarnow I, Olsen LH, et al. Body size, but neither age nor asymptomatic mitral regurgitation, influences plasma concentrations of dimethylarginines in dogs. Res Vet Sci 2006;80:336–42.

53. Grauer GF. Early detection of renal damage and disease in dogs and cats. Vet Clin North Am Small Anim Pract 2005;35:581–96.

54. WSAVA Nutritional Assessment Guidelines Task Force Members, Freeman L, Becarova I, Cave N, et al. WSAVA Nutritional Assessment Guidelines. J Small Anim Pract 2011;52:385–96.

55. Chandler ML, Takishima G. Nutritional concepts for the veterinary practitioner. Vet Clin North Am Small Anim Pract 2014;44:645–66.

56. Prusevich P, Patch D, Obare E, et al. Validation of a novel high throughput immunoassay for the quantitation of symmetric dimethylarginine (SDMA) [AACC 2015 abstract B-048]. Clin Chem 2015;16:S135 (supplement 2015).

57. Patch D, Obare E, Prusevich P, et al. High throughput immunoassay for kidney function biomarker symmetric dimethylarginine (SDMA) [AACC 2015 abstract B-047]. Clin Chem 2015;16:S135 (supplement 2015).
58. Watson ADJ, Lefebvre HP, Elliot J. Using urine specific gravity. International Renal Interest Society Guidelines. 2015. Available at: http://www.iris-kidney.com/education/urine_specific_gravity.html. Accessed March 18, 2016.
59. Lulich JP, Osborne CA, O'Brien TD, et al. Feline renal failure: questions, answers, questions. Compend Contin Educ Pract 1992;14:127–53.
60. Brown SA. Renal dysfunction in small animals. The Merck Veterinary Manual Web site. 2013. Available at: https://www.merckmanuals.com/vet/urinary_system/noninfectious_diseases_of_the_urinary_system_in_small_animals/renal_dysfunction_in_small_animals.html. Accessed March 14, 2016.

Kidney Disease and the Nexus of Chronic Kidney Disease and Acute Kidney Injury

The Role of Novel Biomarkers as Early and Accurate Diagnostics

Murthy Yerramilli, PhD*, Giosi Farace, MSc, PhD, John Quinn, MS, Maha Yerramilli, MS, PhD

KEYWORDS

- Biomarkers • Kidney • Renal • SDMA • CKD • AKI • Diagnostics • SDMA

KEY POINTS

- Chronic kidney disease and kidney injury are interconnected; the presence of one is a risk for the other.
- It is necessary to develop species-specific and target organ–specific biomarkers that result in sensitive and reliable diagnostic tests.
- A combination of diagnostics that assesses kidney function and ongoing disorder (active injury) will give practitioners a complete picture, allowing better patient management, improved care, and better outcomes.
- Symmetric dimethylarginine is a more reliable and earlier marker for chronic kidney disease than creatinine.
- Kidney-specific clusterin, cystatin B, and inosine are all markers for the diagnosis of active kidney injury in both cats and dogs.

KIDNEY DISEASE AND THE NEXUS OF CHRONIC KIDNEY DISEASE AND ACUTE KIDNEY INJURY

The progression of chronic kidney disease (CKD) is characterized by continuously advancing and irreversible loss of kidney function caused by loss of renal architecture and individual nephrons characterized by progressive scarring that ultimately results in structural damage to the kidney.[1,2] General mechanisms include systemic and glomerular hypertension, the renin-angiotensin-aldosterone system (RAAS), podocyte

Disclosure: The authors are employees of IDEXX Laboratories.
IDEXX Laboratories, Research & Development, 1-IDEXX Drive, Westbrook, ME 04092, USA
* Corresponding author.
E-mail address: Murthy-Yerramilli@idexx.com

loss, dyslipidemia, and proteinuria. CKD is a silent disease that can remain asymptomatic until an advanced stage. Underlying CKD is one of the most important predictors of vulnerability toward acute kidney injury (AKI) after exposure to risk factors such as nephrotoxic drugs or major surgeries.

AKI is characterized by abrupt deterioration in kidney function and major causes include nephrotoxic drugs such as nonsteroidal antiinflammatory drugs (NSAIDs) and chemotherapeutics, infections, vasculitis, surgery, neoplasia, and blockage of urinary tract by kidney stones. After AKI, renal function could be fully recovered in surviving patients; there could be incomplete recovery resulting in CKD; there could be exacerbation of preexisting CKD, accelerating its progression; or there may also be complete nonrecovery needing permanent renal replacement therapy.[3–5]

For a long time, CKD and AKI have been seen as two distinct diseases in isolation. Lately, multiple epidemiologic and outcome analysis studies in humans have suggested that the two diseases are not distinct entities but are closely associated and interconnected with common risk factors and disease modifiers (**Fig. 1**). CKD is a risk factor for AKI and vice versa. Persistent or repetitive injury over a period of time could progress CKD.[6–8] This latest understanding brings new perspectives to the diagnosis and monitoring of kidney diseases, highlighting the need for a panel of appropriate biomarkers that reflect functional as well as structural damage and recovery, predict potential risk, and provide prognosis. The utility of these biomarkers should go beyond diagnostic applications and provide insights into whether the disease is active (ie, continuously progressing) or pathologically stable. Such diagnostic tools have the potential to change long-held clinical practice patterns and therapeutic approaches, and help unravel elusive mechanisms concerning the nature of progressive versus stable kidney disease. Early and accurate diagnosis could provide opportunities for timely and effective interventions and prevention of further disease progression.

BIOMARKERS

A biomarker is defined as a physical, functional, or biochemical indicator of a physiologic or disease process that has diagnostic and/or prognostic utility with the ability to

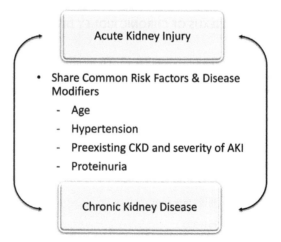

Fig. 1. Nexus between CKD and acute kidney injury.

be measured accurately and reproducibly. The present role of biomarkers is rapidly expanding beyond diagnosing progression and regression of diseases. Biomarkers are becoming indispensable in accelerating drug discovery and development, in understanding the efficacy and toxicity of therapies, and in shortening the duration of clinical trials by creating measurable and objective intermediate end points rather than long-term hard end points such as survival time.[9–12] The journey of a biomarker from bench to clinic is long and difficult, as shown in **Fig. 2**.

There are a variety of biomarkers discovered and reported on regular basis, but very few of them reach the clinics. There are several requirements and strict criteria that a biomarker needs to meet to be an ideal marker and adopted into clinical practice.[13] Some of these features are presented in **Fig. 3**.

CREATININE AS A KIDNEY FUNCTION BIOMARKER AND FALSE RESPONSES

Serum creatinine has been the standard-of-care test for kidney function and disease for about 100 years. It is a breakdown product of muscle metabolism and correlates with muscle mass.[14–16] As a result, kidney function is overestimated in cachectic low-muscled animals, whereas it may result in false diagnoses of kidney dysfunction in heavily muscled animals. Creatinine metabolism must reach and remain at a steady state to reflect kidney function, and this hampers detection of small losses of renal function. In addition, differences that depend on gender, age, and race have been observed in human patients. Because of these limitations, severe loss of kidney

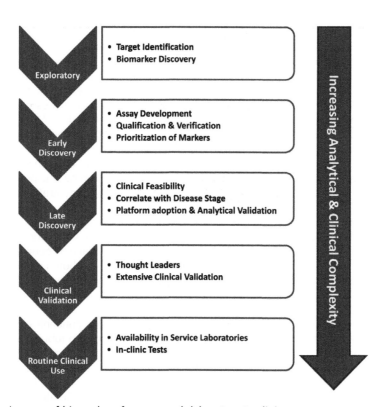

Fig. 2. Journey of biomarkers from research laboratory to clinic.

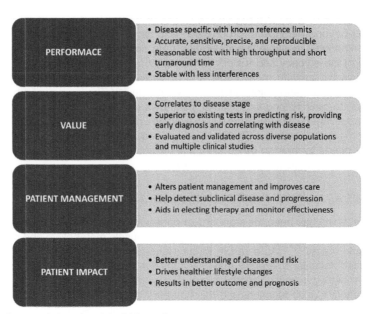

Fig. 3. Characteristics of an ideal biomarker.

function may occur before significant changes in creatinine level are observed.[17] However, trending within the reference range has been shown to improve the clinical performance of creatinine measurements. There are also several issues associated with the analytical measurement of the creatinine level using the Jaffe reaction, the most commonly used method, including significant interference from endogenous compounds, such as ascorbate, pyruvate, glucose, bilirubin, and ketoacids, that cause overestimation of creatinine. Hemolysed samples can also cause issues because of the increased release of the noncreatinine chromogens listed earlier.[18] Lipemic and icteric samples can interfere with the optical measurement and thus falsely lower the creatinine result obtained. It has been shown that clinically relevant drug concentrations (eg, cephalosporins, aminoglycosides, trimethoprim, and phenacemide) caused false increases in creatinine levels. The effect of these drugs was proportional to the serum drug concentration and additive to the baseline concentration of serum creatinine.[19,20]

It has also been shown that serum creatinine level increases after ingestion of cooked meat products in humans and dogs, and that this increase occurs independently of glomerular filtration rate (GFR).[21,22] In dogs, serum creatinine concentrations increased on average 0.4 mg/dL and were increased for several hours after feeding. Most of the commercially available pet foods and treats contain cooked meats; hence care should be taken in interpreting increased creatinine concentrations in nonstarved animals.

There are multiple biological processes that affect creatinine concentrations independent of kidney function, including hydration status, changes in tubular secretion, and alterations in transport.[17,23–27] In hypertonic dehydration, depletion of total body water leads to hypernatremia in the extracellular compartment. This process draws fluid from the intracellular compartment together with creatinine. Dehydration therefore leads to increased circulating creatinine concentrations. Creatinine is mostly eliminated when it passes from the blood into the urine through the glomerulus.

However, a significant percentage is secreted through the proximal tubule. In healthy humans this has been estimated to account for 28% to 40% of total excreted creatinine. Tubular secretion of creatinine has been reported in the dog as well. There are also some drugs that can influence biological processes that in turn could affect creatinine concentrations independent of kidney function. The highly prescribed corticosteroid, prednisone, accelerates muscle metabolism, leading to increased creatinine concentrations.[20] Also certain diseases, such as acute pancreatitis, seem to nonspecifically increase creatinine concentrations, potentially caused by dehydration and decreased blood flow.[28,29]

Even with all these significant limitations, creatinine assessment still remains the standard of care for the evaluation of kidney function in both human and veterinary medicine because finding new markers that offer significant performance improvements compared with creatinine has proved to be extremely challenging. Instead of moving toward new markers, human medicine has focused on the development of algorithms (Cockcroft and Gault, Modification of Diet in Renal Disease [MDRD], Chronic Kidney Disease Epidemiology [CKD-EPI]) that account for some of the gender and age issues described earlier; however, there are some serious shortcomings of creatinine that still remain unaddressed, highlighting the limitations of such approaches.[17] No such attempts have been made in veterinary medicine to derive even modest improvements in the clinical performance of creatinine, leaving it as a poor biomarker for kidney function in cats and dogs.

The frustrating inaccuracies associated with creatinine are a serious obstacle to the qualification of new biomarkers when creatinine serves as the reference for comparison. As an example, multiple studies involving biomarkers such as neutrophil gelatinase-associated lipocalin (NGAL) in human medicine might have reached positive outcome had there been a true gold standard for AKI rather than defining AKI as change in serum creatinine level.[30] The dependence on creatinine sets up the new biomarkers for poor accuracy and performance because of either false-positives (true tubular injury but no significant change in serum creatinine) or false-negatives (absence of true tubular injury, but increases in serum creatinine level) caused by prerenal issues or any of the several confounding variables that were discussed earlier. In veterinary medicine, clinicians need to learn from these missteps taken in human medicine and need to be careful when evaluating new biomarkers for active kidney injury. Rather than relying on creatinine, clinicians would be better served by focusing more on the association between new biomarkers and clinical outcomes, treatments, and reduction in adverse outcomes.

RENAL BIOMARKER DISCOVERY

Biomarker discovery is a complex and challenging process.[31] The principal enabling technology is mass spectrometry (MS) combined with disease-associated differential analysis, a widely used approach in which statistically significant differences in the expression of proteins or the production of metabolites between disease and control cohorts identify potential biomarkers. Any biological fluids from clinically well-characterized populations can be used in the discovery process. However, serum is preferred because it is considered the most comprehensive circulating representative of the proteome and metabolome of all body tissues and of both physiologic and pathologic processes. Also, the accessibility and vast clinical laboratory infrastructure that is already in place for the analysis of serum once biomarkers reach the clinic makes it the most suitable biological sample. However, this process needs to address the complexity that comes from the presence of tens of thousands of proteins, peptides, and metabolites with abundances spanning several orders of magnitude; for example, from albumin to thyroxine.

The process and the work flow used in the discovery of the markers discussed in this article is presented in **Fig. 4**. Serum and urine samples from clinically well-characterized healthy and disease cohorts of dogs were analyzed using a combination of advanced technologies and processes involving liquid chromatography mass spectroscopy (LCMS), bioinformatics, and data analytics identifying differentially expressed metabolites and proteins as potential biomarkers.

As examples, this research approach identified symmetric dimethylarginine (SDMA) as an early marker for kidney function, along with urinary clusterin and cystatin B and serum cystatin B and inosine as markers of active kidney injury. The biology and the performance of these markers are discussed individually in this article.

KIDNEY-SPECIFIC BIOMARKERS

Biomarkers are not always specific to the organ of interest because some protein markers are secreted by multiple tissues. As an example, clusterin messenger RNA is ubiquitous in all animal tissues and is abundant in liver, stomach, brain, and testes.[32] Similarly, NGAL is expressed and secreted by immune cells, hepatocytes, adipocytes, epithelial cells, liver, lung, colon, and renal tubular cells in various pathologic states.[33] Alkaline phosphatase is another example that is secreted by multiple tissues, and it is used to assess liver function.[34] However, the current diagnostic methods measure both liver and bone alkaline phosphatase levels. These isoforms are both products of the same gene, and the only difference is the posttranslational glycosylation, which means that use of this marker to monitor either bone metabolism or liver dysfunction can be compromised if a simple sandwich enzyme-linked immunosorbent assay (ELISA) approach is adopted that measures all isoforms.

Hence it is important to measure proteins specifically from the target organ or disorder to avoid false diagnoses. This specificity could be accomplished by targeting subtle differences such as posttranslational modifications (PTMs) that are specific to the disease process in order to develop accurate diagnostics, as described later for kidney-specific urinary clusterin (**Fig. 5**).

SYMMETRIC DIMETHYLATED ARGININE
Discovery

Symmetric dimethylated arginine (SDMA) and asymmetrical dimethylated arginine (ADMA) were first isolated from human urine in 1970 by Kakimoto and Akazawa.[35] They found that the excretion of these compounds was not from dietary sources and thought it to be from an endogenous source. In 1992, Vallance and colleagues[36]

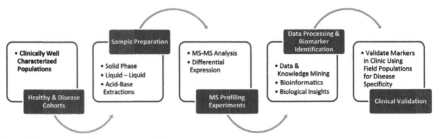

Fig. 4. Biomarker discovery workflow.

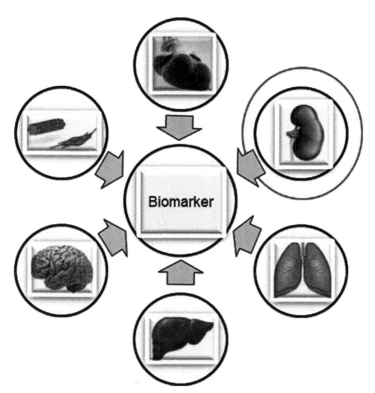

Fig. 5. Concept of organ-specific biomarkers.

reported an 8-fold increase in combined ADMA and SDMA levels in the serum of hemodialysis patients. Marescau and colleagues,[37] in 1997, reported that the concentrations of SDMA in both serum and urine correlated with the degree of renal insufficiency in nondialyzed patients with CKD and first suggested that serum SDMA was a good indicator for the onset of renal dysfunction.

Biochemistry

Arginine is a conditional essential amino acid and most animals make their own. Posttranslational modification of protein arginine groups occurs in the mitochondria involving the enzyme protein arginine methyltransferase, which results in 2 structural isomers, SDMA and ADMA.[38] N-monomethyl arginine (NMMA) is the intermediate form of both dimethylated isomers; the structures of arginine and its methylated derivatives are shown in **Fig. 6**. Arginine methylation primarily occurs in histones for the purpose of transcriptional regulation. In general, asymmetric methylation of the arginine (ADMA) activates transcription, whereas symmetric methylation (SDMA) is a repressive signal.[39] Proteolysis of these methylated proteins results in the release of SDMA and ADMA into the cytoplasm and then from the cell into the circulation via the y$^+$ cationic transporters.[40]

Although ADMA has been shown to be an endogenous inhibitor of nitric oxide synthase (NOS) and a marker for cardiovascular disease, SDMA does not interfere with NOS activity[36] or arginine transport at physiologic concentrations.[41] Approximately 80% of circulating ADMA is eliminated through enzymatic pathways,[42] making it a poor marker for renal function. However, SDMA is strictly eliminated through the

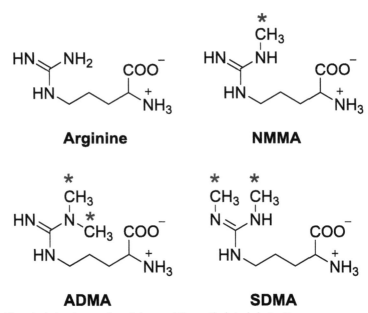

Fig. 6. Chemical structures of arginine and its methylated derivatives.

kidneys by renal filtration and excretion, and so circulating concentrations are primarily affected by changes in GFR and thus correlate with kidney function.[43]

Further evidence supporting that SDMA has no physiologic role was shown when GFR, cardiac function, and blood pressure were found to be unchanged in mice that received chronic infusions of SDMA for 28 days. Also, no renal histopathologic changes were observed, thus strengthening the idea that SDMA does not play a role in renal impairment.[44]

SYMMETRIC DIMETHYLATED ARGININE AS A MARKER FOR RENAL FUNCTION

SDMA was shown to correlate well with creatinine and renal insufficiency in a rodent model using Sprague-Dawley rats and Swiss mice in which insufficiency was induced by ligating branches of renal arteries or by removing the right kidney.[45] In a similar canine model in which dogs underwent either heminephrectomy or ligation of the left renal artery and subsequent contralateral nephrectomy, circulating SDMA levels were shown to increase as renal mass was reduced.[46]

SDMA was determined in a study of 257 people, consisting of healthy controls and patients with CKD on dialysis and patients who had undergone kidney transplant. SDMA levels were significantly increased in patients with CKD compared with the control population. Dialysis-dependent patients had even higher concentrations of circulating SDMA, which returned to baseline posttransplant.[47]

Multiple additional studies have further established SDMA as a more specific, sensitive, and accurate marker of renal function compared with serum creatinine.[25,48–50]

CORRELATION WITH GLOMERULAR FILTRATION RATE

GFR is the gold standard in determining kidney function in people and animals. However, GFR cannot be measured directly and instead is measured through the urinary or plasma clearance of various small molecules, including inulin and iohexol. The plasma clearance methods for determining a measured GFR (mGFR) require a bolus injection of the small molecule and multiple, precisely timed measurements of the marker molecule from blood collections documenting elimination of the marker, making the process expensive and inconvenient. In human medicine, various formulas to account for the impact of race and gender on the creatinine concentration are widely used to calculate an estimated GFR (eGFR); however, they are not routinely used in veterinary practice.

Serum SDMA concentration has been shown to correlate well with mGFR in people, establishing it as an endogenous marker of GFR. Studies comparing mGFR with SDMA have included endogenous creatinine clearance, and inulin and iohexol clearance.[43,51] In 2006, Kielstein and colleagues[43] provided an extensive summary of a meta-analysis of 18 studies of SDMA predictions of kidney function involving 2136 human patients. SDMA concentrations correlated highly with inulin clearance as an estimate of mGFR.

The first evidence for using SDMA to assess renal disease in dogs using a remnant kidney model was published in 2007 and showed a strong correlation of SDMA with mGFR by inulin clearance.[46] More recently, a linear relationship was shown between GFR and SDMA levels in a population of cats[52,53] and in carrier females and affected males from a colony of dogs with X-linked hereditary nephropathy[54] compared with mGFR using iohexol clearance.

In another study involving client-owned cats with CKD, SDMA concentrations were shown to increase and were correlated with serum creatinine.[55] In addition, a study evaluating hyperthyroid cats showed that SDMA level correlated better than serum creatinine level with mGFR estimated by iohexol clearance before starting diet therapy and at 6 months of follow-up.[56]

SYMMETRIC DIMETHYLATED ARGININE AS AN EARLY AND RELIABLE RENAL BIOMARKER IN CATS AND DOGS

In cats[53] and dogs,[54,57] SDMA has been shown to be an earlier marker of kidney dysfunction than creatinine, which is known to increase only after significant loss of renal function. A recently published retrospective study in cats found that an increase in SDMA above the upper reference limit of normal corresponded with an average 40% loss in mGFR from baseline; however, in some cases changes in mGFR as low as 25% were detected by increases in SDMA level. In this population the increased SDMA level diagnosed CKD an average of 17 months earlier than creatinine.[53] **Fig. 7** shows a representative case of a cat from Hall and colleagues,[53] in which SDMA level increased above the upper reference limit 9 months earlier than creatinine.

In this feline study,[53] serum SDMA had a sensitivity of 100%, specificity of 91%, positive predictive value (PPV) of 86%, and negative predictive value (NPV) of 100% when using a 30% decrease from median mGFR (by iohexol) of colony cats as the reference limit to confirm decreased renal function. The specificity and PPV of SDMA were affected by what were considered as 2 false-positives. In both of these cases, SDMA level was increased above the reference interval but mGFR was only decreased by 25% below the median reference; this might mean that SDMA testing was able to detect CKD even earlier in these cats. Meanwhile, in this same study, serum creatinine had a sensitivity of only 17%, specificity of 100%, PPV of 100%, and NPV of only 70%.

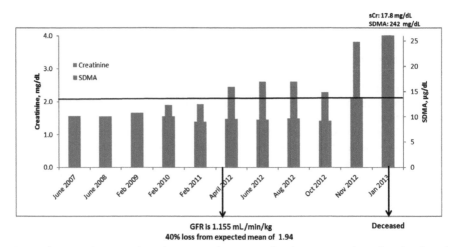

Fig. 7. The typical progression of SDMA and creatinine levels in a normal cat that developed CKD. The red bars are the SDMA concentrations and the blue bars are creatinine. The line represents the upper reference limit for both markers.

In a similar retrospective study in dogs with CKD, SDMA level increased an average of 9.8 months earlier than serum creatinine and was significantly correlated with mGFR. **Fig. 8** shows one of the dogs from the study[58] in which SDMA level increased above the upper reference limit at least 20 months earlier than creatinine.

In a prospective study involving male dogs affected with X-linked hereditary nephropathy and unaffected male littermates, SDMA remained unchanged in unaffected dogs, whereas it increased during disease progression, correlating strongly with a decrease in GFR in affected dogs. SDMA identified, on average, less than 20% decrease in GFR, which was significantly earlier than recognized with serum creatinine.[54]

Preliminary results suggest that increased serum SDMA concentrations above its upper reference limit and its ratio with creatinine may have prognostic value in dogs

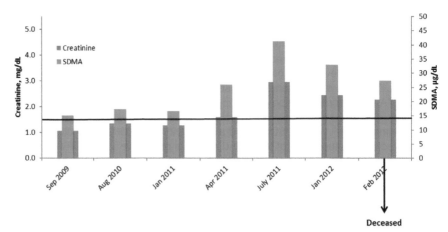

Fig. 8. The typical progression of SDMA and creatinine levels in a normal dog that developed CKD. The red bars are the SDMA concentrations and the blue bars are creatinine. The line represents the upper reference limit for both markers.

and cats with CKD.[59] Results from the same study have also suggested that a new biochemical pathway involving the enzyme AGXT2 may be resulting in discordance between creatinine and SDMA clearance. The enzyme AGXT2 is a transaminase present in glomeruli and catalyzes the conversion of glyoxylate to the essential amino acid glycine. The enzyme uses beta aminoisobutyric acid (BAIB), which is a catabolic end product of the pyrimidine degradation pathway, as an amine donor. Disorders such as inflammation, fibrosis, and neoplastic infiltration can damage cells, resulting in the loss of this enzyme, and as a result the enzyme substrates, glyoxylate and BAIB, accumulate in the kidney. Glyoxylate is converted to oxalate and can lead to the formation of oxalate nephroliths, whereas BAIB is strongly cationic and can bind to the negatively charged basement membrane, altering its polarity. Although the clearance of neutral molecules such as creatinine is not affected by this change in polarity, the clearance of SDMA, which is extremely cationic, is affected and this results in increased concentrations in circulation and thus may provide new diagnostic insights. However, these findings are preliminary and require additional and detailed studies in a clinical setting.[59]

SPECIFICITY OF SYMMETRIC DIMETHYLATED ARGININE AS A RENAL BIOMARKER

Multiple studies in different clinical scenarios have established SDMA as an extremely specific and sensitive biomarker of renal function. A major shortcoming of creatinine is its dependence on muscle mass, because it is the major metabolite of muscle breakdown. As a result, its levels can be falsely increased in heavily muscled animals and it can underestimate kidney function in these patients.[60,61] In addition, cachectic patients who are losing muscle mass or geriatric animals with low muscle mass may have falsely low levels of creatinine, thus causing an overestimation of kidney function.

In a prospective study of cats,[60] the correlation of muscle mass with creatinine and SDMA levels was investigated. GFR was determined in order to understand true kidney function in these animals and changes in body mass and composition were assessed by dual-energy X-ray absorptiometry, leading to the determination of total mass, fat mass, and lean muscle mass. Cats were grouped into those less than 12 years old and those greater than 15 years old.

Table 1 shows that, as the cats aged, total lean muscle mass and GFR decreased in group B compared with group A. Creatinine also decreased as the cats aged, even though GFR decreased, meaning that creatinine level moved in the wrong direction, showing that it is affected by decreased lean muscle mass. In contrast, SDMA level increased, thus truly reflecting decreased renal function and signifying that it is unaffected by changes in muscle mass.

In a similar prospective study of dogs, body composition was again determined by dual-energy X-ray absorptiometry, and the correlations between lean mass, creatinine level, and SDMA level were studied over 6 months (**Fig. 9**). Lean muscle

Table 1				
Effect of lean body mass and GFR on creatinine and SDMA in cats				
Group	Age (y)	GFR (mL/min/kg)	Total Muscle Lean Mass (kg)	Creatinine Level (mg/dL)	SDMA Level (μg/dL)
A	<12 (n = 11)	1.56	4.01	1.55	15.7
B	>15 (n = 10)	1.29	2.58	1.31	22.3

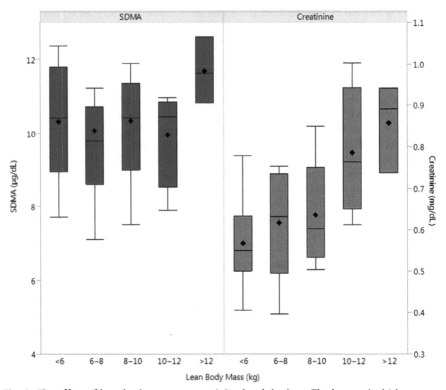

Fig. 9. The effect of lean body mass on creatinine levels in dogs. The box and whiskers cover the 10th and 90th percentiles of the population at each lean body mass category with the point representing the mean for each group. As the lean body mass increases, SDMA level (box and whiskers on left hand side) is unchanged, whereas creatinine level (box and whiskers on right hand side) increases.

mass and age were significantly correlated with creatinine, whereas SDMA was not.[61]

The population mean for SDMA in healthy humans,[62] cats,[53] and dogs[54] is 9.6, 9.8, and 9.6 μg/dL respectively. Considering the significant differences in size and lean body mass, the virtually identical population mean concentrations further suggest that SDMA is a true filtration marker uninfluenced by extrarenal factors such as age, gender, and muscle. Note that Singer[63] showed that the differences in GFR across mammals are not significant when normalized to their metabolic rates.

Increased SDMA level reflects reduced renal function, so increased SDMA concentrations are found in multiple disorders when compounded by reduced renal function.

In a human acute inflammatory response model, SMDA levels were determined in patients, without the confounding effects of multiple organ failure, and showed no significant changes caused by inflammation.[64] In patients with sepsis caused by leptospirosis, studies showed no significant difference in SDMA levels compared with those in patients without sepsis. Increases in SDMA levels only occurred when concurrent AKI was observed.[65]

Hepatorenal syndrome (HRS) is a major complication of end-stage cirrhosis in human patients and is characterized by functional renal failure. SDMA concentrations were found to be elevated in these patients compared with those with cirrhosis but there was no renal failure. Thus, renal dysfunction is a main determinant of increased SDMA in patients with HRS, and SDMA level is not influenced by liver disease.[66]

Prolonged supplementation with L-arginine in women with preeclampsia produced no changes in circulating SDMA concentrations.[67] The authors have measured arginine levels using LCMS in normal canine and feline populations and showed that the SDMA is not affected by serum arginine concentrations (**Fig. 10**).

In human patients with stroke, SDMA was shown to be a highly sensitive and specific marker of renal function and a prognostic indicator of mortality.[68] Increased SDMA concentrations are associated with CKD and worse long-term prognosis in patients with myocardial infarction. Researchers concluded that SDMA accumulation from reduced renal clearance reflects renal dysfunction. CKD is a known independent risk factor for adverse outcome in cardiac patients. There is good correlation between SDMA level and eGFR in this population. SDMA is a stronger predictor of cardiac events exacerbated by renal dysfunction compared with serum creatinine–calculated eGFR because SDMA level more accurately reflects filtration rate than serum creatinine level, and thus SDMA better identifies patients with a worse prognosis.[69] The authors have measured N-terminal pro–brain natriuretic peptide (NTproBNP) in nearly 300 dogs, including healthy and cardiac patients, and found no correlation between the cardiac marker and SDMA (**Fig. 11**). Increased SDMA concentrations were observed only in dogs that had compromised renal function.

The risk of CKD and AKI is a common problem in patients with cancer because of the toxicity of the chemotherapeutics, which limits treatment. With the greater incidence of cancer and particularly hematological malignancies, new therapies are being developed with increased urgency. This work will undoubtedly lead to an increased prevalence of kidney impairment and injury, which highlights the need for more effective and sensitive diagnostic biomarkers and tests. Although about 40% of human patients with lymphoma are known to have compromised kidney function, only 8% of the affected patients are diagnosed by creatinine alone, whereas the remaining 32% require biopsies[70–73] for diagnostic accuracy. In France, the IRMA studies (Insuffisance Rénale et Médicaments Anticancéreux [Renal Insufficiency and Anticancer Medications]) studies have reported a prevalence of reduced GFR (<90 mL/min/1.73 m²) in about 52% of a cohort of 5000 patients with different types of solid tumors. According to the international definition and stratification of human CKD, the prevalence of stages 3 to 5, excluding dialysis, was also high at about 12% in this population.[74] There are several recognized causes of kidney impairment in cancer, including medications, volume depletion, tumor lysis syndrome, obstruction, cancer infiltration, and

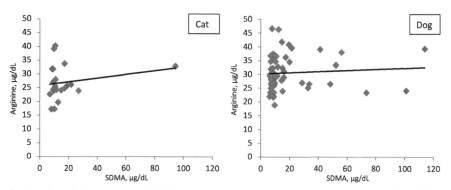

Fig. 10. Correlation between SDMA and arginine levels in cats and dogs showing that SDMA level is not influenced by the circulating arginine concentration.

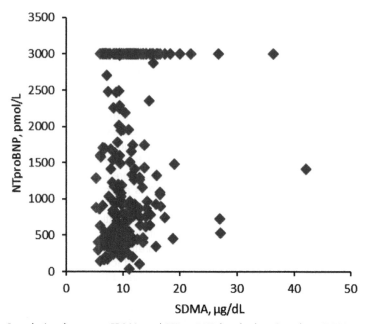

Fig. 11. Correlation between SDMA and NTproBNP levels showing that SDMA concentrations are not dependent on circulating NTproBNP concentrations.

sepsis. The ineffectiveness of creatinine is likely caused by reduced production as a result of cachexia, reduced protein intake, and medications to mention few. Although such detailed information is nonexistent for veterinary patients at this time, there is no reason to think the situation is any different.

It is possible that increased protein turnover in malignancies may lead to increased production of dimethylarginines, including both ADMA and SDMA. However, in a study that included different types of human hematological malignancies, ADMA but not SDMA was shown to have significantly increased concentration in the population with malignancies compared with the control group.[75] Mean plasma levels of SDMA were not different between the two groups (**Table 2**), further suggesting that any observations of increased SDMA levels in such disorders are likely caused by impaired kidney function. This finding supports the hypothesis described earlier that, as cells become malignant, increased protein turnover leads to increased ADMA production as a result of transcriptional activation via asymmetric methylation of the arginine.

Despite a wealth of evidence over the last 45 years in the form of experimental and clinical studies showing that SDMA level is a better measure of kidney function than creatinine level, a lack of a convenient analytical method has slowed the routine

Table 2
ADMA and SDMA in control and human patients with malignances

Analyte	Mean Plasma Levels in Group with Malignancies	Mean Plasma Levels in Control Group	P Value
ADMA (μmol/dL)	32	12.8	<.001
SDMA (μmol/dL)	10.7	9.6	.637

adoption of SDMA into clinics. Until recently, the measurement of SDMA level was performed primarily using the expensive and complex technique of mass spectroscopy. However, as of July 2015, a more convenient and accessible clinical chemistry assay has been developed and marketed for routine veterinary diagnostics by IDEXX. The International Renal Interest Society (IRIS) has recently recognized SDMA as a biomarker for kidney function in dogs and cats.[76]

IMPACT OF EARLY NUTRITIONAL INTERVENTIONS

Early diagnosis of CKD allows the initiation of renoprotective interventions that could potentially slow the progress or stabilize the disease. Dietary modifications are easy to implement and have high pet owner compliance, and, so far, feeding renal diets to cats and dogs with IRIS CKD stage 2 or higher has been considered the standard of care with strong clinical evidence for its effectiveness. Proven dietary modifications include decreased protein, phosphorous, and sodium, along with soluble fiber, omega 3 and 6 fatty acids, and antioxidants.[2,77]

A recent study of geriatric client-owned cats with early stage kidney disease, consistent with IRIS CKD stage 1, found that cats that were given a renal diet were more likely to maintain their serum SDMA concentrations than cats that continued to consume foods of the owner's choice. These results suggest that nonazotemic cats with increased serum SDMA levels (early renal insufficiency) fed a food designed to promote healthy kidneys are more likely to show stable renal function compared with cats fed owner's-choice foods. However, cats not receiving a renoprotective diet are more likely to show progressive renal insufficiency.[78]

In a similar study involving geriatric dogs with kidney disease consistent with IRIS stage 1, only dogs consuming the renal diet showed significant decreases in serum SDMA and Cr concentrations (both $P \leq .05$) across time. Compared with baseline, dogs that received the renal diet for 6 months showed decreases in serum SDMA level in 8 out of 9 cases, whereas of those that remained on owner's-choice foods for 6 months, approximately 50% increased their serum SDMA and Cr concentrations. These results suggest that nonazotemic dogs with early renal insufficiency and increased serum SDMA level are more likely to show improved kidney function when put on renal diets.[79]

URINARY CLUSTERIN

Clusterin, also known as apolipoprotein J, is a highly glycosylated extracellular chaperone.[80–82] It is expressed from a broad spectrum of tissues and is part of many physiologic processes, including sperm maturation, lipid transportation, complement inhibition, tissue remodeling, membrane recycling, and stabilization of stressed proteins, and is an inhibitor of apoptosis.[83–91] Although urinary clusterin concentrations are increased in kidney tubular damage, serum clusterin concentrations are affected in several physiologic and pathophysiologic processes, including sperm development, Alzheimer disease, atherosclerosis, and cancer.[92–94] Urinary clusterin as a marker of renal damage has been evaluated in a population of dogs with leishmaniasis, in which a statistically significant increase in clusterin concentrations was observed.[95] A second study evaluated clusterin levels in beagles with AKI induced by gentamycin, and the results showed a significant increase in clusterin concentrations following the drug-induced injury.[96]

Clusterin exists in two forms: secreted and nuclear. Although secretory clusterin delays apoptosis, nuclear clusterin triggers cell death. The secreted form consists of two 40-kDa chains derived from a single polypeptide precursor, alpha (amino acid residues 206–427) and beta (amino acid residues 1–205), which are connected by 5 symmetric disulfide bonds.[97] The secreted form also undergoes significant PTMs, including N-glycosylation. These PTMs are specific to the disease process and also to the tissue of origin.

Urinary clusterin is part of the US Food and Drug Administration and International Council on Harmonisation of Technical Requirements for Registration of Pharmaceuticals for Human Use (ICH) renal biomarker panels for drug development and toxicity.[98] A differential expression experiment consisting of healthy and kidney disease cohort dogs as described earlier also identified clusterin as a marker of kidney injury.

There are several immunoassays that have been developed and marketed for measuring clusterin levels in various body fluids, including plasma, serum, and urine. Urinary clusterin has most characteristics required of a biomarker of kidney damage or disease. It is expressed in urine at low to undetectable levels in the healthy kidney, and its levels increase significantly in response to an injury. In addition, urinary clusterin levels have been found to decrease in response to recovery from kidney injury.

Serum concentrations of clusterin (60–100 μg/mL) are 1000-fold higher than the urinary concentrations (<100 ng/mL) in healthy humans and dogs. Contamination of a urine sample with blood at levels as low as 0.2% (v/v) could lead to false-positives. This problem is more acute in veterinary medicine, because of infection, trauma, neoplasia, inflammation, and accidental contamination during catheterization and cystocentesis, with recognition that 33% of canine and 54% of feline urine samples submitted to a commercial reference laboratory have some level of blood contamination. The blood contamination brings nonspecific clusterin isoforms into the urine, and hence it is important to ensure that only kidney-specific clusterin is measured.

To show the complications of false-positive results from contamination by nonspecific clusterin, the clusterin concentration was determined in a control canine urine sample using a commercial kit and then spiked with normal canine serum (0.002% to 10% v/v). The resulting mixtures were analyzed and the results obtained are shown in **Table 3**.

At contamination levels of more than 0.5%, the clusterin concentration is above the upper reference limit of 70 ng/mL for the assay, resulting in a false-positive result.[99]

The urine from healthy canines was examined by urinalysis dipstick (IDEXX Laboratories) for the presence of blood. Urinary clusterin levels were measured using a commercially available two-site immunoassay kit according to the manufacturers' instructions (Biovendor Research and Diagnostic Products). As shown in **Table 4**,

Table 3 Negative impact on urinary clusterin quantitation when whole blood is spiked into control urine as determined with a commercial assay		
Sample	Whole-blood Contamination (%)	Clusterin (ng/mL)
Negative Urine	0	13.0
0.01-μL Spike	0.01	16.4
0.5-μL Spike	0.05	36.8
1-μL Spike	0.1	50.3
5-μL Spike	0.5	257.4
10-μL Spike	1	539.0
50-μL Spike	5	1321.3
100-μL Spike	10	2370.8

Table 4
Negative impact on urinary clusterin quantitation in normal canine urines contaminated with whole blood as determined with a commercial assay

Sample	Biovendor Clusterin Assay	Urine Dipstick Blood Pad Result
1	<LOQ	Negative
2	<LOQ	Negative
3	29	Negative
4	<LOQ	Negative
5	1045	3
6	1015	3
7	760	3
8	65,000	3

Abbreviation: LOQ, lower than the limit of quantitation.

healthy canines with no detectable blood in their urine had levels of clusterin within the reference range (70 ng/mL); however, those having blood contamination (samples 5–8) had clusterin levels 10 to 100 times above the normal reference range and would result in strong false-positives.

To accurately measure the clusterin levels associated with active kidney injury it is therefore necessary to measure only the kidney-specific isoform. An in vitro cellular model was developed that mimics the proximal tubule using cultured canine kidney cells. Stressing these cells with nephrotoxic gentamicin (**Fig. 12**) provided kidney-specific clusterin mimicking the time-dependent in vivo physiologic response in a dog given gentamicin. Meanwhile, the plasma isoform was purified from canine whole blood. By screening with lectins, a family of proteins that recognize different sugar moieties, the glycosylation pattern of the two isoforms was found to be different.

A sandwich format immunoassay was developed using the lectin that showed the highest affinity for kidney-specific clusterin isolated from the in vitro model together

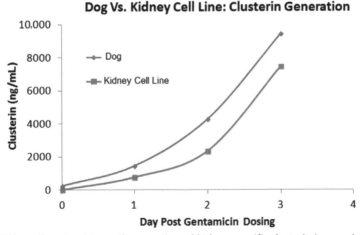

Fig. 12. Effect of gentamicin on the secretion of kidney-specific clusterin in a canine kidney cell line (*squares*) and in vivo in a dog (*diamonds*).

with a-specific monoclonal antibody raised against clusterin. To show the specificity of the kidney-specific clusterin immunoassay (KSCI), fresh whole blood or plasma from a healthy dog was spiked into buffer and analyzed using both the KSCI and the Biovendor assay.

As shown in **Fig. 13**, clusterin was detected at significantly high concentrations in both matrices by the commercial assay but not the KSCI. Taking into consideration that a high percentage of urine samples from healthy dogs and cats have blood contamination, the only way to accurately measure clusterin level is to use a KSCI.

Kidney-specific clusterin level was measured in urine from a canine gentamicin model (**Fig. 14**) and the urines of dogs presenting to a clinic with inflammatory or ischemic-induced active kidney injury (**Fig. 15**). In the model system, dogs were given 40 mg/kg gentamicin daily for 5 days. In this dog, serum creatinine was essentially unchanged throughout the study, whereas kidney-specific clusterin level increased rapidly, reaching 5 times baseline when dosing was stopped and peaked at 10 times baseline at day 11. This finding shows that clusterin is an earlier and more sensitive marker than serum creatinine for active kidney injury. In the patient samples there is a clear separation between healthy patients and those diagnosed with active kidney injury.

Preliminary results (not shown) have shown the feasibility of the current kidney-specific urinary clusterin immunoassay for feline samples as well.

In conclusion, kidney-specific clusterin is a sensitive and specific marker for active kidney injury in companion animals.

URINARY AND SERUM CYSTATIN B

The cystatins are a family of protein inhibitors of cysteine proteases and are ubiquitous in mammals. They are composed of 3 main individual families, as shown in **Fig. 16**.[100] All these cystatins share high sequence homology and a common tertiary structure of an alpha helix lying on top of antiparallel beta sheets. Cystatin C, the

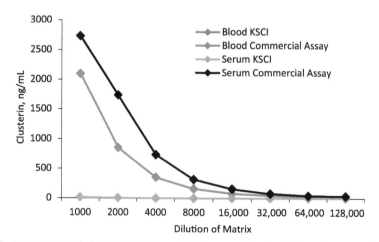

Fig. 13. Comparison of the performance of kidney-specific clusterin and commercial clusterin immunoassays when negative urine was spiked with whole blood and serum. The blue (whole blood) and green (serum) lines are the results from the kidney-specific assay and the red (whole blood) and black (serum) lines are the results from the commercial assay.

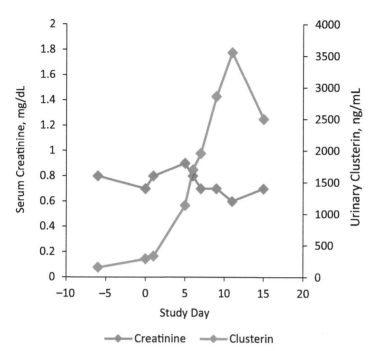

Fig. 14. Kidney-specific urinary clusterin level measured in a dog from the gentamicin model study. Gentamicin was administered daily for 5 days at 40 mg/kg and serum and urine samples were collected daily for 15 days. The blue line is the serum creatinine level and the red line is urinary clusterin.

most familiar of these proteins, along with cystatins D and S are 14 kDa, have 2 disulfide bonds, and belong to family 2. Cystatin C is freely filtered through glomeruli and is considered to be a marker for GFR.[101] Kininogens are much larger and highly glycosylated plasma proteins and are part of family 3. They are composed of a single polypeptide chain and contain 2 inhibitory domains homologous to cystatins of family 2. Kininogens are multifunctional and are involved in multiple biological processes and disorders, including blood coagulation, acute phase response, and cardiac disease.[100]

Cystatins A and B are members of family 1 and are small monomeric proteins of around 11 kDa. They are not glycosylated and do not have the disulfide bridges seen in larger family 2 and family 3 proteins. They also lack signal sequences and so are generally intracellular proteins confined to the cell.[100] Some cystatin B is present in extracellular fluids, and it has been purified from human urine.[102] Cystatin B has been shown to inhibit members of the lysosomal cysteine proteinases, cathepsin family, specifically cathepsins B, H, and L.[100,103–105]

Mutations of cystatin B have been found in progressive myoclonus epilepsy of the Unverricht-Lundborg type (EPM1).[106] EPM1 is a rare autosomal recessive disease that results in neurologic dysfunction that leads to dementia, cerebellar ataxia, and dysarthria.[107,108]

A differential expression experiment consisting of healthy and kidney disease cohort dogs (as described earlier) identified several peptides from cystatin B in the disease cohort. However, the UniProt (Universal Protein Resource) database[109,110] describes a protein that is truncated to 76 amino acids in the cat and 77 amino acids in the dog,

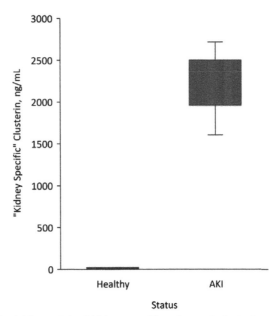

Fig. 15. Box and whiskers plot of kidney-specific urinary clusterin from clinically healthy dogs (n = 7) and dogs with diagnosed AKI (n = 12), showing the ability of the biomarker to differentiate the two populations.

compared with 98 amino acids in other mammalian species, including humans. The missing 22 (cat) and 21 (dog) amino acids represent the N-terminus of the protein and without the intact protein it is not possible to accurately measure concentrations of cystatin B.

Canine cystatin B was purified from canine kidney cells and the full sequence was determined by tryptic digestion followed by LCMS. Through this approach the following sequence shown in **Fig. 17** was identified. A recombinant protein was

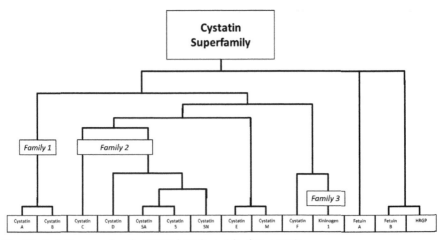

Fig. 16. Cystatin superfamily. HRGP, histidine rich glycoprotein.

Canine Cystatin B: MMCGAPSASQPATADTQAIADQVKAQLEERENKKYTTFKAVTFRSQVVAGTNYFIKVQVDDDEFVHLRVFQSLPHENKPLALSSYQTNKAKHDELAYF
Human Cystatin B: MMCGAPSATQPATAETQHIADQVRSQLEEKENKKFPVFKAVSFKSQVVAGTNYFIKVHVGDEDFVHLRVFQSLPHENKPLTLSNYQTNKAKHDELTYF

Fig. 17. Full amino acid sequence of canine and human cystatin B.

created using this sequence and was shown to be identical to native protein extracted from canine kidney cells using LCMS.

Cystatin B is an intracellular protein and generally not freely circulating in large concentrations. This finding was further confirmed when no protein was found in the supernatant collected from stressed canine kidney cells. However, cystatin B was purified from ruptured canine kidney cells. Therefore, any cystatin B that is detected in serum or urine must result from the rupture and death of tubular epithelial cells. In active kidney injury, apoptosis and necrosis of epithelial cells in the proximal tubule is likely to result in increased serum and urinary cystatin B levels (**Fig. 18**).

Nothing has been published linking cystatin B and kidney disease in companion animals. A recent study in humans[111] for the first time showed alterations in protease profiles of urinary extracellular vesicles from patients with diabetic nephropathy, resulting in the increase in cystatin B levels and showing a link between cystatin B and kidney disease.

Monoclonal antibodies were raised against the recombinant canine cystatin B and their specificity confirmed using Western blot analysis of purified native samples (**Fig. 19**). A sandwich ELISA was also developed using these antibodies.

Cystatin B was measured using the ELISA in serum and urine from a canine gentamicin model (**Fig. 20**) and the urines of dogs presenting to a clinic with inflammatory or ischemic-induced active kidney injury (**Fig. 21**). In the model system, dogs were given 10 mg/kg gentamicin every 8 hours until serum creatinine level reached 1.5 mg/dL. That point was reached on day 8; whereas serum cystatin B level was increased over baseline on day 1. These preliminary results suggest that cystatin B is an earlier marker than creatinine for active kidney injury. In the patient samples with naturally occurring kidney disease there is a clear separation between healthy patients and those diagnosed with active kidney injury. In most of the patients with urinary tract infections (UTIs), cystatin B concentrations were similar to those of healthy dogs.

The feasibility of this assay for feline samples has also been shown. From these early results, cystatin B is emerging as a promising new marker for active kidney injury in both serum and urine, which requires further detailed clinical field studies before the marker can be available for routine use in the clinic.

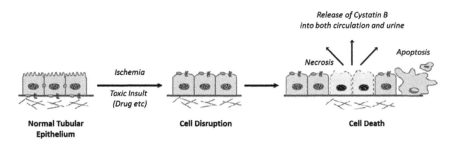

Fig. 18. Potential mechanism of cystatin B release in AKI.

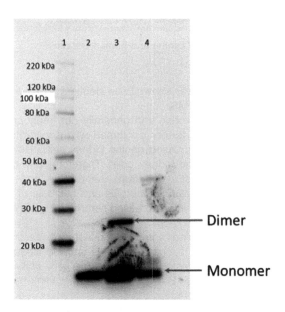

Lane	Sample
1	Molecular Weight Standards
2	Native Sample Prep 1
3	Native Sample Prep 2
4	Native Sample Prep 3

Fig. 19. Western blot of purified cystatin B from 3 different canine urine samples. Lane 1 is the reference molecular weight ladder and lanes 2 to 4 are the canine urine samples. All 3 samples contain the cystatin B monomer, whereas the sample in lane 3 also has some dimeric cystatin B.

SERUM INOSINE

Lately the role of adenosine metabolism, signaling, and receptor binding in processes related to renal fibrosis and kidney injury, such as ischemia, hypoxia, and apoptosis, has attracted substantial attention.[112,113] ATP is the energy source of the cell, and its levels decrease during cellular energy demand. ATP is sequentially hydrolyzed to ADP, to AMP, and then to adenosine. The extracellular actions of adenosine are mediated by the binding of the nucleotide to 4 types (A_1R, $A_{2a}R$, $A_{2b}R$, and A_3R) of G protein–coupled adenosine membrane receptors.

It is suggested that endogenous adenosine is formed by renal tubular epithelial cells.[114] Inhibition of cellular uptake of adenosine increases the interstitial adenosine concentrations, leading to decreased circulating concentrations and resulting in a significant decrease in renal blood flow and GFR. This process suggests that the renal hemodynamics depend on the adenosine concentrations in the interstitium. The interstitial concentrations of adenosine are generally low but significantly increase during hypoxia and inflammation through the hydrolysis of ATP and subsequent release from injured or apoptotic cells.[115]

It has been shown in a canine hypoxia model that the accumulated interstitial adenosine is converted mainly into inosine by adenosine deaminase.[116] Increased circulating concentrations of plasma adenosine result in renal vasodilator response in most parts of the renal vasculature, including larger renal arteries, juxtamedullary

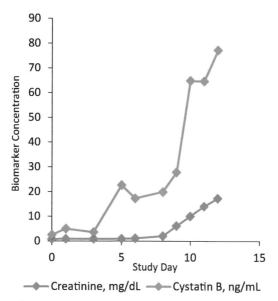

Fig. 20. Kidney-specific serum cystatin B levels measured in a canine gentamicin model. Gentamicin was given at 10 mg/kg every 8 hours until creatinine (*blue*) reached 1.5 mg/dL. Kidney-specific cystatin B level (*red*) increased several days earlier.

afferent arterioles, efferent arterioles, and medullary vessels. However, the efferent arteriole closer to the glomerulus responds to adenosine with vasoconstriction.

It was shown that adenosine is deaminated to inosine in the isolated basolateral membrane (BLM) of kidney proximal tubules by adenosine deaminase. It further has been shown that the inosine reduced Na^+-ATPase activity significantly by inhibiting the sodium pump mediated by the A_1 receptor/Gi/cyclic AMP pathway. Our biomarker discovery research has identified inosine as a biomarker for AKI through the differential expression technique described earlier in this article. The plasma and serum concentrations of inosine decreased rapidly and significantly following nephrotoxin exposure in canine gentamicin (**Fig. 22**)[117] and dichromate models of AKI (**Fig. 23**). The results suggested that inosine is not only one of the most sensitive biomarkers to injury but that it also responds to mark the recovery from the injury by the restoration to the normal circulating concentrations. It is likely that injury to the tubular epithelial cells by these nephrotoxins resulted in the loss of adenosine deaminase activity preventing the conversion of adenosine to inosine, leading to depletion of circulating inosine.

NEUTROPHIL-ASSOCIATED LIPOCALIN

Neutrophil-associated lipocalin (NGAL) (also known as 24p3, SIP24, lipocalin 2, or siderocalin) is a 24-kDa protein that binds iron-containing ligands (siderophores). It was originally discovered in human neutrophils,[118] but is found in several different tissues, including skin, alveolar and oral mucosa, adipose tissue, and proximal and distal tubules.[33] It is markedly induced in injured epithelial cells, including kidney, colon, liver, and lung, and in neoplasia. Its primary function is not clear but is probably associated with its ability to bind extracellular iron. It can bind siderophores produced by

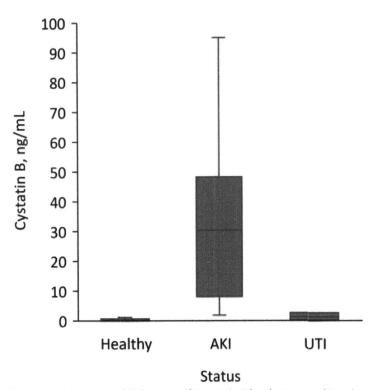

Fig. 21. Box and whiskers plot of kidney-specific cystatin B levels measured in urines of dogs that were diagnosed as either being healthy (n = 14), having an AKI (n = 16), or having a urinary tract infection (UTI) (n = 13). The plot shows that urinary cystatin B can differentiate dogs with AKI from the healthy and UTI populations.

both prokaryotes and eukaryotes. The binding of prokaryotic siderophores elicits a bacteriostatic effect by sequestering iron, whereas binding eukaryotic siderophores helps shuttle iron across cellular membranes used in cellular proliferation and differentiation.[30]

There is growing evidence and support for the use of NGAL as an AKI biomarker within the human medical community, with several studies showing increased plasma levels and serum and urinary NGAL concentrations in AKI events secondary to cardiac surgery, contrast-induced nephropathy, and kidney transplant.[30] In dogs, several studies have found that NGAL concentration is increased in AKI earlier than serum creatinine.[119,120]

Several potential issues have been noted for NGAL that could limit its adoption as a kidney marker. It has been observed that NGAL seems to perform best in homogenous patient populations with temporally predictable forms of AKI, and that there are significant correlations with age and gender.[30,33,121] Also, serum NGAL level has been found to correlate with alanine transaminase, aspartate transaminase, cholesterol, and high-sensitivity C-reactive protein. Circulating concentrations of NGAL may also be influenced by coexisting conditions such as CKD, chronic hypertension, systemic infections, inflammation, anemia, and hypoxia.[122]

Significant upregulation is observed in common inflammatory diseases such as eczema, periodontitis, and ulcerative colitis, and in metabolic disorders such as

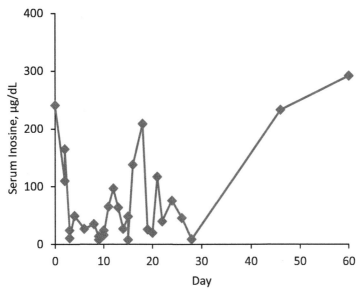

Fig. 22. Serum inosine concentration in a canine gentamicin model. The dog was given 8 mg/kg gentamicin for the first 7 days of the study and then 10 mg/kg until serum creatinine level increased 50% from day 0; this occurred on day 16. The increasing and decreasing concentrations of the biomarker during the study represent injury and recovery cycles.

obesity and type II diabetes in human patients. It is also overexpressed in several solid tumor malignancies, including skin, thyroid, breast, liver, and stomach.[33] In addition, urinary NGAL concentrations also seem to be heavily correlated with serum creatinine level, GFR, and proteinuria.[122]

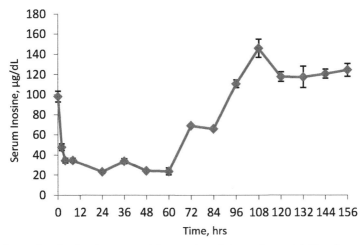

Fig. 23. Serum inosine levels measured in a canine dichromate model. The dog was given dichromate before time = 0 hours and samples were taken every 12 hours for 7 days. As dichromate was cleared from the circulation the biomarker concentration returned to baseline, indicating recovery of kidney function.

OTHER RENAL BIOMARKERS

Several other novel renal biomarkers have been described in human medicine, including cystatin C, kidney injury molecule-1, retinol binding protein, trefoil factor 3, insulinlike growth factor binding protein-7, and tissue inhibitor of metalloproteinase-2.[123–125] However, there is very limited information about their applicability to veterinary medicine at this time.

SUMMARY

Active injury and chronic disease are interconnected syndromes and not two distinct, and different, entities (see Larry D. Cowgill, David J. Polzin, Jonathan Elliott, et al: "Is Progressive Chronic Kidney Disease a Slow Acute Kidney Injury?," in this issue). Preexisting CKD is a risk factor for active injury and AKI is a risk factor for the initiation and progression of CKD.

Creatinine has been the standard of care for the past 100 years but it is only relevant after 75% of kidney function is lost, and it provides little information about ongoing active injury in the patient. Therefore, there is a need in both human and veterinary medicine for biomarkers that diagnose, predict risk and prognosis, and measure recovery following therapeutic interventions.

As described earlier, small molecules and protein biomarkers can be generated from multiple tissues and metabolic pathways that have no involvement in kidney disease, leading to potential nonspecificity issues. The only way to overcome this problem is to develop analytical methods/tests that specifically measure biomarkers generated by the kidney. It is also important that biomarkers are not influenced by extrarenal factors such as age, gender, breed, muscle mass, and hydration status.

Often decisions about the usefulness of biomarkers are made using reagents and test kits that have been developed for human diagnostics and that may either have poor reactivity toward the canine and feline markers or be overly affected by the sample matrices, leading to inaccurate clinical conclusions. Therefore, it is necessary to develop species-specific diagnostic tests that provide accurate measurements for veterinary patients.

As presented in this article, serum SDMA is an earlier biomarker than serum creatinine for diagnosing and monitoring CKD in cats and dogs on an average of 17 and 10 months, respectively, allowing more time for practitioners to positively intervene. Further, unlike creatinine, SDMA is not influenced by muscle mass, age, and breed. The commercially available IDEXX SDMA assay is specifically developed for veterinary applications and validated for both cats and dogs.

This article presents multiple examples of this approach using advanced analytical tools, including LCMS and bioinformatics, to identify canine clusterin and canine cystatin B from well-characterized clinical samples and then obtain native proteins from canine kidney cells. These purified proteins are then being used to develop *kidney-specific* diagnostic assays.

The combination of diagnostics that assess kidney function (SDMA) and ongoing pathology in patients (active injury markers) gives practitioners a complete toolkit to better manage patients, improve care, and achieve better outcomes.

REFERENCES

1. Thomas R, Abbas K, John RS. Chronic kidney disease and its complications. Prim Care 2008;35(2):329–44, vii.

2. Polzin DJ. Evidence-based step-wise approach to managing chronic kidney disease in dogs and cats. J Vet Emerg Crit Care (San Antonio) 2013;23(2):205–15.

3. Alge JL, Arthur JM. Biomarkers of AKI: a review of mechanistic relevance and potential therapeutic implications. Clin J Am Soc Nephrol 2015;10:147–55.

4. Linda R. Acute kidney injury in dogs and cats. Vet Clin Small Anim 2011;41:1–14.

5. Segev G, Nivy R, Kass P, et al. A retrospective study of acute kidney injury in cats and development of a novel clinical scoring system for predicting outcome for cats managed by hemodialysis. J Vet Intern Med 2013;27(4):830–9.

6. Manjeri AV, Karen AG, Rongpei L, et al. Acute kidney injury: a springboard for progression in chronic kidney disease. Am J Physiol Renal Physiol 2010;298:F1078–94.

7. Hsu CY, Ordonez JD, Chertow GM, et al. The risk of acute renal failure in patients with chronic kidney disease. Kidney Int 2008;74:101–7.

8. Chawla LS, Eggers PW, Star RA, et al. Acute kidney injury and chronic kidney disease as interconnected syndromes. N Engl J Med 2014;371(1):58–66.

9. Strimbu K, Tavel JA. What are biomarkers? Curr Opin HIV AIDS 2010;5(6):463–6.

10. Hawkridge AM, Muddiman DC. Mass spectrometry-based biomarker discovery: toward a global proteome index of individuality. Annu Rev Anal Chem (Palo Alto Calif) 2009;2:265–77.

11. Drucker E, Krapfenbauer K. Pitfalls and limitations in translation from biomarker discovery to clinical utility in predictive and personalised medicine. EPMA J 2013;4:7.

12. Konvalinka A, Scholey JW, Diamandis EP. Searching for new biomarkers of renal diseases through proteomics. Clin Chem 2012;58(2):353–65.

13. Rollins G. A look at emerging cardiac biomarkers: what type of analyte will be the most informative? Clinical Laboratory News 2012;38:1.

14. Narayanan S, Appleton HO. Creatinine: a review. Clin Chem 1980;26(8):1119–26.

15. Perrone RD, Madias NE, Levey AS. Serum creatinine as an index of renal function: new insights into old concepts. Clin Chem 1992;38(10):1933–53.

16. Baxmann AC, Ahmed MS, Marques NC, et al. Influence of muscle mass and physical activity on serum and urinary creatinine and serum cystatin C. Clin J Am Soc Nephrol 2008;3(2):348–54.

17. Dalton RN. Serum creatinine and glomerular filtration rate: perception and reality. Clin Chem 2010;56(5):687–9.

18. Peake M, Whiting M. Measurement of serum creatinine – current status and future goals. Clin Biochem Rev 2006;27:173–84.

19. Hyneck ML, Berardi RP, Johnson RM. Interference of cephalosporins and cefoxitin with serum creatinine determination. Am J Hosp Pharm 1981;38:1348–52.

20. Andreev E, Koopman M, Arisz L. A rise in plasma creatinine that is not a sign of renal failure: which drugs can be responsible? J Intern Med 1999;246:247–52.

21. Preiss DJ, Godber IM, Lamb EJ, et al. The influence of cooked-meat on estimated glomerular filtration rate. Ann Clin Biochem 2007;44:35–42.

22. Watson AD, Church DB, Fairburn AJ. Postprandial changes in plasma urea and creatinine concentrations in dogs. Am J Vet Res 1981;42(11):1878–80.

23. Thijssen S, Zhu F, Kotanko P, et al. Comment on "Higher serum creatinine concentrations in black patients with chronic kidney disease: beyond nutritional status and body composition." Clin J Am Soc Nephrol 2009;4:1011–3.

24. Atherton JC, Green R, Thomas S. Effects of 0.9% saline infusion on urinary and renal tissue compositions in the hydropaenic and hydrated conscious rat. J Physiol 1970;210:45–71.

25. Dixon JJ, Lane K, Dalton RN, et al. Symmetrical dimethylarginine is a more sensitive biomarker of renal dysfunction than creatinine. Crit Care 2013;17(Suppl 2): P423.

26. O'Connell JMB, Romeo JA, Mudge GH. Renal tubular secretion of creatinine in the dog. Am J Physiol 1962;203(6):985–90.

27. Sun H, Frassetto L, Benet LZ. Effects of renal failure on drug transport and metabolism. Pharmacol Ther 2006;109:1–11.

28. Lankisch PG, Weber-Dany B, Maisonneuve P, et al. High serum creatinine in acute pancreatitis: a marker for pancreatic necrosis? Am J Gastroenterol 2010;105(5):1196–200.

29. Beben T, Rifkin DE. GFR estimating equations and liver disease. Adv Chronic Kidney Dis 2015;22:337–42.

30. Devarajan P. Review: neutrophil gelatinase-associated lipocalin: a troponin-like biomarker for human acute kidney injury. Nephrology (Carlton) 2010;15:419–28.

31. Rifai N, Gillette MA, Carr SA. Protein biomarker discovery and validation: the long and uncertain path to clinical utility. Nat Biotechnol 2006;24:971–83.

32. Rosenberg ME, Silkensen J. Clusterin: physiologic and pathophysiologic considerations. Int J Biochem Cell Biol 1995;27(7):633–45.

33. Chakraborty S, Kaur S, Guha S, et al. The multifaceted roles of neutrophil gelatinase associated lipocalin (NGAL) in inflammation and cancer. Biochim Biophys Acta 2012;1826(1):129–69.

34. Griffiths J, Black J. Separation and identification of alkaline phosphatase isoenzymes and isoforms in serum of healthy persons by isoelectric focusing. Clin Chem 1987;33(12):2171–7.

35. Kakimoto Y, Akazawa S. Isolation and identification of N-G, N-G- and N-G, N'-G-dimethyl-arginine, N-epsilon-mono-, di-, and trimethyllysine, and glucosylgalactosyl- and galactosyl-delta-hydroxylysine from human urine. J Biol Chem 1970; 245(21):5751–8.

36. Vallance P, Leone A, Calver A, et al. Accumulation of an endogenous inhibitor of nitric oxide synthesis in chronic renal failure. Lancet 1992;339(8793):572–5.

37. Marescau B, Nagels G, Possemiers I, et al. Guanidino compounds in serum and urine of nondialyzed patients with chronic renal insufficiency. Metabolism 1997; 46(9):1024–31.

38. Tang J, Frankel A, Cook RJ, et al. PRMT1 is the predominant type I protein arginine methyltransferase in mammalian cells. J Biol Chem 2000;275(11):7723–30.

39. Bedford MT, Richard S. Arginine methylation: an emerging regulator of protein function. Mol Cell 2005;18(3):263–72.

40. Caplin B, Leiper J. Endogenous nitric oxide synthase inhibitors in the biology of disease: markers, mediators and regulators? Arterioscler Thromb Vasc Biol 2012;32(6):1343–53.

41. Tojo A, Welch WJ, Bremer V, et al. Colocalization of demethylating enzymes and NOS and functional effects of methylarginines in rat kidney. Kidney Int 1997; 52(6):1593–601.

42. Achan V, Broadhead M, Malaki M, et al. Asymmetric dimethylarginine causes hypertension and cardiac dysfunction and is actively metabolized by dimethylarginine dimethylaminohydrolase. Arterioscler Thromb Vasc Biol 2003;23(8):1455–9.

43. Kielstein JT, Salpeter SR, Bode-Böger SM, et al. Symmetric dimethylarginine (SDMA) as endogenous marker of renal function – a meta analysis. Nephrol Dial Transplant 2006;21(9):2445–51.

44. Veldink H, Faulhaber-Walter R, Park JK, et al. Effects of chronic SDMA infusion on glomerular filtration rate, blood pressure, myocardial function and renal histology in C57BL6/J mice. Nephrol Dial Transplant 2013;28(6):1434–9.

45. Al Banchaabouchi M, Marescau B, Possemiers I, et al. NG NG-dimethylarginine and NG, NG-dimethylarginine in renal insufficiency. Pflugers Arch 2000;439(5): 524–31.

46. Tatematsu S, Wakino S, Kanda T, et al. Role of nitric oxide-producing and -degrading pathways in coronary endothelial dysfunction in chronic kidney disease. J Am Soc Nephrol 2007;18(3):741–9.

47. Fleck C, Janz A, Schweitzer F, et al. Serum concentrations of asymmetric (ADMA) and symmetric (SDMA) dimethylarginine in renal failure patients. Kidney Int 2001;59(Suppl 78):S14–8.

48. Oner-Iyidogan Y, Oner P, Kocak H, et al. Dimethylarginines and inflammation markers in patients with chronic kidney disease undergoing dialysis. Clin Exp Med 2009;9(3):235–41.

49. Fleck C, Schweitzer F, Karge E, et al. Serum concentrations of asymmetric (ADMA) and symmetric (SDMA) dimethylarginine in patients with chronic kidney diseases. Clin Chim Acta 2003;336(1–2):1–12.

50. Payto DA, El-Khoury, JM, Bunch DR, et al. A-105: SDMA outperforms serum creatinine-based equations in estimating kidney function compared with measured GFR. AACC 2014 Annual Meeting & Clin Lab Expo. Chicago, July 27–31, 2014.

51. Schwedhelm E, Böger RH. The role of asymmetric and symmetric dimethylarginines in renal disease. Nat Rev Nephrol 2011;7(5):275–85.

52. Braff J, Obare E, Yerramilli M, et al. Relationship between serum symmetric dimethylarginine concentration and glomerular filtration rate in cats. J Vet Intern Med 2014;28(6):1699–701.

53. Hall JA, Yerramilli M, Obare E, et al. Comparison of serum concentrations of symmetric dimethylarginine and creatinine as kidney function biomarkers in cats with chronic kidney disease. J Vet Intern Med 2014;28(6):1676–83.

54. Nabity NB, Lees GE, Boggess MM, et al. Symmetric dimethylarginine assay validation, stability, and evaluation as a marker for the detection of chronic kidney disease in dogs. J Vet Intern Med 2015;29(4):1036–44.

55. Jepson RE, Syme HM, Vallance C, et al. Plasma asymmetric dimethylarginine, symmetric dimethylarginine, L-arginine and nitrite/nitrate concentrations in cats with chronic kidney disease and hypertension. J Vet Intern Med 2008; 22(2):317–24.

56. Vaske HH, Armbrust L, Zicker SC, et al. Assessment of renal function in hyperthyroid cats managed with a controlled iodine diet. Int J Appl Res Vet M 2016; 14:38–48.

57. Yerramilli M, Yerramilli M, Obare E, et al. ACVIM abstract NU-42: symmetric dimethylarginine (SDMA) increases earlier than serum creatinine in dogs with chronic kidney disease (CKD). J Vet Intern Med 2014;28(3):1084–5.

58. Hall JA, Yerramilli M, Obare E, et al. Serum concentrations of symmetric dimethylarginine and creatinine in dogs with naturally occurring chronic kidney disease. J Vet Intern Med 2016;30(3):794–802.

59. Yerramilli M, Yerramilli M, Obare E, et al. Prognostic value of symmetric dimethylarginine to creatinine ratio in dogs and cats with chronic kidney disease. J Vet Intern Med 2015;29(4):1274.

60. Hall JA, Yerramilli M, Obare E, et al. Comparison of serum concentrations of symmetric dimethylarginine and creatinine as kidney function biomarkers in healthy geriatric cats fed reduced protein foods enriched with fish oil, L-carnitine, and medium-chain triglycerides. Vet J 2014;202(3):588–96.

61. Hall JA, Yerramilli M, Obare E, et al. Relationship between lean body mass and serum renal biomarkers in healthy dogs. J Vet Intern Med 2015;29(3):808–14.

62. El Khoury JE, Bunch DR, Reineks E, et al. A simple and fast liquid chromatography-tandem mass spectroscopy method for the measurement of underivatized L-arginine, symmetric dimethylarginine and asymmetric dimethylarginine and establishment of reference ranges. Anal Bioanal Chem 2011; 402(2):771–9.

63. Singer MA. Of mice and men and elephants: metabolic rate sets glomerular filtration rate. Am J Kidney Dis 2001;37(1):164–78.

64. Blackwell S, O'Reilly DS, Reid D, et al. Plasma dimethylarginines during the acute inflammatory response. Eur J Clin Invest 2011;41(6):635–41.

65. Lukasz A, Hoffmeister B, Graft B, et al. Association of angiopoietin-2 and dimethylarginines with complicated course in patients with leptospirosis. PLoS One 2014;9(1):e87490.

66. Lluch P, Mauricio MD, Vila JM, et al. Accumulation of symmetric dimethylarginine in hepatorenal syndrome. Exp Biol Med (Maywood) 2006;23(1):70–5.

67. Rytlewski K, Olszanecki R, Korbut R, et al. Effects of prolonged oral supplementation with L-arginine on blood pressure and nitric oxide synthesis in preeclampsia. Eur J Clin Invest 2005;35(1):32–7.

68. Lüneburg N, von Holten RA, Töpper RF, et al. Symmetric dimethylarginine is a marker of detrimental outcome in the acute phase after ischaemic stroke: role of renal function. Clin Sci (Lond) 2012;122(3):105–11.

69. Meinitzer A, Kielstein JT, Pilz S, et al. Symmetrical and asymmetrical dimethylarginine as predictors for mortality in patients referred for coronary angiography: the Ludwigshafen Risk and Cardiovascular Health Study. Clin Chem 2011;57(1): 112–21.

70. Khalil MA, Latif H, Rehman A, et al. Acute kidney injury in lymphoma: a single centre experience. Int J Nephrol 2014;2014:272961.

71. Lahoti A, Kantarjian H, Salahudeen AK, et al. Predictors and outcome of acute kidney injury in patients with acute myelogenous leukemia or high-risk myelodysplastic syndrome. Cancer 2010;116(17):4063–8.

72. Sellin L, Friedl C, Klein G, et al. Acute renal failure due to a malignant lymphoma infiltration uncovered by renal biopsy. Nephrol Dial Transplant 2004;19:2657–60.

73. Luciano RL, Brewster UC. Kidney involvement in leukemia and lymphoma. Adv Chronic Kidney Dis 2014;21(1):27–35.

74. Launay-Vacher V, Aapro M, De Castro G Jr, et al. Renal effects of molecular targeted therapies in oncology: a review by the cancer and the Kidney International Network (C-KIN). Ann Oncol 2015;26:1677–84.

75. Szuba A, Chachaj A, Wróbel T, et al. Asymmetric dimethylarginine in hematological malignancies: a preliminary study. Leuk Lymphoma 2008;49(12):2316–20.

76. Available at: http://iris-kidney.com/guidelines/staging.aspx. Accessed September 03, 2016.

77. Elliot DA. Nutritional management of chronic renal disease in dogs and cats. Vet Clin North Am Small Anim Pract 2006;36(6):1377–84.

78. Hall JA, MacLeay J, Yerramilli M, et al. Positive impact of nutritional interventions on serum symmetric dimethylarginine and creatinine concentrations in client-owned geriatric cats. PLoS One 2016;11:e0153653.

79. Hall JA, MacLeay J, Yerramilli M, et al. Positive impact of nutritional interventions on serum symmetric dimethylarginine and creatinine concentrations in client-owned geriatric dogs. PLoS One 2016;11(4):e0153653.

80. Wyatt AR, Yerbury JL, Wilson MR. Structural characterization of clusterin-chaperone client protein complexes. J Biol Chem 2009;284(33):21920–7.

81. Poon S, Rybchyn MS, Esterbrook-Smith SB, et al. Mildly acidic pH activates the extracellular molecular chaperone clusterin. J Biol Chem 2002;277:39532–40.

82. De Silva HV, Stuart WD, Park YB, et al. Purification and characterization of apoli-poprotein J. J Biol Chem 1990;265(24):14292–7.

83. Blaschuk O, Burdzy K, Fritz I. Purification and characterization of cell-aggregating factor (clusterin), the major glycoprotein in ram testis fluid. J Biol Chem 1983;258(12):7714–20.

84. Griswold MD, Roberts K, Bishop P. Purification and characterization of a sulph-ated glycoprotein secreted by Sertoli cells. Biochemistry 1986;25:7265–70.

85. Sylvester SR, Skinner MK, Griswold MD. A sulfated glycoprotein synthesized by Sertoli cells and by epididymal cells is a component of the sperm membrane. Biol Reprod 1984;31:1087–101.

86. Calero M, Tokuda T, Rostagno A, et al. Functional and structural properties of lipid-associated apolipoprotein J (clusterin). Biochem J 1999;344:375–83.

87. Burkey BF, de Silva HV, Harmony JA. Intracellular processing of apolipoprotein J precursor to a mature heterodimer. J Lipid Res 1991;32:1039–48.

88. Murphy BF, Kirsabaum L, Walker ID, et al. SP-40,40 a newly identified normal human serum protein found in the SC5b-9 complex of complement and in the immune deposits in glomerulonephritis. J Clin Invest 1988;81:1858–64.

89. Wilson MR, Roeth PJ, Easterbrook-Smith SB. Clusterin enhances the formation of insoluble immune complexes. Biochem Biophys Res Commun 1991;177(3): 985–90.

90. Viard I, Wehrli P, Jornot L, et al. Clusterin gene expression mediates resistance to apoptotic cell death induced by heat shock and oxidative stress. J Invest Dermatol 1999;112(3):290–6.

91. Leskov KS, Klokov DY, Li J, et al. Synthesis and functional analyses of nuclear clusterin, a cell death protein. J Biol Chem 2003;278:11590–600.

92. Patel NV, Wei M, Wong A, et al. Progressive changes in regulation of apolipopro-teins E and J in glial cultures during postnatal development and aging. Neurosci Lett 2004;371:199–204.

93. Choi-Miura NH, Oda T. Relationship between multifunctional protein clusterin and Alzheimer disease. Neurobiol Aging 1996;15(5):717–22.

94. Rodriguez-Pineiro AM, De la Cadena MP, Lopez-Saco A, et al. Differential expression of serum clusterin isoforms in colorectal cancer. Mol Cell Proteomics 2006;5:1647–57.

95. Zhou X, Ma B, Lin Z, et al. Evaluation of the usefulness of novel biomarkers for drug induced acute kidney injury in the beagle dogs. Toxicol Appl Pharmacol 2014;280:30–5.

96. Garcia-Martinez JD, Tvarijonaciciute A, Ceron JJ, et al. Urinary clusterin as a renal marker in dogs. J Vet Diagn Invest 2015;24(2):301–6.

97. Choi-Miura NH, Kahashi Y, Nakano Y, et al. Identification of the disulfide bonds in human plasma protein SP-40, 40 (apolipoprotein-J). J Biochem 1992;112: 557–61.

98. Available at: http://c-path.org/. Accessed September 3, 2016.
99. Quinn J, Zieba M, Yerramilli M. ACVIM abstract NU-13: effect of blood contamination in canine urine on the performance of a commercial immunoassay for the acute kidney injury (AKI) marker: urinary clusterin (UCLUS). J Vet Intern Med 2015;29(4):1214.
100. Ochieng J, Chaudhuri G. Cystatin superfamily. J Health Care Poor Underserved 2010;21(Suppl 1):51–70.
101. Hoek FJ, Kemperman FA, Krediet RT. A comparison between cystatin C, plasma creatinine and the Cockcroft and Gault formula for the estimation of glomerular filtration rate. Nephrol Dial Transplant 2003;18(10):2024–31.
102. Abrahamson M, Barrett AJ, Salvesen G, et al. Isolation of six cysteine proteinase inhibitors from human urine. Their physicochemical and enzyme kinetic properties and concentrations in biological fluids. J Biol Chem 1986;261:11282–9.
103. Green GD, Kembhavi AA, Davies ME, et al. Cystatin-like cysteine proteinase inhibitors from human liver. Biochem J 1984;218:939–46.
104. D'Amico A, Ragusa R, Carousa R, et al. Uncovering the cathepsin system in heart failure patients submitted to left ventricular assist device (LVAD) implantation. J Transl Med 2014;12:350.
105. Jarvinen M, Rinne A. Human spleen cysteine proteinase inhibitor. Purification, fractionation into isoelectric variants and some properties of the variants. Biochim Biophys Acta 1982;708:210–7.
106. Pennacchio LA, Lehesjoki AE, Stone NE, et al. Mutations in the gene encoding cystatin B in progressive myoclonus epilepsy (EPM1). Science 1996;271: 1731–4.
107. Koskiniemi M, Donner M, Majuri H, et al. Progressive myoclonus epilepsy: a clinical and histopathological study. Acta Neurol Scand 1974;50:307–32.
108. Berkovic SF, Andermann F, Carpenter S, et al. Progressive myoclonus epilepsies: specific causes and diagnosis. N Engl J Med 1985;315:296–305.
109. Available at: http://www.uniprot.org/uniprot/F1PS73. Accessed February 29, 2016.
110. Available at: http://www.uniprot.org/uniprot/M3X7X2. Accessed February 29, 2016.
111. Musante L, Tataruch D, Gu D, et al. Proteases and protease inhibitors of urinary extracellular vesicles in diabetic nephropathy. J Diabetes Res 2015;2015: 289734.
112. Veena SR, Peter JC, Stephen IA, et al. The role of adenosine receptors A2A and A2B signaling in renal fibrosis. Kidney Int 2014;86:685–92.
113. Assaife-Lopes N, Wengert M, de Sá Pinheiro AA, et al. Inhibition of renal Na+-ATPase activity by inosine is mediated by A1 receptor-induced inhibition of the cAMP signaling pathway. Arch Biochem Biophys 2009;489:76–81.
114. Spielman WS, Arend LJ. Adenosine receptors and signaling in the kidney. Hypertension 1991;17:117–30.
115. Eltzschig HK. Adenosine: an old drug newly discovered. Anesthesiology 2009; 111:904–15.
116. Nishiyama A, Kimura S, He H, et al. Renal interstitial adenosine metabolism during ischemia in dogs. Am J Physiol Renal Physiol 2001;280:F231–8.
117. Palm CA, Segev G, Cowgill LD, et al. Urinary clusterin and serum inosine: biomarkers for early identification of acute kidney injury in dogs. J Vet Intern Med 2014;28(4):1346–74.
118. Devarajan P. Neutrophil gelatinase-associated lipocalin (NGAL): a new marker of kidney disease. Scand J Clin Lab Invest Suppl 2008;241:89–94.

119. Segev G, Palm C, LeRoy B, et al. Evaluation of neutrophil gelatinase-associated lipocalin as a marker of kidney injury in dogs. J Vet Intern Med 2013;27(6):1362–7.
120. Palm CA, Segev G, Cowgill LD, et al. Urinary neutrophil gelatinase-associated lipocalin as a marker for identification of acute kidney injury and recovery in dogs with gentamicin-induced nephrotoxicity. J Vet Intern Med 2016;30(1):200–5.
121. Mårtensson J, Bellomo R. The rise and fall of NGAL in acute kidney injury. Blood Purif 2014;37:304–10.
122. Lippi G, Aloe R. Neutrophil gelatinase associated lipocalin (NGAL): analytical issues (review). Ligand Assay 2013;18:332–6.
123. de Geus HR, Betjes MG, Bakker J. Biomarkers for the prediction of acute kidney injury: a narrative review on current status and future challenges. Clin Kidney J 2012;5:102–8.
124. Sirota JC, Klawitter J, Edelstein CL. Biomarkers of acute kidney injury. J Toxicol 2011;2011:328120.
125. Vijayan A, Faubel S, Askenazi DJ, et al. Clinical use of the urine biomarker [TIMP-2] × [IGFBP7] for acute kidney injury risk assessment. Am J Kidney Dis 2016;68(1):19–28.

Is Progressive Chronic Kidney Disease a Slow Acute Kidney Injury?

Larry D. Cowgill, DVM, PhD[a],*, David J. Polzin, DVM, PhD[b],*,
Jonathan Elliott, MA, Vet MB, PhD, Cert SAC, MRCVS[c],
Mary B. Nabity, DVM, PhD[d], Gilad Segev, DVM[e],
Gregory F. Grauer, DVM, MS[f], Scott Brown, VMD, PhD[g],
Cathy Langston, DVM[h], Astrid M. van Dongen, DVM[i]

KEYWORDS

- Progressive chronic kidney disease • Kidney biomarkers • IRIS CKD stage 1
- IRIS AKI grade I

KEY POINTS

- Novel kidney biomarkers can expose subtle and subclinical kidney disease that may otherwise remain undiscovered with conventional diagnostic assessment.

Continued

Disclosure: Dr L.D. Cowgill has served as a paid consultant for IDEXX Laboratories and CEVA Animal Health. He is a member of the Inernational Renal Interest Society and has received gift funding from IDEXX Laboratories to support his research. Dr J. Elliott has served as a paid consultant for Bayer Animal Health, Boehringer Ingelheim, Elanco Animal Health, Idexx Ltd, CEVA Animal Health, Orion Inc, Nextvet Ltd, and Waltham Centre for Pet Nutrition. He receives research grant funding from CEVA Animal Health, Elanco Animal Health, Zoetis Animal Health, Royal Canin, and Waltham Centre for Pet Nutrition. He is a member of the International Renal Interest Society. Drs D.J. Polzin, M.B. Nabity, G. Segev, G.F. Grauer, S. Brown, C. Langston, and A. M. van Dongen have nothing to disclose.
[a] Department of Medicine and Epidemiology, School of Veterinary Medicine, University of California, Davis, 2108 Tupper Hall, Davis, CA 95616, USA; [b] Department of Veterinary Clinical Sciences, College of Veterinary Medicine, University of Minnesota, 1352 Boyd Avenue, C-325, St Paul, MN 55108, USA; [c] Department of Comparative Biomedical Sciences, Royal Veterinary College, University of London, Royal College Street, London NW1 0TU, UK; [d] Department of Veterinary Pathobiology, College of Veterinary Medicine & Biomedical Sciences, Texas A&M University, College Station, TX, USA; [e] Small Animal Internal Medicine, Koret School of Veterinary Medicine, The Hebrew University of Jerusalem, P.O. Box 12, Rehovot 76100, Israel; [f] Department of Clinical Sciences, College of Veterinary Medicine, Kansas State University, Manhattan, KS 66506, USA; [g] Department of Physiology and Pharmacology, College of Veterinary Medicine, The University of Georgia, Athens, GA 30602-7388, USA; [h] Department of Veterinary Clinical Sciences, The Ohio State University College of Veterinary Medicine, Columbus, OH, USA; [i] Department of Clinical Sciences of Companion Animals, PO Box 80.154, Utrecht NL 3508 TD, The Netherlands
* Corresponding author
E-mail addresses: ldcowgill@ucdavis.edu; polzi001@umn.edu

Continued

- Active kidney injury biomarkers have the potential to establish a new understanding of traditional views of chronic kidney disease (CKD), including its early identification and possible mediators of its progression.
- Sensitive and specific biomarkers are likely to lead to insights into clinical kidney disease and facilitate new diagnostic and therapeutic approaches.
- Therapeutic approaches may be monitored to biomarker endpoints and logically adjusted or extended until the biomarker activity is nullified.

THE 2015 INTERNATIONAL RENAL INTEREST SOCIETY NAPA MEETING

In May 2015, the International Renal Interest Society (IRIS), a veterinary society established to advance the scientific understanding of kidney disease in small animals, sanctioned the 2015 IRIS Napa Meeting. The meeting was conceived as a highly focused strategic planning forum composed of many of the profession's recognized leaders in nephrology[a] to direct recognition and innovative solutions to evolving critical issues in veterinary nephrology. The theme of the meeting was, Re-evaluation and Understanding of IRIS CKD Stage1 and AKI Grade I Kidney Disease as Predictors of Progressive Kidney Disease. Since the inception of the IRIS CKD staging and acute kidney injury (AKI) grading systems to categorize and stratify kidney disease in animals,[1,2] there has been confusion and misunderstanding of the value and clinical utility of these early (nonazotemic) categories. The clinical relevance of these categories has been questioned, as has the justification to embed asymptomatic and nonazotemic patients in the overarching understanding of kidney disease. A significant focus of the Napa Meeting reflected on the relevance of early kidney disease and the importance of its recognition to the subsequent fate and outcomes of kidney disease discovered by conventional practices and methodologies.

The recognition of early, asymptomatic kidney disease is generally established on the basis of directed screening of at risk animals or as an incidental observation from routine testing of animals for other purposes. Which criteria define which animals to screen? Which evaluations are most accurate and sensitive on a screening panel? Is there value to establishing evidence-based risk assessment algorithms that generate a risk score providing cost-effective predictions to guide practice patterns for screening CKD Stage 1 and/or AKI Grade I? Answers to these questions will help establish the diagnostic and clinical significance of Stage 1 and Grade I kidney disease.

Currently, kidney disease is documented and stratified by use of function markers that may reflect slow states of transition or steady state conditions. Conventional practice patterns rely on urine specific gravity, proteinuria, serum creatinine, and symmetric dimethylated arginine (SDMA) to reflect CKD that may be static (nonprogressive) or may be active and variably progressive. Serum creatinine has been relied on for at least a century to predict the adequacy or inadequacy of kidney function with relative utility.[3] More recently, SDMA has become available to complement some of the shortcomings of creatinine, but additional time is required to duly establish its role and acceptance. (See Roberta Relford, Jane Robertson, Celeste

[a] Napa Scientific Panel: Larry D. Cowgill (Cochair), David Polzin (Cochair), Gilad Segev, Greg Grauer, Astrid van Dongen, Jonathan Elliott, Cathy Langston, Mary Nabity, and Scott Brown. IDEXX Sponsorship Team: Roberta Relford, Jane Robertson, Murthy Yerramilli, Jason Lee, Troy Goddu, Leif Lorentzen, Donald McCarann, and Lori Jackowitz.

Clements' article, "Symmetric Dimethylarginine: Improving the Diagnosis and Staging of Chronic Kidney Disease in Small Animals"; and Murthy Yerramilli, Giosi Farace, John Quinn, et al: "Kidney Disease and the Nexus of Chronic Kidney Disease and Acute Kidney Injury: The Role of Novel Biomarkers as Early and Accurate Diagnostics," in this issue). Despite familiarity with creatinine for the diagnosis of kidney disease, its utility has been constrained by the misperception it is blinded to early and subclinical kidney dysfunction and its excessively broad reference range for dogs and cats.[3] IRIS CKD Stage 1 encompasses the normal reference range for creatinine, which creates confusion identifying this stage as CKD. Documented CKD often is associated with the bias that the disease is advanced at the time of diagnosis, and the kidney fate is predetermined. A patient recognized in a more advanced stages of kidney disease, however, by logical extension must have started from or passed through a lesser category of kidney disease prior to its later recognition. Kidney disease that progresses from IRIS CKD Stage 1 to higher stages likely has undergone an episodic or ongoing active process promoting the progressive erosion of steady state function.

A functional diagnostic marker may fail to detect the underlying active component if offset by renal reserve, or if it is matched by compensatory adaptation of the residual kidney mass. Only when active injury outpaces repair or compensatory adaptation does the progression become evident.[4] Equally important, many animals with recognized CKD maintain static or have nonprogressive kidney function over extended periods of time.[5,6] These patients may justify different diagnostic, monitoring, and therapeutic attention. An important outcome of the Napa Meeting was establishment of a strategic hypothesis for the recognition and understanding of early (IRIS CKD Stage 1) kidney disease. Specifically, this hypothesis underscored the likelihood for underlying active kidney injury contributing to the risk for progression of CKD or lack of an active component leading to stable kidney function.

The Napa Meeting explored potential relationships between CKD and AKI. Both IRIS CKD Stage 1 and IRIS AKI Grade I represent early kidney disease states, which may not be recognized until they proceed to a more advanced classifications. If progressive CKD is associated with active episodic or ongoing injury to the kidney, and if AKI is linked to progressive CKD (discussed later), could both these disease syndromes be explained by the same pathologic process or processes progressing concurrently at different rates to establish both categories? Should early CKD and AKI be viewed as interconnected rather than separate clinical conditions? To this issue, the following questions relative to early CKD and early AKI were proposed by the participants:

1. Are IRIS CKD Stage 1 and IRIS AKI Grade I similar processes developing at different rates, or are they separate processes that should be viewed as interconnected? Is progressive CKD a slow-moving AKI?
2. Is IRIS CKD Stage 1 an active condition leading to progressive CKD or an inactive condition associated with stable kidney disease?
3. Is IRIS AKI Grade I a marker that could proceed to a rapidly progressive AKI or a slowly progressive CKD?
4. Are there better future definitions for IRIS CKD stage 1?

The answers to these questions forecast the need to develop diagnostics to better distinguish active versus the absence of active kidney injury and progressive versus static CKD and to document the pattern(s) and causes of progressive CKD. If early kidney disease (IRIS CKD Stage 1) could be identified as active or inactive, there would be potential to alter the management and monitoring of patients to minimize its progression to more advanced stages.

IS THERE A NEED TO DISTINGUISH TWO SPECIFIC TYPES OF KIDNEY DISEASE: ACUTE VERSUS CHRONIC?

Historically, kidney disease has been broadly defined into 2 seemingly distinct categories, CKD and AKI.[7–9] Each category of disease has distinctive features and has been defined by unique categorization schemes, the IRIS CKD staging system for CKD and the IRIS AKI grading system for AKI.[1,2] CKD is perceived as slow in onset, characteristically progressive over time, and irreversible, whereas AKI develops rapidly and maintains the potential for repair and return of kidney function. Recently, these categories of kidney disease have been shown to interrelate, and their distinctions have become blurred at their interface. CKD is a known risk factor for the development of AKI, and AKI is recognized increasingly as a potential mediator for progressive CKD and end-stage kidney disease.[9,10]

CKD is defined by sustained functional and/or structural damage to the kidneys over a course greater than 2 to 3 months.[1,7] Decreasing kidney function recognized by reductions in glomerular filtration rate (GFR) or estimation of GFR by increasing serum creatinine or SDMA are the most common features identifying CKD in animals.[7,11] (See also Roberta Relford, Jane Robertson, Celeste Clements' article, "Symmetric Dimethylarginine: Improving the Diagnosis and Staging of Chronic Kidney Disease in Small Animals," in this issue). CKD is established initially by a singular or a combination of insults to the kidney that result in structural or functional damage to renal parenchyma that is repaired incompletely and promotes variable kidney dysfunction.

Progression, or sustained worsening of kidney function over time, is a hallmark of CKD in most animals, but its pathogenesis remains elusive and likely is multifactorial. Equally elusive is the explanation why some animals with CKD maintain stable kidney function and apparently fail to progress. These differences in behavior may hold clues to explain the mechanisms of progressive CKD as well as therapeutic targets and intervention points to halt the process. Multiple risk factors for developing CKD have been documented, including age, hypertension, proteinuria, infectious agents, endocrine disease, breed predilections, AKI, and heart disease, among others. Progressive CKD is a natural consequence of an inability to resolve these risks or other comorbidities in animals with established CKD. Identification of progressive CKD in the absence of these identifiable comorbidities or after resolution of initial insults has been more intangible.

To date, the timely recognition of animals with progressive CKD and those with static CKD has been constrained by the lack of early diagnostic predictors. Serum creatinine and SDMA are static markers of kidney mass reflecting steady state predictions of kidney function, which may include renal reserve and compensatory adaptations to ongoing nephron loss in addition to discrete reductions of functional kidney mass. Neither of these static (functional) kidney markers is sufficiently sensitive to signal early, subtle, and potentially ongoing kidney injury, which may evolve slowly with a resultant decrease in functional renal mass. Other predictors of progression need discovery and validation. Proteinuria has been associated consistently with risks for progression in both human and animal patients with CKD. Urinary protein excretion has been shown to correlate with progressive CKD in cats and dogs, but the urine protein:creatinine ratio has low specificity for CKD progression, and it is unclear if proteinuria is a marker for progression or participates in its development.[12] Currently, there are few criteria in veterinary patients to project the risk for progression of CKD. Prediction models in human patients are similarly problematic and subject to bias.[13]

Sustained and overt damage to the glomerulus or tubulointerstitium from primary diseases, like hypertension, glomerulonephritis, and chronic pyelonephritis, which are not fully resolved, promote an expected progressive damage and an expected loss of functional kidney mass. The risks, patterns, and mechanisms for progression from seemingly occult CKD remain unknown. Progression of CKD to end-stage kidney disease could occur stepwise from sporadic active insults, which are either overt or subclinical and of similar or differing etiologies. These episodic injuries could promote cumulative damage resulting in further dysfunction and concurrent reduction of GFR and GFR markers (**Fig. 1**). Alternatively, metabolic or signaling disruptions to kidney structures intrinsically associated with the establishment of CKD or AKI could promote ongoing stresses or disordered metabolism within the residual renal mass, which perpetuates sustained injury with a varying time course and further loss of kidney parenchyma and function. The respective prevalence and influences of these alternative pathways is unknown. Similarly, the underlying mechanisms participating in progression have been hypothesized widely but remain largely undefined.[13,14] Regardless of which pattern or mechanism of CKD progression prevails in an individual patient, all seem to share a common feature of active stress or injury to the residual structures of the kidney.

There is accumulating evidence from a variety of models of AKI proposing a sequence of effective adaptive or maladaptive events in cellular repair that likely influence the prevention or predisposition to progressive CKD.[4,9,10,15–21] After an acute insult, injured tubular epithelial cells may become fatally injured and undergo necrosis or apoptosis, proliferate and regenerate the damaged epithelium, or undergo failed regeneration but survive cell death in a state of cell-cycle G2/M arrest.[4,9,10,17–19,22] Arrested cells reprieved from apoptosis, however, fail to participate in regenerative repair and up-regulate maladaptive signaling pathways for myofibroblast proliferation and fibrosis in the interstitium predisposing to progression of CKD. Tubular epithelia subjected to more severe or repeated injury, sustained or ongoing injury, or epithelia that are more senescent also are more susceptible to cell-cycle arrest.[10,17,18,20]

These observations provide a speculative foundation for progression of CKD that may involve recurrent or sustained injury to the kidneys, which promotes active interstitial inflammation and fibrosis. These events remain clinically occult and undetected until there is a quantum decrement in functional renal mass ultimately detectable by traditional (functional) clinical markers. Triggers for sustained or active injury could

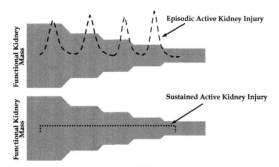

Fig. 1. Schematic illustration of progressive CKD causing a decrease or worsening in functional kidney mass (or GFR) over time in response to stepwise or episodic insults to the kidney (*upper panel*) or subsequent to sustained active kidney injury resulting from intrinsic stress or disordered metabolism associated with the established CKD (*lower panel*).

include unresolved primary disease (eg, glomerulonephritis), comorbid conditions (eg, systemic hypertension, heart disease, and regional ischemia), chronic medications (eg, angiotensin-converting enzyme inhibitors, diuretics, antibiotics, and nonsteroidal anti-inflammatory drugs), chronic inflammation, chronic immune stimulation, recurrent infection, and proteinuria, among other predispositions.

Independent of the nature of the insult to the kidney, a common theme for CKD progression seems to be active and ongoing stress, metabolic dysregulation, and loss of morphologic and functional integrity of the tubular epithelium leading to interstitial inflammation and fibrosis. The tubular epithelial focus prevails whether the insult is preglomerular hemodynamic changes predisposing to subtle hypoxia; sustained glomerular disease promoting vascular rarefaction, proteinuria, and reduced ultrafiltrate; tubular stress or inflammation; or postrenal events associated with outflow obstruction.[10,14,18,23]

A prevailing stress to tubular epithelia is persistent and severe exposure to protein escaping glomerular permselectivity. An excessive protein load can dysregulate the normal cubilin and megalin receptor-mediated endocytosis of protein by proximal tubular cells and predispose these cells to atrophy and apoptosis.[23] In addition, excessive reabsorption of protein and protein-bound substances, including fatty acids, may promote cellular stress responses that activate a variety of genes promoting proinflammatory cytokines, autophagy, and activated immune responses. Consequently, there is compelling evidence that proteinuria per se propagates a maladaptive cycle of tubular injury, epithelial degeneration, and scarring in the adjacent interstitium.[23]

Recent experimental studies using both ischemia-reperfusion and toxic models of AKI, have provided an enhanced understanding how active, potentially sustained, and ongoing stresses to tubular epithelia can promote progressive cellular maladaptation and inflammatory and fibrotic consequences in the tubulointerstitium. These active cellular events are temporally disassociated from worsening GFR or markers of kidney function.[19,24] Despite their high metabolic activity and oxygen requirements, the inner cortex and outer medullary segments of the kidney exist in a state of tenuous oxygenation, which is highly regulated in health but subject to profound inadequacy with vascular compromise, hypoperfusion, and relative hypoxia. With either subtle or profound tubulointerstitial injury, this tenuous vasculature can be secondarily compromised further disrupting oxygen delivery and the balance between tubular energy demands and oxygen availability. Kidney injury can be directed specifically to the vasculature promoting endothelial cell activation, leukocyte and platelet aggregation, and compromised perfusion and oxygen delivery to the tubular epithelium. More importantly, tubular epithelial injury subsequent to oxidative stress activates vasoconstrictive signals, promoting a vicious cycle of heightened ischemia, progressive vascular rarefaction, and stimulation of growth factors, which signal interstitial fibrosis and progressive hypoxia.[10,14,17–20]

Cellular stress of various causes also stimulates a diverse spectrum of directed pathways leading to dysregulated apoptosis, local inflammatory responses, and/or interstitial fibrosis, which have been associated with progressive CKD.[10,14,17–20] One of these maladaptive cellular responses is associated with accumulation of inappropriately processed or unfolded proteins in the endoplasmic reticulum (ER).[19,25] Cellular adaptations to ER dysregulation are initiated to adjust the translation, translocation, folding, and degradation of ER proteins as protective mechanisms, but they simultaneously promote cellular autophagy.[19,25] Autophagy is a cellular clean-up process in which damaged cytosolic constituents and organelles are encapsulated in autophagosomes and degraded for reutilization in cytosolic lysosomes. Autophagy is a protective adaptation to protect the cell from death. In experimental models of kidney diseases, however, the misfolded protein-induced dysfunction of the ER and mitochondria can stimulate proinflammatory responses via nuclear factor-κB upregulation and mediation of transcription of target genes for inflammatory interleukins, tumor necrosis factor α, and adhesion molecules.[19,25] Sustained or severe cellular stresses overstimulate these adaptive responses and activate downstream signaling pathways for apoptosis of the disrupted cell.

These observations illustrate that diverse and seemingly uncoordinated events or reactions often are channeled through common metabolic junctions to promote a common or universal cellular response. Similarly, the kidney responds to many overt stresses and injuries with a series of adaptive reactions fundamentally intended to reestablish cellular integrity and promote cell survival. When the stress or injury is sustained or insurmountable, however, these same cellular responses may become maladaptive or the cell is programmed to die.[4,17] These latter responses are expressed clinically as acute kidney injury with variable recovery, kidney death, or more subtly as progressive chronic kidney disease. If the kidney recovers, many of these adaptive cellular responses become pathways for the transition of overt acute kidney injury to progressive chronic kidney disease. A majority of models highlighting this progression have focused on the continuum from AKI to CKD.[4,9,10,15–22,24] As an overview, in many circumstances, the apparent recovery from an AKI, which by all clinical indications is resolved, leaves behind pathophysiologic embers that smolder asymptomatically to sustain tubular and vascular injury, which slowly and progressively erode functional renal mass. The erosion is perpetuated by proinflammatory messengers that at first are deemed adaptive but ultimately may become maladaptive.

IDENTIFICATION OF PROGRESSIVE CHRONIC KIDNEY DISEASE: THE SEARCH FOR ACTIVE INJURY MARKERS

In distinction to the AKI to CKD scenario (discussed previously), progressive CKD is recognized in a majority of animals in the absence of an overt AKI. The progression is variable over time and recognized primarily by worsening changes in markers of steady state kidney function, like serum creatinine or SDMA, resulting in increased CKD stage over time. An animal with a serum creatinine of 1.8 mg/dL, previously classified as IRIS CKD Stage 2, who subsequently is recognized with a serum creatinine of 3.5 mg/dL and classified as IRIS CKD Stage 3, must have experienced interim kidney injury resulting in the progression. Where there is less attention to trending kidney function markers or staging of CKD, the progressive nature of CKD may be signaled by the appearance and worsening of overt clinical features of kidney dysfunction, including inappetence, weight loss, polydipsia, polyuria, micturition disorders, lethargy, and vomiting. In further distinction to the AKI to CKD scenario, many animals are identified with CKD of unknown etiology and no precedent acute injury in which kidney function and health seem stable for extended periods of time. To date it is unknown why some animals manifest progression and some do not, and in the absence of overt and persistent kidney disease (eg, pyelonephritis, glomerulonephritis, nephrolithiasis, hypertension, and nephrotoxic drugs), there are no diagnostic features of CKD that forecast which individual animals are predisposed to progression and which are not.

Also unknown is the pattern or nature of the injury promoting progression. For some animals, progression may be provoked by sequential episodic bouts of kidney damage that remain subclinical and undetected (see **Fig. 1**). These episodes may escape functional detection and remain unrecognized clinically until the episodic damage exceeds the renal reserve capacity or compensatory adaptations of the kidneys.[4,26] At this stage, there is evident worsening of steady state function markers and progressive increases in CKD stage. Alternatively or in combination with episodic damage, underlying mechanisms promoted by the existing CKD or an ongoing but low-grade AKI may perpetuate cellular stresses or insults that direct sustained injury to the kidney. Again, this ongoing damage may remain undetectable until parenchymal loss exceeds functional compensations. Either of these potential patterns of progression may be too subtle to be recognized by clinical features or evidence of ill health. Similarly, current definitions of AKI grade and CKD stage may be too insensitive to reveal ongoing or episodic active kidney injury until there has been a finite change in static kidney function predicted with currently available tests. Unfortunately, static kidney function tests only detect the impact of these active processes after substantial functional or structural damage has occurred.[4,27]

A sensitive and specific predictor that discriminates whether a patient is likely to progress or remain stable with CKD would provide tremendous diagnostic and therapeutic advantage.[4,19,26] For patients with identified progressive CKD, this could provide earlier opportunity to seek subclinical conditions, which might be injuring the kidneys and institute more timely monitoring of the disease. It also would provide an opportunity to initiate therapies that might ameliorate progression or development of clinical signs as well as indicate the effectiveness of therapeutic interventions. If a therapeutic regimen failed to convert the patient to a nonprogressive status, there might be justification to modify the therapy before additional loss of kidney function occurred.

There has been growing interest and research in human nephrology directed at discovering biomarkers that would predict the early onset of AKI.[4,27–29] Similar efforts are underway in veterinary medicine and show great promise.[30–38] (See also Murthy Yerramilli, Giosi Farace, John Quinn, et al: "Kidney Disease and the Nexus of Chronic Kidney Disease and Acute Kidney Injury: The Role of Novel Biomarkers as Early and Accurate Diagnostics," in this issue). An AKI biomarker should be detectable in urine and/or plasma such that it can be assessed routinely and serve as an indicator of kidney function or dysfunction or response to injury. The ideal marker should reflect kidney specific events, be unique and specific to the kidney, and reflect very early and potentially sustained phases of the pathogenesis and repair processes. Additionally, the ideal marker should reflect the extent of these ongoing processes, their location, changes in these processes in response to therapeutic intervention over time, and potentially the etiologic insult. A singular biomarker is highly unlikely to be able to distinguish both processes associated with induction of the AKI and also events associated with repair of the injury. The absence of a biomarker associated with active injury, however, may predict resolution of the active phase. More realistically, a panel of biomarkers predictive of differing phases of induction, maintenance, and repair of AKI might serve these ideal goals.

CANDIDATE BIOMARKERS FOR ACTIVE KIDNEY INJURY

Novel AKI biomarkers have been screened and selected for their prediction of early and sensitive alterations of normal cellular processes in the kidney and historically have been exploited for their potential to detect early AKI.[4,27–29] This restricted focus to AKI, however, constrains their broader and potentially important application to CKD. Kidney-specific biomarkers that localize to functional renal tubular epithelia (or other kidney-specific loci) and respond to diverse stresses or disruption of normal cellular function have potential to signal the early, specific, and sensitive existence of kidney injury and are perhaps better termed, *active kidney injury biomarkers*. An active kidney injury biomarker could expose ongoing or progressive kidney injury in advance of conventional diagnostic methods that document consequent alterations in GFR or substantive loss of functional parenchyma over time.

With this perspective, static CKD may be redefined as a stable, unchanging state of long-standing and irreversible loss of varying degrees of kidney parenchyma and function associated with the absence of detectable active kidney injury. It would be characterized by stable biochemical markers of kidney function (eg, serum creatinine and/or SDMA concentration) over a prolonged but variable period of time of perhaps greater than 5 to 6 months. Progressive CKD, on the other hand, could represent a state of long-standing and irreversible loss of variable degrees of kidney parenchyma and function associated with persistent or intermittent active kidney injury over an arbitrary 2-month to 4-month interval. The implied active injury, albeit subtle or occult, secondarily generates cumulative damage to the kidney and an ongoing loss of structural kidney parenchyma and function. These ongoing pathologic processes ultimately are detected by conventional biochemical markers of kidney function and increases in CKD stage. Evidence of serum creatinine and/or SDMA trending upward is the current standard for identifying progressive CKD, but these changes can be slow to develop and detect injury after it has already reduced kidney function (**Fig. 2**). Detection of biomarkers associated with active kidney injury in animals with CKD has the potential to predict or identify those patients whose underlying kidney disease is ongoing and likely to progress in advance of biochemical markers whose short-term values reflect static kidney function.

Many candidate serum and urinary biomarkers have been assessed in human medicine,[11,20,22,26,27,29] and many of the promising markers are now being evaluated and validated in animals.[30,38] (See also Murthy Yerramilli, Giosi Farace, John Quinn, et al: "Kidney Disease and the Nexus of Chronic Kidney Disease and Acute Kidney Injury: The Role of Novel Biomarkers as Early and Accurate Diagnostics," in this issue). Some of the most promising candidates include urinary proteins that reflect functions or cellular processes specific to the kidney that are disrupted by pathophysiologic events secondary to injury or cellular stress. Retinol binding protein (RBP), cystatin C, cystatin B, kidney injury molecule-1 (KIM-1), neutrophil gelatinase-associated lipocalin (NGAL), interleukin-18, liver-type fatty acid–binding protein tissue inhibitor metalloproteinase-2, and insulin-like growth factor–binding protein 7 are among the most actively pursued.[11,20,26,27,29,30,38] (See also Murthy Yerramilli, Giosi Farace, John Quinn, et al: "Kidney Disease and the Nexus of Chronic Kidney Disease and Acute Kidney Injury: The Role of Novel Biomarkers as Early and Accurate Diagnostics," in this issue).

RBP is a 21-kDa protein produced in the liver and serves as the principal carrier of vitamin A in the circulation. When not complexed to larger plasma proteins, free RBP is freely filtered by the glomerulus and subsequently reabsorbed by megalin-mediated endocytosis and catabolized by the proximal tubular epithelium. With proximal tubular dysfunction, RBP can escape reabsorption and appear abnormally in urine.[30,39] This linkage to tubular dysfunction has established RBP as a candidate for early identification of kidney injury. RBP has been evaluated in dogs associated with a variety AKI models, and its appearance precedes routine clinical predictors as an early marker of AKI. Urinary RBP is only loosely associated, however, with proximal tubular dysfunction and is nonspecific for active injury to the tubular epithelium.[30,39]

Cystatin C is a 13-kDA cysteine protease inhibitor constitutively produced by most cells and subsequently circulated in blood after release from the cells. It is freely filtered across the glomerulus and subject to proximal tubular reabsorption from the

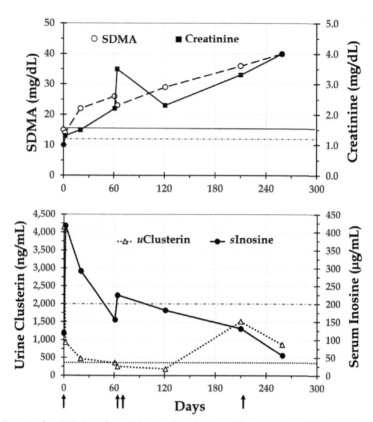

Fig. 2. Progressive CKD in a dog with mitral and tricuspid valvular insufficiency and regurgitation and right-sided congestive heart failure, ascites, and increased intra-abdominal pressure. Both N-terminal prohormone of brain natriuretic peptide (NT-proBNP) and cTroponin I (not shown) were markedly elevated consistent with heart failure. (*Upper panel*) Changes in serum creatinine (*solid squares*) and IDEXX SDMA (*open circles*) over time illustrating progressive worsening of kidney function. The solid and dashed horizontal lines represent the upper reference range for creatinine and IDEXX SDMA, respectively. (*Lower panel*) Associative changes in the active kidney injury biomarkers, urine clusterin (*u*Clusterin) (*open triangles*) and serum inosine (*s*Inosine) (*closed circles*), to periodic abdominocentesis (*arrows*) and decreased intra-abdominal pressure. The mixed dashed horizontal line represents the lower reference threshold for serum inosine and the dotted horizontal lines represents the upper reference range for urine clusterin. Note the marked improvement in both urinary clusterin and serum inosine subsequent to institution of medical therapy and abdominocentesis (*arrows*) on day 0. Although improved, both markers demonstrate only transient resolution of the ongoing kidney injury, which progresses over time and between abdominocentesis procedures as the congestive heart failure progresses. The biomarker-predicted active injury is further associated with the progressive CKD.

filtrate and degradation in the proximal epithelia. Like RBP, dysfunction of megalin-mediated endocytosis from acute injury or decreased reabsorptive capacity results in urinary detection of cystatin C and its increased renal excretion.[30] Cystatin C has been proposed as an early predictor of kidney dysfunction. It also lacks specificity, however, for active kidney injury, is not uniquely produced by kidney cells, and, as for any freely filtered protein, is confounded by excessive proteinuria, which might promote its urinary excretion without substantive active or ongoing tubular injury.

Despite the interest and efforts to validate KIM-1 as an AKI biomarker in human pa-tients,[11,20,22,26,27,29] in preliminary investigations, there has been no success (working with the developers) to detect KIM-1 in dogs with any of the available human, primate, or rodent assays for KIM-1 (Drs Carrie Palm and Larry D. Cowgill, personal communi-cation, 2014).

NGAL is a 24-kDa protein initially identified bound to gelatinase in specific granules of neutrophils. Subsequently, NGAL expression has been demonstrated by a variety of epithelia and specifically is up-regulated more than 10-fold in renal tubular epithelia within the first few hours after ischemic, obstructive, and toxic kidney injuries in human patients with AKI, naturally acquired kidney disease in dogs, and experimental models of AKI in dogs.[22,27,28,30–38,40] Recent studies in dogs with experimental gentamicin-induced AKI and in dogs with naturally acquired AKI, demonstrated NGAL sensitivities and specificities approaching 95% or greater for the early detection of AKI.[32,33] A commercially available assay for detection of canine NGAL is available (Abbott Labora-tories, Abbott Park, Illinois) and has been validated for early detection of AKI. Although urinary NGAL currently is promising, it lacks uniqueness with regard to its cellular origins and specificity for kidney injury, and it can be influenced by comorbid diseases.

Other promising biomarkers include serum inosine, urinary clusterin, and urinary cystatin B, which are under active evaluation in a variety of dog and cat models of AKI, naturally acquired active kidney injury, and progressive CKD. (See Murthy Yerramilli, Giosi Farace, John Quinn, et al: "Kidney Disease and the Nexus of Chronic Kidney Disease and Acute Kidney Injury: The Role of Novel Biomarkers as Early and Accurate Diagnostics," in this issue). The attraction of these novel bio-markers is their exclusive origins to renal tubular epithelia, integral association with cellular activities coupled to stress or damage, and highly specific analytical evalua-tion. As such, these markers offer the potential sensitivity and specificity to forecast active and sustained disruption of normal cellular processes as harbingers of subse-quent loss of steady state kidney functions or residual renal mass. Although the clinical directive for these kidney-specific biomarkers is to facilitate the diagnosis of early AKI, preliminary studies have documented their sensitivity for kidney disease beyond AKI. Their potential extends to document subclinical yet active and ongoing kidney injury associated with concurrent urinary diseases or other systemic illness that may have an impact on the kidney secondarily. For future diagnostics, individual markers or a panel of novel markers could provide the potential to recognize subtle and often sub-clinical kidney disease that would otherwise remain undiscovered until more substan-tial injury and dysfunction triggers alterations in conventional diagnostics. Even more importantly, active kidney injury biomarkers have potential to establish a new under-standing of traditional views of CKD, including early identification and possible medi-ators of its progression. Novel, kidney-specific biomarkers will likely establish a completely new and sophisticated paradigm in the approach to the understanding, diagnostic evaluation, and treatment of kidney disease in dogs and cats. Despite their initial attraction, the value and clinical utility of any novel kidney biomarker to forecast outcomes or direct treatment must be founded on the basis of well-designed and pro-spective controlled longitudinal studies of patients with CKD.

POTENTIAL APPLICATION OF NOVEL ACTIVE INJURY KIDNEY BIOMARKERS TO FORECAST EARLY KIDNEY INJURY
Early Recognition of Acute Kidney Injury

Urinary NGAL has been shown to be a sensitive and early predictor of AKI in dogs with both experimentally induced and naturally occurring AKI and may precede detection of kidney disease by serum creatinine or SDMA by more than a week[31–33,36] (**Fig. 3**). In dogs with naturally acquired urinary tract disease, urinary NGAL was a highly sensitive and specific predictor of AKI, including dogs categorized as IRIS AKI Grade I.[32]

In collaboration with IDEXX Laboratories, one of the authors (Larry D. Cowgill) similarly has evaluated the diagnostic performance of serum inosine, urinary clusterin, and urinary cystatin B in a gentamicin-induced model of AKI in dogs. (See Murthy Yerramilli, Giosi Farace, John Quinn, et al: "Kidney Disease and the Nexus of Chronic Kidney Disease and Acute Kidney Injury: The Role of Novel Biomarkers as Early and Accurate Diagnostics," in this issue). In this model, each of these novel biomarkers demonstrated a robust response or change within 72 to 120 hours from the induction of gentamicin documenting early and ongoing active injury. Each marker forecast the active kidney injury 7 to 10 days before any identifiable change in serum creatinine or SDMA. (See Murthy Yerramilli, Giosi Farace, John Quinn, et al: "Kidney Disease and the Nexus of Chronic Kidney Disease and Acute Kidney Injury: The Role of Novel Biomarkers as Early and Accurate Diagnostics," in this issue). These preliminary observations have provided optimism they may serve as unique diagnostic tools to disclose kidney injury at a time when it is otherwise diagnostically camouflaged.

Active Kidney Injury in Urinary Tract Infection

In a previous study evaluating the specificity of urinary NGAL as a predictor of AKI in dogs, a significant increase in its urinary expression was observed in dogs with lower urinary tract disease (infection, neoplasia, and urolithiasis) compared with healthy dogs.[32] Because NGAL was identified originally as a component of neutrophil granules and is up-regulated in response to inflammatory signals, it was tenable

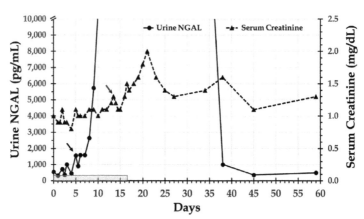

Fig. 3. Changes in urine NGAL (*solid circles and curve*) and serum creatinine (*solid triangles and dashed curve*) in an experimental model of gentamicin nephrotoxicity in a dog. Gentamicin was injected subcutaneously twice daily for 16.5 days (*shaded area*) until the serum creatinine increased by 50%. Urinary NGAL predicted the active kidney injury by day 5 (*solid arrow*) whereas the AKI was not recognized until day 14 by IRIS AKI guidelines (*open arrow*). Note the discontinued left axis as urinary NGAL increased by more than 480 times the baseline concentration to a peak value to 264,000 pg/mL at day 19 before decreasing to the baseline over the subsequent 26 days. (*Data from* Palm CA, Segev G, Cowgill LD, et al. Urinary neutrophil gelatinase-associated lipocalin as a marker for identification of acute kidney injury and recovery in dogs with gentamicin-induced nephrotoxicity. J Vet Intern Med 2016;30:200–5).

neutrophil-associated inflammation that could have been the source of urinary NGAL in these dogs.[41] It is difficult, however, to exclude the presence of subclinical kidney involvement in this lower urinary tract cohort. The increased urinary NGAL expression may have forecasted kidney involvement that was otherwise subclinical and undetectable.

To gain preliminary insight into these alternative possibilities, in collaboration with Drs Shelly Vaden and Murthy Yerramilli, one of the authors (Larry D. Cowgill) recently has screened urine from 36 dogs with documented urinary tract infection for the presence of urinary cystatin C, urinary NGAL, and urinary clusterin as predictors of concurrent active kidney injury. No dog had clinical evidence of AKI although 6 dogs (17%) had historical CKD. The urine was considered positive for active kidney injury if at least 2 of 3 biomarkers were above the normal threshold or if urinary clusterin (of renal tubular origin) alone was above the reference threshold. For the 30 dogs with no documented CKD, 43% demonstrated biomarker predicted active kidney injury, 37% had no biomarker predicted active kidney injury, and 20% demonstrated equivocal biomarker activity (**Table 1**, excludes the equivocal group). Although these data are preliminary and require additional prospective evaluation and validation of the long-term outcomes of these cases, they might suggest a large proportion of dogs with active urinary tract infection may simultaneously have upper tract kidney involvement promoting subclinical and otherwise undetectable active injury. Identification of active kidney injury concurrent with lower urinary tract disease may suggest the kidneys are concurrently infected and potentially a source for recurrent infection of the lower urinary tract. If not infected, the active injury may involve alternative mechanisms associated with lower tract infection and pose a risk for erosion of renal reserve and progressive CKD. If these findings are confirmed by further validation studies, it suggests a new paradigm and significance to urinary tract infection and portends new diagnostic and therapeutic responsibilities.

Table 1
Blood and urine analytes from 30 dogs with documented urinary tract infection and no evident kidney involvement

Test (Units; Reference Range)	No Biomarker Evident Kidney Injury (n = 11)	Biomarker Predicted Kidney Injury (n = 13)
Clinical parameters median (range)		
Creatinine (mg/dL; 0.5–1.5)	0.9 (0.4–1.2)	0.9 (0.4–1.2)
BUN (mg/dL; 9–31)	14.0 (3–21)	21 (8–75)
IDEXX SDMA (μg/dL <14)	8.0 (6–16)	12.0 (7–17)
Uprot/creat (<0.5)	0.26 (0.04–0.89)	1.46 (0.02–8.85)
Urine specific gravity	1.017 (1.006–1.032)	1.025 (1.013–1.042)
uWBC (/hpf; 0–5)	10 (0 to >500)	0 (0–20)
uRBC (/hpf; 0–5)	15 (0 to >500)	0 (0–15)
Urinary niomarkers, median (range)		
uCystatin C (ng/mL, <300)	57 (1–115.7)	370 (29 to >2500)
uNGAL (ng/mL, <10)	2.6 (1.6–5.8)	40.4 (0.26–220.1)
uClusterin (ng/mL, <600)	97 (0–274)	2010 (119–2527)

Abbreviations: BUN, blood urea nitrogen; uClusterin, urine clusterin; uCystatin C, urine cystatin C; uNGAL, urine NGAL; Uprot/creat, urine protein/creatinine ratio; uRBC, urine red blood cell count; uWBC, urine white blood cell count.

Active Kidney Injury in Acute and Chronic Cardiorenal Syndrome

Acute and chronic cardiorenal disorders are another clinical arena in which the kidney may be subjected to subclinical and potentially sustained active injury secondarily to disease, failure, or management of primary cardiovascular disease. Severe and persistent heart failure is commonly associated with progressive CKD that may be punctuated by episodes of acute kidney decompensation concurrent with decompensation of cardiac function or escalation of drug therapy (see **Fig. 2**). Active kidney injury biomarkers may facilitate recognition of the incipient kidney damage. This would permit more conscientious management of the cardiac disease and proactive preservation of kidney function and protection from kidney injury with its management (**Fig. 4**).

Fig. 2 illustrates the influence of progressive venous congestion on the kidneys (congestive nephropathy) subsequent to right heart failure and the development of ascites and increased intra-abdominal pressure. With abdominocentesis the intra-abdominal pressure and congestion are relieved temporarily with an associated dramatic improvement of the active injury markers (urine clusterin and serum inosine) with the initial abdominocentesis. Although improved, the markers further illustrate the ongoing kidney injury associated with ongoing cardiac disease and progressive congestion between abdominocentesis procedures and their prediction of the progressive CKD.

IS PROGRESSIVE CHRONIC KIDNEY DISEASE A SLOW-MOVING ACUTE KIDNEY INJURY? A NEW LOOK AT CHRONIC KIDNEY DISEASE

As discussed and illustrated previously, novel kidney biomarkers can expose subtle and subclinical kidney disease that may otherwise remain undiscovered with conventional diagnostic assessment. More importantly, active kidney injury biomarkers have potential to establish a new understanding of our traditional views of CKD, including its early identification and possible mediators of its progression. In a recent evaluation of urinary NGAL in dogs with kidney disease, there was significantly greater NGAL excretion in dogs with CKD than noted for healthy control dogs or those with lower urinary tract disease.[32] The urinary NGAL excretion was clearly less than in dogs with AKI, but this observation suggested some degree of active injury may be ongoing in these dogs absent the typical presentation of acute-on-chronic disease. Similar findings were reported for serum NGAL in dogs with CKD, in which serum NGAL was significantly higher than control dogs and increased with IRIS CKD Stage. Changes in serum NGAL are less specific, however, than urine NGAL for predicting AKI.[34]

Progressive CKD generally develops in dogs with heart disease as the heart disease transitions from compensated to incipient or overt failure or with escalation in cardiac therapy. Concurrent with this transition in cardiac function, there is expression of active kidney injury markers (predictive of an IRIS AKI Grade I or IRIS CKD Stage 1 injury), which precedes the temporal progression to more advanced CKD Stages (see **Fig. 2**). Absent active injury, kidney function typically remains stable (**Fig. 5**). Similarly, as suggested in **Table 1**, animals with urinary tract infection and identifiable active kidney injury biomarkers might be classified as IRIS AKI Grade I or CKD Stage 1 (depending on the duration of infection and initial creatinine concentration) based on biomarker expression but by most other criteria would otherwise have unrecognized kidney disease. With persistent expression of active injury kidney biomarkers, there would ultimately be the expectation for transition to higher grades or stages of kidney disease and the detection of progressive CKD over time.

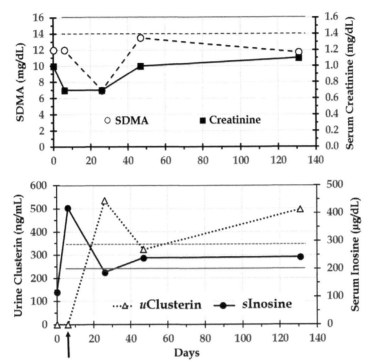

Fig. 4. Changes in conventional function test and novel active kidney injury markers in a dog with progressive valvular heart disease and impending cardiac failure. Cardiac therapy including furosemide and ACE inhibition was started on Day 0. By Day 6, the dog's cardiac signs had improved. However, 12 hours after discharge for a progress check on day 6, the dog was represented to the emergency service for acute respiratory signs and heart failure secondary to a ruptured chordae tendineae requiring a rapid escalated the cardiac medications (*arrow*). (*Upper panel*) Changes in serum creatinine (*solid squares*) and IDEXX SDMA (*open circles*) over time. The solid and dotted horizontal lines represent the upper reference range for creatinine and IDEXX SDMA, respectively. (*Lower panel*) Associative changes in the active kidney injury biomarkers, urine clusterin (*u*Clusterin) (*open triangles*) and serum inosine (*s*Inosine) (*closed circles*) over time. The solid line represents the lower reference threshold for serum inosine, and the dotted horizontal line the upper reference range for urine clusterin. The initial decrease in serum inosine suggest active kidney injury in response to the impending cardiac failure. The initial medical management for incipient congestive heart failure resulted in a marked improvement (increase) in serum inosine as a measure of resolving active kidney injury/stress between day 0 and day 6. The subsequent acute decompensated heart failure and escalation of the medical management (*arrow*) promoted biomarker-predicted active kidney injury (decreased serum inosine and increased urinary clusterin), which persisted at a low level with compensation of the heart failure. The active kidney injury was not detected by serum creatinine or IDEXX SDMA.

With this overview, a hypothesis has been proposed that progressive CKD may result from clinically occult or overt acute insults to the kidneys, which are episodic or sustained in character (a slow-moving or sustained AKI) subsequent to exposure to diverse processes including metabolic and/or physiologic stresses. Documentation of active and especially persistently active kidney injury may be predictive of patients who are at risk for progression of CKD. Patients in whom evidence of active kidney injury is absent are more likely to maintain stable kidney function. To support this

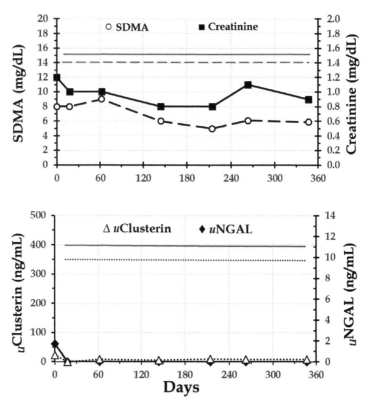

Fig. 5. Changes in conventional markers of kidney function and novel active kidney injury markers in a dog with compensated mitral valvular heart disease. (*Upper panel*) Changes in serum creatinine (*solid squares*) and IDEXX SDMA (*open circles*) over time. The solid and dotted horizontal lines represent the upper reference range for creatinine and IDEXX SDMA, respectively. (*Lower panel*) Associative changes in the active kidney injury biomarkers, urine clusterin (*u*Clusterin) (*open triangles*), and urine NGAL (*u*NGAL) (*closed diamonds*) over time. The solid and dotted horizontal lines represent the upper reference ranges for urine NGAL and urine clusterin, respectively. Note with stable and compensated heart failure, there is remarkable stability of kidney function and no biomarker-predicted active kidney injury over an extended period of time.

hypothesis, prospective studies involving canine and feline patients with well-characterized CKD are needed. The advent of active kidney injury biomarkers is likely to provide a renewed perspective and clinical significance to both IRIS CKD Stage 1 and IRIS AKI Grade I classifications. Although patients with these classifications are nonazotemic and generally asymptomatic, detectible active kidney injury markers may provide justifiable criteria for them to be classified with early kidney disease, thus distinguishing them from animals with normal kidneys. IRIS CKD Stage 1 and IRIS AKI Grade I classifications identified based on biomarker criteria warrant heightened clinical significance as a recognizable gateway to more advanced kidney disease and progressively worsening kidney function. It is worth noting that the transition from Stage 1 to Stage 2 CKD is associated with proportionally greater loss of functional renal mass than occurs with the transition between more advanced CKD stages. When followed over time or, ideally, coupled with markers of kidney repair, Stage 1 or Grade I classification might be further defined as continued active, resolving, or inactive to guide clinical decision making and therapeutic monitoring.

Sensitive and specific biomarkers are likely to lead to new insights into clinical kidney disease and facilitate new diagnostic and therapeutic approaches. Detection of active kidney injury (whether classified as CKD or AKI) may require a new designation depending on whether a patient's condition resolves, fails to develop progressive clinical manifestations over time, or progresses to overt clinical disease. Given the common pathophysiologic foundations and mediators working in the same cellular milieu, the distinctions between CKD and AKI might be viewed more interactively as a singular process in both early manifestations and advancing stages. It is easy to foresee new opportunities and applications for biomarker diagnostics and their applications for early recognition of kidney injury associated with:

1. Critical care
2. Systemic diseases and their management, including (eg, heart failure, proteinuria, infectious disease, and immune-mediated disease)
3. Anesthesia and invasive procedures.
4. Animals presenting for vague illness
5. Acute-on-chronic kidney disease and progression of CKD

If validated for specificity, sensitivity, and clinical utility, to be useful diagnostically clinicians need to be proactive in testing patients at risk for active kidney injury before the disease is identified by conventional diagnostic parameters or overt clinical signs. The established use of active kidney injury biomarkers will require changes in practice patterns related to CKD and its potential progression. Clinicians by necessity will need to recognize and anticipate the potential risks and clinical circumstances that might predispose to progressive CKD, including comorbid diseases (eg, hypertension, pre-existing kidney disease, heart failure, pancreatitis, heat stroke, and vomiting), medications (eg, angiotensin-converting enzyme inhibitors, diuretics, antimicrobials, and nonsteroidal anti-inflammatory drugs), and diagnostic and therapeutic procedures (eg, anesthesia, surgery, dentistry, and contrast administration).

This potential new diagnostic paradigm also will require an updated consensus for diagnostic and therapeutic responses to Stage 1 or Grade I kidney injury. It promises answers to the questions, which triggers or processes promote progression of CKD? and how can progression be recognized and potentially mitigated at its earliest stage to preserve kidney function? Similarly, therapeutic approaches may be monitored to biomarker endpoints and logically adjusted or extended until the biomarker activity is nullified.

REFERENCES

1. Available at: www.iris-kidney.com. Accessed August 1, 2016.
2. Elliott J, Cowgill L. Diagnostic algorithms for grading of acute kidney injury and staging the chronic kidney disease patient. In: Elliott J, Grauer GF, editors: BSAVA manual of canine and feline nephrology and urology. 3rd edition, in press.
3. Braun JP, Lefebvre HP, Watson AD. Creatinine in the dog: a review. Vet Clin Pathol 2003;32:162–79.
4. Basile DP, Bonventre JV, Mehta R, et al, ADQI XIII Work Group. Progression after AKI: understanding maladaptive repair processes to predict and identify therapeutic treatments. J Am Soc Nephrol 2016;27(3):687–97.
5. Elliott J, Syme HM, Markwell PJ. Acid-base balance of cats with chronic renal failure: effect of deterioration in renal function. J Small Anim Pract 2003;44(6):261–8.

6. Chakrabarti S, Syme HM, Elliott J. Clinicopathological variables predicting progression of azotemia in cats with chronic kidney disease. J Vet Intern Med 2012;26:275–81.

7. Polzin D. Chronic kidney disease. In: Ettinger S, Feldman E, editors. Textbook of veterinary internal medicine. Chichester (United Kingdom): Saunders; 2010. p. 2036–67.

8. Cowgill LD, Langston CE. Acute kidney disease. In: Bartges JW, Polzin DJ, editors. Nephrology and urology of small animals. St Louis (MO): Wiley-Blackwell; 2011.

9. Chawla LS, Eggers PW, Star RA, et al. Acute kidney injury and chronic kidney disease as interconnected syndromes. N Engl J Med 2014;371:58–66.

10. Chawla LS, Kimmel PL. Acute kidney injury and chronic kidney disease: an integrated clinical syndrome. Kidney Int 2012;82:516–24.

11. Lopez-Giacoman S, Madero M. Biomarkers in chronic kidney disease, from kidney function to kidney damage. World J Nephrol 2015;4:57–73.

12. Syme HM, Markwell PJ, Pfeiffer D, et al. Survival of cats with naturally occurring chronic renal failure is related to severity of proteinuria. J Vet Intern Med 2008;20: 528–35.

13. Onuigbo MA, Agbasi N. Chronic kidney disease prediction is an inexact science: the concept of "progressors" and "nonprogressors". World J Nephrol 2014;3: 31–49.

14. Kaissling B, Lehir M, Kriz W. Renal epithelial injury and fibrosis. Biochim Biophys Acta 2013;1832:931–9.

15. Coca SG, Singanamala S, Parikh CR. Chronic kidney disease after acute kidney injury: a systematic review and meta-analysis. Kidney Int 2012;81:442–8.

16. Heung M, Chawla LS. Acute kidney injury: gateway to chronic kidney disease. Nephron Clin Pract 2014;127:30–4.

17. Ferenbach DA, Bonventre JV. Mechanisms of maladaptive repair after AKI leading to accelerated kidney ageing and CKD. Nat Rev Nephrol 2015;11:264–76.

18. Bonventre JV. Primary proximal tubule injury leads to epithelial cell cycle arrest, fibrosis, vascular rarefaction, and glomerulosclerosis. Kidney Int Suppl 2014;4: 39–44.

19. Zuk A, Bonventre JV. Acute Kidney Injury. Annu Rev Med 2016;67:293–307.

20. Chaturvedi S, Ng KH, Mammen C. The path to chronic kidney disease following acute kidney injury: a neonatal perspective. Pediatr Nephrol 2016. [Epub ahead of print].

21. Zager RA. Progression from acute kidney injury to chronic kidney disease: clinical and experimental insights and queries. Nephron Clin Pract 2014;127:46–50.

22. Tan HL, Yap JQ, Qian Q. Acute kidney injury: tubular markers and risk for chronic kidney disease and end-stage kidney failure. Blood Purif 2016;41:144–50.

23. Zoja C, Abbate M, Remuzzi G. Progression of renal injury toward interstitial inflammation and glomerular sclerosis is dependent on abnormal protein filtration. Nephrol Dial Transplant 2015;30:706–12.

24. Kellum JA, Chawla LS. Cell-cycle arrest and acute kidney injury: the light and the dark sides. Nephrol Dial Transplant 2016;31:16–22.

25. Mohammed-Ali Z, Cruz GL, Dickhout JG. Crosstalk between the unfolded protein response and NF-κB-mediated inflammation in the progression of chronic kidney disease. J Immunol Res 2015;2015:428508.

26. Fuhrman DY, Kellum JA. Biomarkers for diagnosis, prognosis and intervention in acute kidney injury. Contrib Nephrol 2016;187:47–54.

27. Alge JL, Arthur JM. Biomarkers of AKI: a review of mechanistic relevance and potential therapeutic implications. Clin J Am Soc Nephrol 2015;10:147–55.

28. Koyner JL, Garg AX, Coca SG, et al, TRIBE-AKI Consortium. Biomarkers predict progression of acute kidney injury after cardiac surgery. J Am Soc Nephrol 2012; 23:905–14.
29. Kashani K, Kellum JA. Novel biomarkers indicating repair or progression after acute kidney injury. Curr Opin Nephrol Hypertens 2015;24:21–7.
30. De Loor J, Daminet S, Smets P, et al. Urinary biomarkers for acute kidney injury in dogs. J Vet Intern Med 2013;27:998–1010.
31. Segev G, Daminet S, Meyer E, et al. Characterization of kidney damage using several renal biomarkers in dogs with naturally occurring heatstroke. Vet J 2015;206:231–5.
32. Segev G, Palm C, LeRoy B, et al. Evaluation of neutrophil gelatinase-associated lipocalin as a marker of kidney injury in dogs. J Vet Intern Med 2013;27:1362–7.
33. Palm CA, Segev G, Cowgill LD, et al. Urinary neutrophil gelatinase-associated lipocalin as a marker for identification of acute kidney injury and recovery in dogs with gentamicin-induced nephrotoxicity. J Vet Intern Med 2016;30:200–5.
34. Ahn HJ, Hyun C. Evaluation of serum neutrophil gelatinase-associated lipocalin (NGAL) activity in dogs with chronic kidney disease. Vet Rec 2013;173:452.
35. Ahn JY, Lee MJ, Seo JS, et al. Plasma neutrophil gelatinase-associated lipocalin as a predictive biomarker for the detection of acute kidney injury in adult poisoning. Clin Toxicol 2016;54:127–33.
36. Lee YJ, Hu YY, Lin YS, et al. Urine neutrophil gelatinase-associated lipocalin (NGAL) as a biomarker for acute canine kidney injury. Vet Res 2012;8:248.
37. Hsu WL, Lin YS, Hu YY, et al. Neutrophil gelatinase-associated lipocalin in dogs with naturally occurring renal diseases. J Vet Intern Med 2014;28:437–42.
38. Hokamp JA, Nabity MB. Renal biomarkers in domestic species. Vet Clin Pathol 2016;45:28–56.
39. Raila J, Brunnberg L, Schweigert FJ, et al. Influence of kidney function on urinary excretion of albumin and retinol-binding protein in dogs with naturally occurring renal disease. Am J Vet Res 2010;71:1387–94.
40. Nabity MB, Lees GE, Cianciolo R, et al. Urinary biomarkers of renal disease in dogs with X-linked hereditary nephropathy. J Vet Intern Med 2012;26:282–93.
41. Decavele AS, Dhondt L, De Buyzere ML, et al. Increased urinary neutrophil gelatinase associated lipocalin in urinary tract infections and leukocyturia. Clin Chem Lab Med 2011;49:999–1003.

Current Understanding of the Pathogenesis of Progressive Chronic Kidney Disease in Cats

Rosanne E. Jepson, BVSc, MVetMed, PhD, FHEA, MRCVS

KEYWORDS

- Chronic kidney disease • Progression • Fibrosis • Mineral and bone disorder
- Parathyroid hormone • Phosphorus • Hypertension
- Renin-angiotensin-aldosterone system

KEY POINTS

- Chronic kidney disease (CKD) is a common condition in mature, senior, and geriatric cats and is characterized by tubulointerstitial inflammation and fibrosis.
- CKD is a complex disease condition, the development of which is likely to be influenced by genetic, environmental, and individual patient factors.
- Factors that have been associated with progressive CKD from experimental and human medicine include hemodynamic adaptations to renal injury, systemic hypertension, activation of the renin-angiotensin aldosterone system, proteinuria, hyperphosphatemia hypoxia, and oxidative stress.
- Irrespective of the inciting injury, the common pathway for the progression of renal injury is via inflammation and fibrosis.
- Understanding factors associated with progression of disease give potential for therapeutic intervention, which may slow advancing disease.

INTRODUCTION

Chronic kidney disease (CKD) is a common condition identified in cats at both general practice and the referral level. The term CKD is used to imply alteration in structure or function of the kidney that has occurred over a period of time, typically 3 months. Many different underlying renal diseases can affect the feline kidney, some localizing to a particular region of the kidney, some being congenital, and others acquired in origin. At least initially, not all of these conditions will result in azotemia and yet they may still fulfill the criteria of CKD, for example, altered tubular function or primary

The author has nothing to disclose.
Department of Clinical Science and Services, Royal Veterinary College, Hawkshead Lane, North Mymms, Hertfordshire AL9 7TA, UK
E-mail address: rjepson@rvc.ac.uk

glomerular disease. However, when examining postmortem tissue from geriatric cats diagnosed with CKD in a first-opinion setting, where the predominant breed examined was either the domestic shorthair or longhair, then specific renal diseases accounted for only ~16% of all CKD.[1] The most common histopathologic findings in the remaining cats were nonspecific tubulointerstitial inflammation, fibrosis, and mineralization referred to as tubulointerstitial nephritis.[1–4] The development and progression of these lesions will be the focus of this article, but given the limited response of the kidney to an inciting injury, tubulointerstitial inflammation and fibrosis are common end pathology for many primary renal diseases.

Early studies suggested that approximately 15% to 30% of cats greater than the age of 15 years show evidence of CKD.[5] However, markers of glomerular filtration rate (GFR) used in clinical practice are insensitive for the detection of early decline in renal function (see Murthy Yerramilli, Giosi Farace, John Quinn, et al: "Kidney Disease and the Nexus of Chronic Kidney Disease and Acute Kidney Injury: The Role of Novel Biomarkers as Early and Accurate Diagnostics"; and Roberta Relford, Jane Robertson, and Celeste Clements' article, "Symmetric Dimethylarginine: Improving the Diagnosis and Staging of Chronic Kidney Disease in Small Animals," in this issue), and it is appreciated that substantial renal abnormality may be present by the time a patient develops azotemic CKD.[2] Such patients may have other evidence that points to the clinical diagnosis of CKD without the requirement for renal biopsy, for example, persistently inadequately concentrated urine or abnormalities identified with diagnostic imaging of the kidney. These patients are recognized within the International Renal Interest Society (IRIS) staging system as having nonazotemic stage 1 or 2 CKD. Recent studies that include these early diagnosed patients suggest that the prevalence of CKD is much higher, and in the study by Marino and colleagues,[6] 80% of cats greater than 15 years old were defined as having CKD.

CAUSE OF FELINE CHRONIC KIDNEY DISEASE

The underlying cause of feline CKD, where the primary histopathologic finding is tubulointerstitial nephritis, is poorly understood. CKD should be considered a complex disease that is likely to be influenced by genetic, individual, and environmental factors.

AGING AND THE KIDNEY

In human medicine, it is known that GFR declines with age as a consequence of renal structural change, tubular dysfunction, and a decrease in the number of functioning nephrons. These changes begin around the age of 30 to 40 years but accelerate after the age of 50 to 60 years.[7–9] Decline in GFR in humans has been reported to be between 0.4 and 1.02 mL/min/y and CKD has been reported to be present in approximately 35% of the general population over the age of 70 years using current criteria.[7,10] These results have led studies to question whether the criteria that are used for the diagnosis and staging of CKD (Kidney Disease Outcomes Quality Initiative guidelines) should be applied equally to young and old alike given that decrease in GFR may be "normal" in old age, and the mortality risk associated with a given stage of CKD may be different between young and older age groups. It can therefore be debated whether a diagnosis of CKD in the elderly truly represents a disease process rather than part of normal aging.[10–13] Although CKD is most often identified in cats over the age of 12 years, there is evidence that tubulointerstitial inflammation may be identified in the renal parenchyma of young cats that have died for other reasons, and as such, it has been proposed that the development of CKD may also be part of a normal aging process in cats.[14]

Aging is a programmed biological process, which is regulated by many genes. It results in impairment to normal adaptive responses and homeostatic mechanisms that make organs susceptible to either internal or external stressors.[10] Transcriptional differences have been identified between the young and the old, affecting many genes.[10] However, there are certain genes, for example, *Klotho* (an aging suppressor gene encoding for α-Klotho) and *SIRT 1* (encoding for sirtuin-1, which is an NAD-dependent histone deacetylase involved in cellular regulation), which may be of particular interest.[10,15] Klotho was first identified in 1997 in a mutant mouse strain that demonstrated an aging phenotype and shortened lifespan.[16] Subsequently its concurrent role in phosphorus homeostasis and kidney disease has made it a gene and molecule of particular interest with relation to CKD and declining renal function with age.[17,18]

Several different mechanisms can contribute to age-related organ dysfunction, including mitochondrial injury, telomere shortening, oxidative stress, profibrogenic and pro-inflammatory mediators, and an imbalance between cell repair and proliferation versus apoptosis and cell death (**Fig. 1**). However, many of these mechanisms occur not only during aging but also as part of an organ's response to injury and as part of the healing process. Cellular senescence occurs as part of the aging process (replicative senescence) and refers to the situation where cells enter a state of replication and growth arrest.[11] Such cells remain viable but show an altered morphology, including increased expression of senescence-associated β-galactosidase (SABG), accumulation of lipofuscin granules, lack of response to mitogenic stimuli, and in some species, for example, humans, replicative senescence is associated with

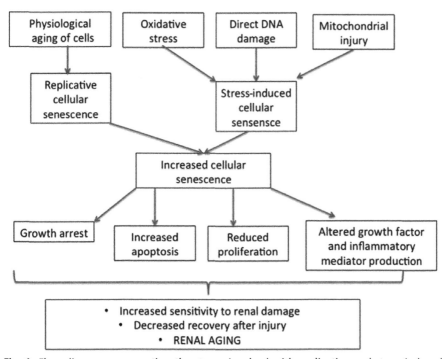

Fig. 1. Flow diagram representing the stages involved with replicative and stress-induced cellular senescence in renal aging.

telomere shortening and reduced telomerase activity.[10] Cellular senescence can also be stimulated by several physiologic stressors, for example, oxidative stress, mitochondrial damage, renin-angiotensin aldosterone system (RAAS) activation, which is referred to as stress-induced premature senescence (SIPS). These stressors may also contribute to telomere shortening.[11] Cellular senescence markers, for example, telomere shortening, SABG, and P16[INK4a] (involved in the SIPS pathway), have been shown to correlate with renal aging in humans, although there are interspecies differences.[19–21] Senescent cells have altered secretion of products such as transforming growth factor-β (TGF-β), epithelial growth factor, insulinlike growth factor, and vascular endothelial growth factor (VEGF). The net effect of these changes is reduced capacity of the kidney to respond to repair and withstand normal stressors, also reducing its ability to recover from periods of, for example, ischemic injury and promotion of inflammation and fibrosis.[11]

In cats, preliminary data evaluating telomere shortening support the concept of an aging process affecting the kidney. Telomere length has been evaluated in renal (proximal [PTC] and distal tubule), hepatic, and dermal tissue from cats with CKD, geriatric and young control cats by telomere fluorescence in situ hybridization with immunostaining in addition to evaluation of SABG.[22] Telomere shortening was evident in PTC of geriatric cats with CKD compared with age-matched and young controls despite no difference in telomere length in skin or liver from the same groups.[22] Significantly increased staining for SABG was also found in renal tissue from cats with CKD compared with the young controls, although the difference between geriatric control cats was not significant.[22] It therefore seems feasible that aging may be a component of the decline in renal function seen in older cats, but it is also likely that other individual and environmental factors contribute to an individual's overall risk of developing CKD.

ASSOCIATION OF CHRONIC KIDNEY DISEASE WITH DEMOGRAPHIC, ENVIRONMENTAL, AND INDIVIDUAL FACTORS

There are relatively few clinical studies that have evaluated phenotypic, environmental, or lifestyle risk factors for the development of feline CKD. However, a recent study indicated that poor body condition, periodontal disease, cystitis, being male neutered rather than female spayed, and anesthesia or documented dehydration in the preceding year were risk factors for CKD.[23] It has been suggested that certain breeds of cats may be predisposed to CKD, for example, Persian, Abyssinian, Siamese, Ragdoll, Maine coon, but the current evidence base for these breed predispositions is low.[5,24,25] Similarly, although the study suggested a predisposition in neutered male cats, other studies have not supported a sex predisposition.

Concern has previously been raised regarding the role that diet may play in the development of CKD in cats. A potassium-depleted high-protein diet has previously been associated with the development of kidney disease, whereas a 2-year study indicated no association between high-salt intake and adverse effect on renal function in older cats.[26,27] A single study has suggested that ad libitum feeding and increased ash intake were associated with CKD compared with control cats, although the study was relatively small.[28] The study by Greene and colleagues[23] did not support an association between diet and development of CKD, such that overall evidence is controversial, and further work is required.

There are many interventions that occur over a cat's lifetime that could impact the future development of CKD; for example, exposure to nephrotoxic drugs or renal toxins, periods of prerenal azotemia, and the requirement for general anesthesia. Such episodes may reflect periods of undetected acute kidney injury (AKI), which may be a stimulus for inflammation and fibrosis (see Larry D. Cowgill, David J. Polzin, Jonathan Elliott, et al: "Is Progressive Chronic Kidney Disease a Slow Acute Kidney Injury?," in this issue). It can be hypothesized that, throughout a cat's lifetime, serial small AKI events could lead to an increased risk of developing CKD.

One further frequent intervention that has been investigated as a potential trigger for the development of CKD is vaccination. For vaccine manufacture, feline viruses (feline herpes virus-1, calicivirus, and panleukopenia virus) are initially propagated using an immortal line of feline-derived tubular epithelial cells, Crandell-Rees feline kidney cells (CRFK). It is impossible for all antigenic components of these cells to be extracted during vaccine purification and manufacture, and therefore, exposure to antigenic components may occur. Administration of certain vaccines could therefore be hypothesized to stimulate antibody production, which may bind feline renal proteins and initiate an inflammatory response. This hypothesis was explored in a series of studies wherein cats were exposed to either CRFK cell lysate or feline viral rhinotracheitis, calicivirus, and panleukopenia (FVRCP) vaccination.[29]

Young cats demonstrated antibody response to both parenteral administration of FVRCP vaccines and CRFK cell lysate, but there was no histopathologic evidence of renal disease after 56 weeks of study.[29] A follow-up study evaluated repeated exposure of previously sensitized cats to CRFK lysate. Although this study was small, there was evidence of tubulointerstitial inflammation in 3 of 6 cats repeatedly inoculated with the CRFK lysate.[30] The antigens have been identified as α-enolase and annexin-A2.[31] However, to date, there have been no published epidemiologic studies that have evaluated vaccination as a risk factor for either the development or the progression of CKD, and any causality between vaccination and naturally occurring CKD remains to be determined.

ASSOCIATION OF THE DEVELOPMENT OF CHRONIC KIDNEY DISEASE WITH CONCURRENT DISEASE

In human medicine, there are several disease conditions that are known to increase an individual's risk of developing CKD, for example, cardiovascular disease, diabetes mellitus, and systemic hypertension. However, the evidence base for concurrent disease influencing the development and progression of CKD in cats is much more limited.

Cardiovascular and Renal Disorder

The term cardiorenal syndrome has been coined in human medicine to express the relationship that exists between *cardiovascular* and renal disease and to define the situation whereby acute or chronic dysfunction in one organ may induce acute or chronic dysfunction in the other.[32] Both cardiac and renal diseases are common in cats, and therefore, these conditions may be diagnosed concurrently. However, there has been very little focus on the interplay between these 2 body systems, which depend on many similar homeostatic mechanisms. The role that cardiovascular disease plays in the development of CKD has not been explored.

A recent consensus group has been established to consider these issues further and to promote research into cardiovascular and renal disorders (CvRD).[33] Potential mechanisms by which CvRD may be detrimental to the kidney include cardiac shock, low cardiac output, and hypotension resulting in reduced renal perfusion, AKI and azotemia, activation of the RAAS, systemic arterial thromboembolism resulting in renal infarction, and passive congestion of the kidney during congestive heart failure. In particular, inciting renal injuries that result in ischemia provide an interesting link to the development of tubulointerstitial inflammation and fibrosis (see Larry D. Cowgill, David J. Polzin, Jonathan Elliott, et al: "Is Progressive Chronic Kidney Disease a Slow Acute Kidney Injury?," in this issue).[34]

Systemic hypertension is a well-recognized risk factor in humans for the development of CKD. Systemic hypertension is identified in approximately 20% of cats diagnosed with CKD, and of cats that have evidence of systemic hypertension, approximately 60% are reported to have underlying azotemic CKD at diagnosis.[35,36] More recently, a study by Bijsmans and colleagues[37] has demonstrated a positive association between age and increasing systolic blood pressure (SBP) and an increased risk of hypertension in those cats with CKD compared with healthy cats. However, in longitudinal population studies, SBP has not been associated with the development of azotemia, the survival of cats with CKD, or having a more progressive phenotype of CKD. The cats in these studies diagnosed with systemic hypertension, however, were always treated with the calcium channel blocker, amlodipine besylate, and therefore the true effect of systemic hypertension on the development and/or progression of CKD may have been masked.[38–40]

Diabetes Mellitus

Unlike in human medicine, to date, no association has been identified between diabetes mellitus and CKD in cats or the development of a diabetic nephropathy, although it remains possible that this reflects the relatively shorter life expectancy of diabetic cats compared with diabetic humans.[23,41]

Hyperthyroidism

Hyperthyroidism is a common condition in the older cat, and therefore, is often diagnosed concurrently with CKD.[42] The effects of hyperthyroidism on renal hemodynamics are well documented from experimental rodent studies, including renal hypertrophy and an increase in GFR that is thought to be predominantly the consequence of RAAS activation secondary to change in β-adrenoceptor activity.[42] Hyperthyroidism has also been implicated in the progression of renal disease, the etiopathogenesis of which is unresolved, but may relate to altered renal hemodynamics, hyperfiltration, and the increased proteinuria identified in hyperthyroidism.[42] Studies have shown that GFR declines after treatment of hyperthyroidism in cats and that, depending on the modality of therapy, between 15% and 49% of hyperthyroid cats will be revealed to be azotemic after treatment.[43,44] However, this is considered to be the consequence of return to euthyroid state rather than direct renal injury. The relative contribution that being hyperthyroid makes to the development or progression of CKD in cats is unknown. Cats with hyperthyroidism have been shown to be more markedly proteinuric, and that this proteinuria resolves with treatment of hyperthyroidism.[45] Proteinuria is present as a consequence of glomerular hypertension, and it can be hypothesized that this, in addition to protein processing by the proximal tubular cells (PTC; see later discussion), may be detrimental to the kidney. However, although proteinuria was significantly associated with all-cause mortality in hyperthyroid cats, it was not associated with development of azotemic CKD.[46] An alternative mechanism that could enable hyperthyroidism to contribute to the development or progression of CKD is hyperparathyroidism, alterations in calcium and phosphorus homeostasis, and the potential for soft tissue, including renal, mineralization. Hyperthyroid cats have been shown to have elevated parathyroid hormone (PTH) and fibroblast growth factor 23 (FGF23) concentrations.[47] However, neither PTH nor FGF23 was significantly associated with the development of azotemia in hyperthyroid cats.[47] The exact role of hyperparathyroidism and disorders of calcium and phosphorus homeostasis and their effect on renal disease in hyperthyroidism remain to be determined.

Upper and Lower Urinary Tract Stone Disease

Both upper and lower urinary tract stone disease are well recognized in the feline literature.[48,49] To date, there are no data specifically evaluating the effect of periods of urethral obstruction as a risk factor for the future development of CKD in cats. However, given that postrenal obstruction is an underlying cause for AKI, it can be hypothesized that any period of urethral obstruction is likely to have a detrimental effect on the kidney. Similarly, in the past decade, there has been increased recognition of cats developing ureterolithiasis and nephrolithiasis, of which approximately 98% of cases are related to calcium oxalate stones.[48–50] It is easy to hypothesize that the acute to chronic injury caused by partial to complete ureteral obstruction may play a role in an individual cat subsequently developing CKD. However, cats with upper urinary tract stones are typically younger (median age 7 years) than cats with CKD, suggesting that this is not going to be the etiopathogenesis for all cats with CKD but should certainly be considered in cats that present with CKD at a younger age.[50] Furthermore, a study by Ross and colleagues[51] evaluated the presence of nephroliths as a risk factor for mortality and progression of CKD but found no association.

Infectious Disease

There has been interest in the potential for infectious disease to contribute to the development of CKD, although evidence for these associations is currently poor.

Urinary tract infections and pyelonephritis

Cats with CKD are at inherent risk of urinary tract infections (UTI) due to reduced host defense mechanisms. UTI are reported to affect between 17% and 33% of cats diagnosed with CKD, a substantial proportion of which may present as asymptomatic bacteriuria.[3,52–54] To date, only the study by Greene and colleagues[23] has specifically evaluated prior episodes of cystitis as a risk factor for CKD in cats, although it was not possible to separate the specific nature of the cystitis in this study, for example, feline lower urinary tract disease versus bacterial cystitis. Nevertheless, the presence of bacterial UTI and the possibility of ascending infections resulting in either acute or chronic pyelonephritis certainly raise concern in relation to acute chronic kidney injury and the progression of CKD. Further work is needed to establish the significance of positive urine cultures in cats with CKD and the role that symptomatic UTI versus asymptomatic bacteriuria plays in the progression of disease.[55]

Feline immunodeficiency virus

Based on the presence of human immunodeficiency–associated interstitial nephritis, several studies have investigated the potential role of feline immunodeficiency virus (FIV).[56] A recent histopathologic study indicated that approximately 50% of cats experimentally infected with FIV demonstrated histopathologic lesions common to patients with HIV nephritis, including mesangial widening, glomerulosclerosis, and immune-mediated glomerulonephritis when compared with controls.[57] Histopathologic lesions were more marked in kidneys from naturally affected cats that were also examined and included additional lesions such as amyloid deposits and interstitial inflammation and fibrosis.[57] However, such cats were older than the experimentally infected cats, and aged-matched controls were not evaluated in this study.[57] To date, epidemiologic studies have not been able to substantiate a clinical association between FIV and CKD.[58,59]

Morbillivirus

Several studies have raised interest in a potential association between CKD and morbillivirus infection (FmoPV), a paramyxovirus identified in cats.[60–64] The virus was shown to have cytopathic effects in FCRK cell lines, and in small numbers of stray cats, there seemed to be a higher prevalence of tubulointerstitial nephritis in seropositive than seronegative cats, although little demographic and phenotypic data were available for either group.[63] FmoPV has also been identified in the urine (10%) and blood (6%) of stray cats in a study performed in Japan, and at a higher prevalence from renal tissue (40%; 4/10) from cats with CKD.[65] In a further study, the prevalence of FmoPV detected in urine by real-time polymer chain reaction (PCR) in client-owned cats was ~15%.[66] However, the prevalence of this virus in cats outside of Japan and China and any true association with the development or progression of CKD remain to be determined.

Leptospirosis

Exposure of cats to leptospirosis is reported, with prevalence ranging from 3% to 35% depending on population and geographic location, although clinically associated disease is rarely reported.[67–70] Experimental studies suggest that cats are largely resistant to acute leptospirosis, although reports of clinical cases suggest that this is a possibility.[68,71] A study by Rodriguez and colleagues[69] has compared seropositivity and urinary PCR between CKD cats and non-age-matched controls. Seropositivity was significantly different between the 2 groups (7.2% non-CKD, 14.9% CKD cats), although PCR results were not.[69] However, a further study demonstrated no significant difference in seroprevalence between azotemic and nonazotemic cats.[72] The exact role that current or prior exposure to leptospire organisms plays in feline CKD therefore requires further study.

Bartonellosis

Potential associations have been made between Bartonella species infection and several different disease conditions, but so far no association has been identified between Bartonellosis and CKD in cats.[73]

Ultimately, irrespective of the underlying cause, CKD is considered to be a progressive disease. The kidney has a limited capacity to respond to an inciting injury with the main pathologic findings and the end-stage pathway being the development of renal inflammation and fibrosis. To date, it is not completely clear whether there is a causal relationship between fibrosis and the development CKD or whether fibrosis is purely a secondary and reparative response. Nevertheless, an understanding of the mechanisms involved in renal inflammation and fibrosis and the factors that contribute to the progression of CKD is important. If the development of CKD cannot be prevented, then the greatest opportunities for intervention lie in early diagnosis and prevention of progression. (See Murthy Yerramilli, Giosi Farace, John Quinn, et al: "Kidney Disease and the Nexus of Chronic Kidney Disease and Acute Kidney Injury: The Role of Novel Biomarkers as Early and Accurate Diagnostics"; and Roberta Relford, Jane Robertson, and Celeste Clements' article, "Symmetric Dimethylarginine: Improving the Diagnosis and Staging of Chronic Kidney Disease in Small Animals," in this issue.)

RENAL INFLAMMATION AND FIBROSIS: THE KIDNEY'S RESPONSE TO INJURY

Healthy renal interstitium is composed of sparse cells (fibroblasts and dendritic cells) embedded in an extracellular matrix (ECM) that is composed of collagen (I, III, VII), fibronectin, and ECM glycoproteins, for example, tenascin. Renal fibrosis usually begins with focal areas of inflammation and activation of mesenchymal cells in response to an inciting injury, progressing to expanding areas of fibrosis and scarring (**Fig. 2**).[74] However, after injury it can be hypothesized that fibrosis may be playing several different roles within the kidney. Intervention to slow or reduce fibrosis could therefore have either negative or positive effects. For example, fibrosis may occur after kidney injury, when renal structural repair is incomplete, with fibrosis acting as an "innocent filler."[75] Alternatively, fibrosis may appear after injury but interfere with the potential for full recovery. In the former scenario, preventing fibrosis would have little impact on the course of disease, whereas in the latter scenario, preventing fibrosis would be important to improve outcome.[75] Fibrosis could also be an intermediate stage, whereby the presence of fibrosis acts as a scaffold for repair. For example, studies of uranyl acetate–induced acute tubular injury suggest that myofibroblasts may emerge after tubular damage, providing a supportive structure, and then regress once regeneration is complete.[76,77] In this situation, prevention of fibrosis would be counterproductive, although the long-term deposition of fibrosis, which does not regress, might be detrimental to the kidney.[75] Although fibrosis may be part of the normal healing process, in CKD, fibrosis may represent a maladapted response of the kidney to injury that fails to terminate (see **Fig. 2**).[78] It is possible that the role of fibrosis may differ between types of renal injury. Tools that modulate fibrosis and evaluate their effect in different disease models would be required to determine whether slowing or preventing fibrosis has clinical benefit.

Renal fibrosis is characterized by an excessive fibrogenic response and expansion of ECM, which destroys the normal renal tissue. Histopathologically, this is

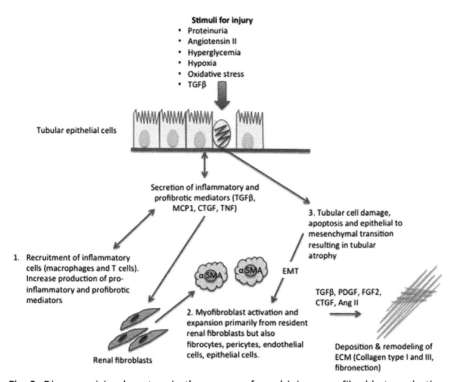

Fig. 2. Diagram giving key steps in the process of renal injury, myofibroblast production, and interstitial inflammation and fibrosis.

characterized by excessive accumulation of ECM, loss of renal microcirculation, infiltration of mononuclear inflammatory cells, tubular atrophy and dilation, and mineralization. In the healthy kidney, fibroblasts play an important role in the homeostasis of ECM secretion and degradation through the production of proteases. However, during fibrosis, fibroblasts become activated and transform to myofibroblasts and subsequently produce excessive quantities of ECM proteins, for example, collagen IV, laminin, fibronectin, elastins, fibrillins, TGF-β-binding proteins, tenascins, and proteoglycans (see **Fig. 2**).

Four major cell types are important for the genesis of progressive renal fibrosis: myofibroblasts, inflammatory cells, microvascular endothelial cells (pericytes), and tubular epithelial cells.[79]

Myofibroblasts

The origin of myofibroblasts in the kidney has been the source of considerable controversy. Based on recent studies, the main source accounting for more than 50% of myofibroblasts is thought to be renal fibroblasts.[80,81] Renal fibroblasts are found in the interstitium of healthy kidneys and are responsible for production of ECM and communicating with endothelial and epithelial cells. Certain subpopulations of renal fibroblasts are responsible for production of erythropoietin (EPO). In fibrosis models (eg, unilateral ureteral obstruction [UUO] and ischemic reperfusion [IR] injury), resident renal fibroblasts and EPO producing fibroblasts undergo a process of transformation to myofibroblasts (**Fig. 3**).[75]

Other sources of myofibroblasts include pericytes, fibrocytes, tubular epithelial cells, and endothelial cells. Pericytes are contractile cells that wrap around microvessels and arise from mesenchymal origin.[82] They play a critical role in the stability and integrity of microvessels and are able to control microcirculation by regulating capillary diameter and hence vascular tone.[82,83] In response to injury, pericytes

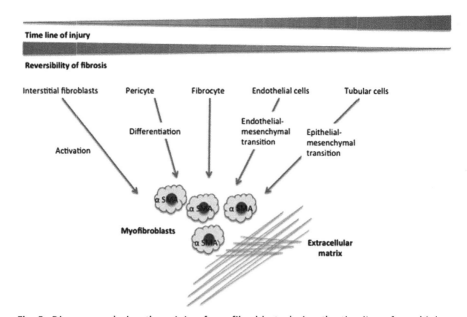

Fig. 3. Diagram exploring the origin of myofibroblasts during the timeline of renal injury.

detach, migrate to the interstitial space, and transform into myofibroblasts (see **Fig. 3**). Pericytes transformation has been demonstrated in experimental models of UUO and IR.[84,85] Myofibroblasts may also originate from fibrocytes (bone marrow–derived myeloid precursor cells) with recent studies suggesting that fibrocytes account for approximately 35% of myofibroblast production.[75,81] Early studies suggested that local renal cells including tubular epithelium might also undergo either epithelial-mesenchymal transition (EMT) and contribute to the myofibroblast population.[86,87] However, conflicting studies have been published using in vivo data, and EMT is likely to represent only a very small (<5%) component of myofibroblast production.[81] Endothelial cells are also capable of EMT with a recent study suggesting they account for approximately 10% of myofibroblast production (see **Fig. 3**).[88,89]

Myofibroblasts have the characteristics of both fibroblasts and smooth muscle cells. Key features include expression of α-smooth muscle actin (α-SMA) and vimentin (intermediate filament protein), abundant rough endoplasmic reticulum, and their ability to secrete pericellular matrix containing collagen and glycosaminoglycans. The recruitment and transdifferentiation of precursors to myofibroblasts can be activated by both local and circulating factors. Important stimuli include autocrine and paracrine growth factors (eg, TGF-β, platelet-derived growth factor [PDGF], VEGF, connective tissue growth factor [CTGF]) of which perhaps the most important is TGF-β. TGF-β production can be stimulated by many factors recognized to promote renal injury, including RAAS, proteinuria, increased single nephron GFR (SNGFR), and oxidative stress.[90–94] Other stimuli for the activation of myofibroblasts include direct interaction with leukocytes/macrophages (see later discussion) and tubular epithelial cells (see later discussion) and local environmental stimuli such as hypoxia and hyperglycemia.

Inflammatory Cells

Inflammatory cells, particularly macrophages, play an important role in inflammation, tissue repair, and fibrosis. Subpopulations of macrophages may be responsible for production of inflammatory mediators, for example, interleukin (IL)-1β, tumor necrosis factor-α (TNF-α), chemokines (Monocyte Chemotactic Protein-1; MCP1), which recruit further inflammatory cells and increase production of TGF-β and PDGF, which promote myofibroblast activation.[78] It has also been speculated that monocytes from the circulation may enter renal tissue and differentiate into fibrocytes (see **Fig. 3**). However, the evidence base for this is largely based on cell culture systems.[75,95,96]

Pericytes

The role of pericytes differentiating to form myofibroblasts has been described earlier. However, pericytes are also important for vascular stability. The loss of pericytes, as they transform to myofibroblasts, contributes to loss of the interstitial capillary network, otherwise known as peritubular capillary rarefaction, and may play a major role in the development of hypoxia, oxidative stress, and progressive tubular cellular injury and fibrosis.[78,79,82,97] Histologic studies evaluating human kidney tissue have demonstrated that areas of renal fibrosis and reduced peritubular capillary density located together.[98,99] Hypoxia is a recognized final common pathway for the progression of CKD (see later discussion).[100,101] In addition, increase in permeability of microvasculature and leakage of plasma proteins such as fibrinogen and albumin into the interstitium may trigger an inflammatory response.[102]

Tubular Epithelial Cells

Tubular epithelial cells have many roles in renal fibrosis. Early in the course of the disease, injured tubular epithelial cells may be a source of inflammatory mediators, for example, cytokines and chemokines (IL-6, MCP-1, TNF-α), which recruit and activate inflammatory cells and promote differentiation of fibroblasts to myofibroblasts.[103] A study by Yang and colleagues[104] demonstrated that tubular epithelial cell cycle arrest in response to toxic, obstructive, and ischemic injury resulted in the development of fibrosis. In response to injury, tubular cells may also increase production of growth factors (eg, TGF- β, PDGF, FGF) and reactive oxygen species (ROS). When secreted either via the paracellular route or to the basolateral membrane into the tubulointerstitium, these factors all have profibrogenic effects.[75,79] Urinary complement factors and cytokines and protein handling by the tubular cells have also been implicated (see later discussion) as stimuli for the release of proinflammatory and profibrotic mediators from tubular cells.[79,105] Later in the disease process, lack of regeneration and loss of tubular epithelial cells may contribute to progression of disease and loss of nephrons.

EVIDENCE OF FIBROSIS IN FELINE CHRONIC KIDNEY DISEASE

The main histopathologic finding reported in older cats with CKD is tubulointerstitial inflammation and fibrosis.[3,4] In human medicine, even in patients with primary glomerular disease, it is tubulointerstitial lesions that correlate most strongly with renal function. Recently, feline studies have compared histopathologic findings with stage of kidney disease and identified that the severity of tubular degeneration, interstitial inflammation, fibrosis, and glomerulosclerosis was more marked in the later IRIS stages of CKD.[2] In a study by Chakrabarti and colleagues,[1] fibrosis was the only histopathologic finding that significantly correlated with severity of azotemia and IRIS stage.

To date, 2 studies have specifically evaluated myofibroblast recruitment in cats with CKD.[106,107] The presence of myofibroblasts in feline renal tissue, identified by the markers α-SMA and tubular and interstitial vimentin, correlated positively with both fibrosis and plasma creatinine concentration.[107] Expression of α-SMA and fibronectin was significantly higher in cats with tubulointerstitial nephritis, particularly in the periglomerular and peritubular areas.[106] It was also evident that α-SMA was expressed at earlier stages of tubulointerstitial nephritis and in some cats before the deposition of ECM.[106]

A limited number of feline studies have also evaluated inflammatory markers that may be stimuli for fibrosis and inflammation, including TGF-β. These studies suggest increased urinary TGF-β in cats with CKD compared with controls and a positive correlation between urinary TGF-β and azotemia.[108,109] However, a conflicting study evaluating active rather than total urinary TGF-β1 found no significant difference between nonazotemic geriatric cats, nonazotemic cats that were known to progress to develop azotemia, and azotemic age-matched cats. However, there was a trend toward increasing active urinary TGF-β in cats that developed azotemia where longitudinal monitoring was available, suggesting that alteration in active urinary TGF-β may be of interest if evaluated serially.[110] A study by Habenicht and colleagues[108] investigated urinary concentrations of IL-8 and MCP-1 as ratios to urine creatinine as potential markers of renal inflammation and injury. No significant difference in MCP-1:creatinine ratio could be detected, although IL-8:creatinine ratios were significantly higher in cats with CKD than control cats. A shortfall of all of these studies is that histopathology has not been routinely available, although, in other species, studies support that the correlation between urinary cytokine levels and renal inflammation is strong.[111]

Transglutaminase 2 (TG-2) has recently been investigated in cats. TG-2 is a calcium-dependent cross-linking enzyme from the transglutaminase family, which plays an important role in stabilizing ECM, thereby promoting ECM deposition and resistance to degradation. There is a strong relationship between TG-2 expression and renal fibrosis in humans with CKD and also rodent models.[112,113] The relationship between TG-2 and renal fibrosis has recently been extrapolated to the cat, wherein TG-2 activity was positively correlated with renal histopathology scoring, plasma creatinine, phosphate, and urea concentrations.[114]

Together these findings begin to support the importance of fibrosis in the pathogenesis of CKD, although further work is required to determine whether fibrosis is detrimental and whether modulating fibrotic pathways holds any clinical benefit.

MECHANISMS OF PROGRESSION AND MALADAPTIVE REPAIR IN CHRONIC KIDNEY DISEASE

In clinical practice, many cats with CKD remain stable for months to years, and median survival times of cats with azotemic IRIS stage 2, 3, and 4 CKD have been reported as 1151, 778, and 103 days, respectively, although there is considerable interindividual variability, and survival times reported are potentially affected by the modalities of therapy, interventions, and resources available.[24,38] However, some cats do demonstrate progressive disease, although the time point at which that progression occurs can be unpredictable.[115] In one study, 29% of cats with IRIS stage 2 disease and 63% of IRIS stage 3 CKD cats progressed to IRIS stage 4 before death.[40] Epidemiologic studies have evaluated factors associated with the development of azotemia, survival of cats with CKD, and also cats that demonstrate a more progressive phenotype of CKD.[24,38–40,116–118] From the experimental and human literature, there are several key pathophysiologic mechanisms that have been implicated in the progression of CKD.

HEMODYNAMIC ADAPTATIONS

In the 1980s, experimental rodent studies were performed that indicated that there was a hemoadaptive response that occurred as a consequence of nephron loss and that resulted in glomerular hypertrophy, hypertension, and hyperfiltration.[119] The net effect of these hemodynamic alterations was maintaining and increasing SNGFR in order to preserve renal function. However, although initially beneficial in terms of maintaining total GFR, ultimately these adaptations were detrimental and a critical point would be reached where self-perpetuating loss of further nephrons would result in progression of disease.[120]

There is evidence from experimental feline studies that similar hemodynamic and structural adaptations occur in cats.[121,122] Early feline renal mass reduction studies documented histopathologic evidence of glomerular lesions, fibrosis, and mineralization, and yet when followed over a year, these cats did not demonstrate the continued progressive decline in GFR that would be anticipated from the rodent studies.[123,124] Micropuncture studies in cats showed that in response to renal mass reduction there was evidence of dilation of preglomerular afferent arterioles, increase in glomerular capillary pressure, and as a consequence, increased effective filtration pressure and SNGFR.[121] Glomerular hypertrophy with a secondary increase in ultrafiltration coefficient, mesangial matrix expansion, and increased proteinuria was also observed.[121] Cats were therefore documented to show similar hemoadaptive and structural changes to those occurring in rodent models, although the changes were, to some extent, dependent on the degree of renal mass reduction. Thus, it has been hypothesized that the predisposition of an individual to progressive CKD may be a balance between adaptive mechanisms preserving GFR versus the development of structural lesions that advance disease.

The role that the hemoadaptive and structural glomerular changes play in naturally occurring feline CKD is more difficult to quantify. Studies evaluating renal abnormality at postmortem examination have scored glomerular lesions that included glomerular hypertrophy, glomerulosclerosis, and obsolescence (global matrix expansion with loss of capillary lumina). Cats with stage 2 CKD demonstrated significantly increased glomerular volume compared with nonazotemic control cats, whereas in stage 3 and 4 CKD cats, glomerular volume was closer to the control population.[1] It was hypothesized that this could be explained if glomerular hypertrophy occurring earlier in the course of CKD as an adaptive process subsequently became maladaptive, resulting in glomerulosclerosis and obsolescence in later stages.

ACTIVATION OF THE RENIN-ANGIOTENSIN-ALDOSTERONE SYSTEM

It is widely accepted that the RAAS is activated in CKD and that both systemic and tissue-specific RAAS systems exist. The kidney contains all the necessary components for local RAAS activation and indeed renal tissue concentrations of angiotensin II (Ang II) are reported to be significantly higher than plasma concentrations.[125,126] As such, quantification of plasma components of RAAS does not necessarily translate to the degree of activation of RAAS within the kidney.[127]

RAAS is particularly important as a modulator of blood pressure and fluid balance through alteration in sodium and water homeostasis as well as being integral to intrarenal hemodynamics and glomerular filtration. Traditionally, the RAAS pathway terminates with conversion of Ang I by angiotensin-converting enzyme (ACE) or alternative pathways (eg, chymase) to Ang II. Ang II mediates its effects predominantly via the type 1 (AT1) receptor, which has a wide distribution throughout the kidney, although type 2 receptors (AT2) are present albeit with a more limited distribution.[125] However, it is now recognized that many further products of both Ang I and Ang II may play important regulatory roles (eg, Ang [1–7]/Mas and Ang IV/AT4 pathways) and may have impact on the pathogenesis of CKD (**Fig. 4**).[125,128,129]

Ang II in particular has been highlighted as an important mediator in the progression of CKD. It acts as a potent vasoconstrictor contributing to the development of glomerular hypertension and hyperfiltration and may modulate the permeability of the glomerular filtration barrier at least partly by altering podocyte interactions.[130–132] Therefore, Ang II can promote renal injury not only through sustained glomerular hypertension and development of glomerulosclerosis but also by promoting proteinuria, which itself may be detrimental to the kidney (see **Fig. 4**; see later discussion).[133] Ang II also has direct fibroproliferative and inflammatory effects by increasing transcription and production of inflammatory and profibrogenic molecules, including TGF-β, hence promoting myofibroblast transformation and fibrosis (see **Fig. 4**).[93] Ang II may play a role in the migration and transformation of pericytes to myofibroblasts and also the differentiation of circulating fibrocytes to fibroblasts. It has been reported to stimulate the production of other growth factors and inflammatory mediators from vascular smooth muscle cells, glomerular endothelium, and mesangial cells (eg, MCP-1 and RANTES) and is a known activator of nuclear factor κβ (NFκβ), which is a key transcription factor in inflammatory disease stimulating upregulation of genes encoding for proinflammatory cytokines.[93,134,135]

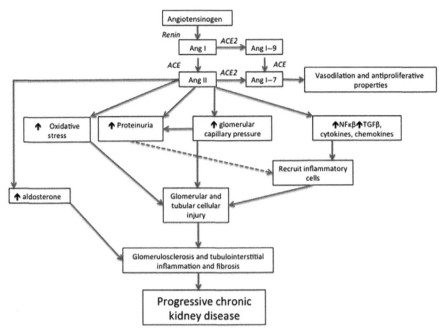

Fig. 4. Flow diagram of the effects of the RAAS on renal fibrosis and progression of kidney disease. Ang 1 to 9, angiotensin 1 to 9; Ang I, angiotensin 1; Ang 1-7, angiotensin 1 to 7.

The vasoconstrictive effects of Ang II on the efferent arteriole result in structural and functional changes to the peritubular microvasculature (see **Fig. 4**). Reduced renal oxygenation due to the effects of vasoconstriction may manifest before the capillary rarefaction, which is identified as part of renal fibrosis.[97,136] In medullary interstitial cells, Ang II has been shown to activate hypoxia-inducible factor (HIF-1α) via ROS generation, and in vivo medullary interstitial cells from kidneys perfused with Ang II stain positively for both HIF-1α and α-SMA. These findings together link Ang II to both hypoxia and oxidative stress–mediated renal fibrosis mechanisms.[137]

Production of aldosterone by the adrenal gland is stimulated by Ang II but may itself have profibrotic effects contributing to the pathogenesis of CKD.[138] Local renal aldosterone production in the renal cortex has been demonstrated in rodent models stimulated by Ang II, decreased sodium intake, and hyperglycemia with the mineralocorticoid receptor identified not only in the distal tubule but also in preglomerular vasculature, in mesangial cells, and on fibroblasts.[139] In vitro studies have shown that mesangial cells significantly increase production of TGF-β and fibronectin in response to aldosterone, an effect that can be mitigated by the aldosterone antagonist, spironolactone.[140] In vivo aldosterone infusion in rats significantly increases urinary TGF-β concentration, and rats that have undergone uninephrectomy and received aldosterone at the same time as AT1 blockade showed increased expression of TGF-β and collagen, supporting that aldosterone is an independent profibrotic mediator.[139,141,142] Aldosterone has also been shown to increase expression of CTGF and to increase production of ROS and inflammatory mediators, such as osteopontin, IL-6, and IL-1.[143,144] Aldosterone may also promote fibroblast growth and proliferation and increase expression of plasminogen activator inhibitor-1, which promotes ECM accumulation.[138,139] Numerous in vivo models of aldosterone inhibition using either the nonselective agent, spironolactone, or the specific aldosterone receptor inhibitor, eplenerone, demonstrate reduction in glomerulosclerosis and interstitial fibrosis.[139]

In human medicine, clinical evidence of the role of RAAS in progression of CKD comes from studies that have evaluated RAAS blockade. Studies investigating both ACE inhibitors (ACEi) and angiotensin receptor blockers (ARB) show improved outcome when these agents are administered for both diabetic- and nondiabetic-related CKD.[145] However, outcomes from these studies have not provided the degree of protection that might be anticipated, and more recent studies have therefore focused on combined ACEi and ARB therapy.[145,146] Although dual therapy may provide further reduction in terms of proteinuria, outcome measures, such as requirement for dialysis, doubling of serum creatinine, and mortality, were not always improved when compared with monotherapy particularly for nonproteinuric patients.[147] There continues therefore to be controversy in terms of optimal therapy for RAAS blockade and whether this should be monotherapy, combined fixed dose, or individualized ACEi/ARB or combined therapy with either aldosterone antagonists or direct renin inhibitors (eg, Aliskiren).[148,149]

There are relatively little data in the literature evaluating RAAS activation in cats with CKD. In experimental feline models of renal mass reduction, significant increases in plasma renin activity (PRA) and aldosterone have been documented.[150–152] In cats that underwent a renal wrap model of renal reduction, increased plasma renin, plasma aldosterone, systemic hypertension, proteinuria, and more marked histopathologic changes were reported.[151] These findings supported RAAS activation in association with this feline experimental model of renal mass reduction, although this may not be directly translated to naturally occurring disease.

A small number of studies have investigated intrarenal RAAS in cats with naturally occurring CKD by immunohistochemistry.[153–155] The first study by Mitani and colleagues[154] evaluated expression of renin and Ang II in feline kidneys. Renin was identified in the afferent arteries and Ang II in the proximal tubules and mononuclear cells. No association was identified between immunostaining of renin with severity of azotemia or histopathologic lesions, but tubular and interstitial Ang II immunostaining correlated with glomerulosclerosis and tubulointerstitial inflammation. The second study by Mitani and colleagues[155] evaluated ACE and ACE2 (mediates production of Ang1-7/Mas pathway) expression. ACE was identified predominantly in the proximal tubules whereas ACE2 was identified in proximal tubules and weaker staining in the distal nephron. Unlike in dogs, there was no association between immunostaining of ACE or ACE2 with histopathology scores, although sample numbers were small. Further work and larger studies are required to confirm the association between altered expression of these components of RAAS with severity and progression of CKD.

Several studies have evaluated plasma components of RAAS in cats with naturally occurring CKD, some of which were also hypertensive, and results have been variable.[156–158] A study investigating PRA and aldosterone concentration in normotensive azotemic CKD and nonazotemic age-matched controls found no significant difference between these groups.[157] Experimental feline studies have demonstrated that administration of ACEi alters renal hemodynamics and reduces proteinuria with the latter observation also observed in cats with naturally occurring CKD.[150,159–161] However, to date, the survival advantage that might be anticipated from administration of an ACEi has not been demonstrated.[159] Clinical equivalency in terms of antiproteinuric effect has been documented between the ARB, telmisartan, and ACEi, but results of on-going studies to evaluate the effect of this alternative approach on RAAS inhibition and progression of renal disease, renal associated mortality, and survival are required.[162] Overall, given the expanding evidence base from in vitro and in vivo experimental studies and from human medicine, it seems likely that RAAS is an important player in the pathogenesis of feline CKD. However, the optimal way to inhibit RAAS to improve outcome remains to be determined.

SYSTEMIC HYPERTENSION

Systemic hypertension has been accepted for many decades in human medicine as a factor implicated in both the development and the progression of kidney disease.[163–165] Early experimental rodent models demonstrated that with reduced renal function, preglomerular vasodilation occurs, permitting override of myogenic renal autoregulation, transfer of elevated systemic pressures to the glomerular capillaries resulting in glomerular hypertension, and glomerulosclerosis.[166] Histopathologic lesions associated with hypertension in the kidney include artherosclerosis (arterial intimal thickening, medial hypertrophy, and duplication of the internal elastic lamina), glomerulosclerosis, and tubular atrophy, which, together in human medicine have been termed arterionephrosclerosis. Systemic hypertension and glomerular hypertension have also been associated with more marked proteinuria both in experimental rodent studies and in human studies.[166,167]

The evidence for systemic hypertension contributing to the development or progression of feline CKD is unclear. In feline experimental renal mass reduction models, systemic hypertension has been associated with histopathologic changes.[151] However, epidemiologic studies evaluating factors associated with the development of azotemia, the survival of cats with CKD, and having a more progressive phenotype of CKD have not identified blood pressure as a risk factor.[38–40] A conflicting factor in all of these studies, however, is that cats diagnosed with systemic hypertension received antihypertensive therapy, and therefore, it is not possible to say whether an association would have been identified had untreated cats been included. Cats with systemic hypertension are more proteinuric than normotensive cats with equivalent stage of CKD.[38] A study evaluating factors associated with the survival of cats with systemic hypertension evaluated time-averaged blood pressure as a variable, giving information about degree of control of SBP despite all cats receiving antihypertensive therapy. When cats were divided into quartiles based on their time-averaged SBP, those in the upper quartile would still have been considered hypertensive despite antihypertensive therapy. Nevertheless, only proteinuria was significantly associated with survival.[36] This association between proteinuria and survival raises questions regarding the role that systemic hypertension plays in the progression of CKD in cats and whether proteinuria might not be the more important factor.

A histopathologic study performed by McLeland and colleagues[2] demonstrated no difference in severity of vascular lesions (vascular hyperplasia, arteriosclerosis, glomerulosclerosis) between hypertensive and normotensive cats with naturally occurring CKD. However, not all cats in this study had blood pressure data available, and only 12 cats were diagnosed ante-mortem with systemic hypertension. A further study by Chakrabarti and colleagues[1] with blood pressure data on 69 cats of which 34 had a diagnosis of systemic hypertension also evaluated post-mortem renal abnormality. The most common hypertension-associated lesion identified was hyperplastic arteriosclerosis in 3% of normotensive and 29% of hypertensive cats, and in a multivariable model, mean glomerular score and hyperplastic arteriosclerosis were significantly and independently associated with time-averaged blood pressure. As for previous studies, all cats in this study diagnosed with systemic hypertension received antihypertensive therapy with amlodipine besylate. Nevertheless, the median time-averaged blood pressure of those cats diagnosed with systemic hypertension that demonstrated hyperplastic arteriosclerosis was 171 mm Hg versus 152 mm Hg for those without.[1] There was, however, no association between time-averaged blood pressure and tubulointerstitial inflammation or fibrosis, and it is difficult to fully interpret the relative effect of blood pressure on these histopathologic changes versus the effect that administration of amlodipine besylate, and afferent arteriolar vasodilation in the face of inadequate blood pressure control, may have played.

Given the associations that have been made in experimental models of hypertension, it is reasonable to perceive that the kidney should be considered a target organ of systemic hypertension and that appropriate antihypertensive therapy should be administered accordingly. The role that systemic hypertension plays in the progression of CKD remains to be fully determined but will prove challenging to evaluate in clinical patients whereby withholding antihypertensive therapy is not ethically justified. Further studies are also warranted to further investigate the role of proteinuria in hypertensive CKD patients and to determine whether blood pressure alone or in combination with proteinuria would be a better end target.

PROTEINURIA

Proteinuria as a consequence of glomerular hypertension, hyperfiltration, and change in permselectivity of the glomerular filtration barrier is proposed to promote an apoptotic response in tubular cells, alter phenotype of tubular cells, and contribute to the development of tubulointerstitial inflammation and fibrosis.[168] In health, filtered proteins are reabsorbed by megalin and cubulin-mediated endocytosis in the proximal tubules such that the magnitude of proteinuria is low.[169] However, the process of protein presentation and reabsorption by the PTC is not considered benign.[168]

For over a decade, there has been evidence from in vitro studies that proteins, such as albumin (delipidated or lipidated), immunoglobulin G, and transferrin, presented to the apical surface of PTC grown in monolayers, upregulate the gene expression and production of vasoactive (eg, endothelin-1), proinflammatory (MCP-1, RANTES, IL-8), and profibrotic factors (eg, TGF-β). Important intermediate mediators have been identified to include NF$\kappa\beta$ and ROS, and megalin has been implicated as a central element linking protein absorption and the intracellular pathways that upregulate gene expression.[105,168] Basolateral release of these modulators raises the potential that in vivo release would potentiate tubulointerstitial inflammation, fibrosis, ECM deposition, and progression of CKD.

There has been debate regarding exactly which protein molecules are most potent in terms of stimulating the inflammatory response and also whether it is protein alone or in association with their fatty-acid binding capabilities (eg, oleic and linoleic acid) that is most important in stimulating this response. Controversy also exists as to whether the concentrations of proteins used in these in vitro studies correspond to or exceed the protein concentration of ultrafiltrate in vivo, and therefore, whether results are directly applicability particularly to patients with primary tubular disease. Rodent models of proteinuria were used to substantiate the role of proteinuria as a stimulus for an inflammatory and profibrotic response demonstrating upregulation of many of the inflammatory mediators, for example, MCP-1, osteopontin, NF$\kappa\beta$, and that these changes lead to inflammatory cell recruitment to the tubulointerstitial space.[170,171] These changes could be abrogated by administration of antiproteinuric therapy, for example, ACEi.[172,173]

Complement activation is a powerful mechanism that can promote both proinflammatory and profibrotic effects via the classical or alternative pathway in the kidney. There is evidence that both intrarenal and filtered C3, an essential factor of both the classical and the alternative pathways of complement activation, may promote formation and insertion of the C5b-9 membrane attack complex.[174,175] Studies in proteinuric rodent models have shown that C3 colocalizes to the apical surface of PTCs in advance of the recruitment of inflammatory cells and that these changes can be mitigated by administration of ACEi.[176]

However, other perhaps less well-documented effects of proteins on the PTC have been reported. A study by Cao and colleagues[177] indicated that high concentrations of albumin presented to PTC stimulated activation of renal RAAS. Studies support that accumulation of nonesterified fatty acids and long-chain acyl-coA transported into the tubule bound to albumin may accumulate in PTC and be a stimulus for PTC apoptosis.[168] In vitro studies using cell culture of both human and rodent PTC have shown that albumin can directly lead to cellular apoptosis via a caspase-9-mediated mitochondrial pathway and that megalin may be an important receptor for this pathway.[178,179] In vivo, proteinuria has been associated with tubular atrophy and number of apoptotic cells, but such studies have primarily been performed in disease conditions or models of marked proteinuria (eg, Heymann nephritis and focal segmental glomerulosclerosis).[180,181] Further work is therefore required to determine the significance of this mechanism in primary tubular disease conditions. In human medicine, numerous studies of both diabetic and nondiabetic CKD have demonstrated that proteinuria is associated with faster GFR decline and progression to end-stage renal disease with evidence that antiproteinuric therapy with an ACEi or ARB can slow this decline, although as described above, dual therapy does not always enhance outcome.[145,147]

For cats, where the primary histopathologic lesion is tubulointerstitial nephritis, the magnitude of proteinuria is typically low with reported median urine protein to creatinine ratios in IRIS stage 2, 3, and 4 CKD being 0.15, 0.22, and 0.65, respectively.[38] In feline CKD, proteinuria has been significantly associated with the development of azotemia, having a progressive phenotype of CKD, and survival of cats with both CKD and hypertension.[36,38–40] In histopathologic studies of feline kidney tissue at post mortem, proteinuria has been significantly associated with the severity of tubular degeneration, inflammation, fibrosis, tubular epithelial cell necrosis, and decreased amount of normal renal parenchyma.[1,2] However, although both ACEi and ARB significantly reduce the magnitude of proteinuria in cats, the benefit in terms of slowing progression of CKD or improving survival has yet to be demonstrated.[159,162] On the basis of data from experimental studies, proteinuria is a key player in the pathogenesis of interstitial inflammation and fibrosis. However, further work is still required to demonstrate in feline medicine the causative association between proteinuria and progression of disease.

HYPERPHOSPHATEMIA

Hyperphosphatemia as a consequence of decreased renal excretion has been associated with progression of renal disease in human studies.[182] Early studies showed that diets with excessive phosphorus supplementation predisposed to histopathologic lesions within the kidney, including necrosis of the convoluted tubules, calcification, and an increase in ECM.[183,184] Conversely, experimental models of renal disease, including the dog, have shown that phosphate restriction is beneficial in reducing renal injury.[185,186] The proposed pathogenesis for phosphate being detrimental to the kidney is incompletely understood, and many key mechanisms have been proposed. The most frequently cited is that hyperphosphatemia predisposes to renal mineralization, which subsequently promotes inflammation and fibrosis. Alternative proposed mechanisms include an association between hyperphosphatemia and vascular calcification, leading to vascular stiffness with subsequent effects on endothelial cell function.[187-190] These alterations in renal microvascular may be contributory to areas of ischemia and hypoxia, which are known stimuli for renal fibrosis (see later discussion).[190] Phosphate may also affect several other key pathways that have been associated with renal disease progression, including cellular apoptosis, cellular senescence, and oxidative stress.[18,191,192] Extracellular phosphate concentrations have also been associated with increased production of profibrotic mediators and may have a direct stimulatory effect on RAAS.[193-195]

There is some evidence supporting the role of phosphorus in the pathogenesis of feline CKD. Early studies evaluating phosphate-restricted diets showed that cats on restricted diets had reduced evidence of renal histopathologic lesions (calcification, fibrosis, and inflammatory cell infiltration) compared with cats on a high-phosphorus diet.[123] Clinical epidemiologic studies have identified phosphorus to be a risk factor for the survival of cats with CKD and also to be associated with a more progressive phenotype of disease.[24,40] To date, one feline study has evaluated post-mortem renal histopathologic findings with pre-mortem phosphate concentrations and identified a significant association with interstitial fibrosis but not with renal mineralization.[1] More recently, epidemiologic studies have focused on the role of other molecules involved in phosphorus homeostasis with both PTH and FGF23 being associated with the development and survival of cats with CKD.[116-118] Perhaps the most convincing evidence that there is likely to be a role for phosphorus homeostasis in the progression of CKD comes from the studies that have demonstrated improved survival in those cats that are fed a phosphate-restricted diet with evidence of modulation of these important regulatory hormones.[115,196,197]

HYPOXIA

Hypoxia has been promoted as another mechanism contributing to the development and progression of CKD. Many different potential mechanisms may contribute to hypoxia.[198] The total blood supply to the kidney is high, representing approximately 20% of cardiac output. However, the presence of the counter-current multiplier system within the kidney and oxygen diffusion shunt means that the renal medulla operates at low oxygen tensions. The high metabolic demand of PTCs means that they may be particularly susceptible to reduced availability of oxygen, a mechanism that is used for beneficial effect as a driving factor for the production of erythropoieitin.

In the kidney, afferent arterioles divide to give rise to glomerular capillaries, which fuse to become the efferent arteriole. Efferent arterioles enter the peritubular complex of capillaries and provide oxygen and nutrients to the tubular cells. Early in the course of CKD, alteration in glomerular structure and the development of glomerulosclerosis may alter the delivery of blood from the glomerulus to peritubular capillaries, limiting the blood supply to renal tissue. Hemoadaptive alterations, driven at least in part by activation of the RAAS (see earlier discussion) and Ang II, result in relative vasoconstriction of the efferent arterioles.[136] The benefit of this may be an increase in glomerular capillary pressure and filtration, but this hemodynamic alteration has secondary consequences on the supply of blood and hence oxygen from the efferent arteriole to the peritubular capillary network and may result in hypoxia.[136]

Delivery of oxygen to tubular cells depends on diffusion. In health, when there is little distance between the peritubular capillaries and tubular epithelial cells, oxygen is delivered efficiently. However, once there is evidence of tubulointerstitial inflammation and fibrosis, the distance for oxygen molecules to traverse increases, contributing to hypoxia. Furthermore, loss of interstitial microvascular and capillary rarefaction may reduce blood supply to regions of the kidney.[100,198]

As part of the normal physiologic response to hypoxia, cells undergo adaptations in gene expression in order to try to counteract the effect of low oxygen. This response typically involves stimulation of HIF-1 and HIF-2.[199] In the kidney, the primary form of HIF expressed in the tubules and interstitial cells is HIF-1α, whereas HIF-2α is identified in mesangial cells, endothelial cells, and fibroblasts. The HIF-α subunits are degraded by an oxygen-dependent mechanism; this means that in periods of hypoxia HIF-α subunits accumulate and form heterodimers with HIF-β subunits. These heterodimers are able to bind to hypoxia response elements associated with key genes that counteract the effects of hypoxia, for example, EPO, VEGF, which stimulates angiogenesis, heme oxygenase, which is involved in heme metabolism, nitric oxide synthase, and cyclo-oxygenase-2, which both have vasodilator properties.[199–201]

Hypoxia itself has also been shown to be a fibrogenic stimulus to tubular epithelial cells, fibrocytes, and endothelial cells.[202] Hypoxia has been shown to stimulate tubular epithelial cells to undergo EMT and activate fibroblasts to increase production of ECM.[203,204] Some tubular epithelial cells that are exposed to hypoxia develop mitochondrial derangements that result ultimately in cellular apoptosis. A secondary consequence of loss of normal renal parenchyma is a decrease in the availability of fibroblasts for the production of EPO, which later in the disease course of CKD may result in anemia. Anemia in CKD may therefore also contribute to reduced oxygen delivery and hypoxia. Overall, therefore, the hemodynamic and structural lesions that occur in CKD contribute and promote hypoxia, which is in itself a driving factor contributing to renal fibrosis and generating a vicious cycle for disease progression (**Fig. 5**).[198]

In cats, there is relatively little information directly relating to hypoxia and its association with the development and progression of CKD. Epidemiologic studies have identified packed cell volume and anemia as being risk factors for the survival of cats with CKD, and anemia is clinically appreciated to contribute to reduction in quality of life.[24,205] In a more recent study, low packed cell volume was an independent predictor of progression of CKD in cats with IRIS stage 2 CKD.[40] Together, these studies give preliminary evidence that anemia, which could certainly contribute to renal hypoxia, is a negative prognostic indicator in terms of progression of disease and survival.

More recently, studies have evaluated urinary VEGF:creatinine concentrations as a method of assessing response to hypoxia within the kidney. Results from these studies so far have been conflicting. A study by Habenicht and colleagues[108] demonstrated significantly lower urinary VEGF:creatinine ratio in cats with CKD compared with healthy controls which could be hypothesized to suggest inadequate response of the kidney to the hypoxic environment. Further work is necessary to clarify the extent to which plasma VEGF concentrations might contribute to urinary VEGF concentrations and to establish further robust markers that may be informative in terms of the role of hypoxia in the progression of CKD in cats.

OXIDATIVE STRESS

Renal oxidative stress occurs when there is an imbalance between the production of ROS (eg, superoxide, hydroxyl radical, and hydrogen peroxide) and availability of

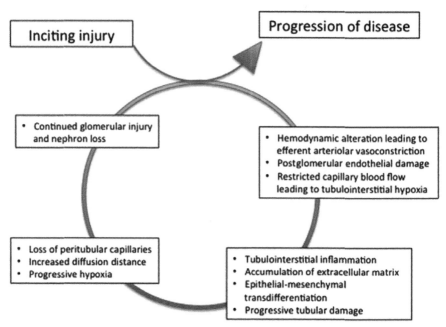

Fig. 5. The role of hypoxia in progression of CKD.

antioxidant defense mechanisms (eg, superoxide dismutase, catalase, glutathione peroxidase, and glutathione). ROS are highly reactive molecules, which can cause damage to DNA, lipid, protein, and carbohydrate, resulting ultimately in structural and functional cellular damage that leads to apoptosis and necrosis, stimulating inflammation and fibrosis. This imbalance is a situation that is referred to as oxidative stress.[206]

Renal cells, particularly tubular cells, have a high metabolic activity and therefore have a high production rate of ROS. The major site of production of ROS is the mitochondria, although endoplasmic reticulum, peroxisome, and lysosomes may also contribute.[207] Oxidative stress occurs in CKD when hyperfiltration and hyperfunctioning of remaining nephrons lead to increased production of ROS, which influence downstream cellular signaling pathways in the kidney to promote renal cell apoptosis, cellular senescence, a decrease in the regenerative capacity of the cells, and fibrosis.[90,208] In particular, ROS have been shown to stimulate NFκβ, which is integral in cellular pathways that promote fibrosis. These factors have deleterious effects in terms of both renal disease progression and reducing renal function. Other factors, such as aging, proteinuria, RAAS activation and Ang II, hyperphosphatemia, inflammation, regions of ischemia and hypoxia, and uremic toxins, can also contribute to the generation of ROS.[206,209]

Assessment of oxidative stress in clinical patients is challenging, and evaluation of biomarkers for oxidative stress is often used in place of direct assessment. These biomarkers may be informative in terms of lipid peroxidation (eg, isoprostanes, malondialdehyde, thiobarbituric acid reactive substances), protein oxidation (eg, protein carbonyls, advanced glycation end products, oxidized low-density lipoproteins), direct measurement of ROS (eg, hydrogen peroxide, DNA or RNA damage) or may be through evaluation of antioxidant mechanisms (eg, catalase, glutathione, reduced-oxidized glutathione [GSH:GSSD], glutathione peroxidase, superoxide dismutase).[206]

In human medicine, studies have shown an increase in oxidative stress markers with advancing stage of CKD.[210,211] However, the response to provision of antioxidants (eg, α-tochopherol, ω-3 fatty acids, n-acetyl cysteine, allopurinol, co-enzyme Q_{10}) has been variable, and a recent *Cochrane Review* found no evidence that antioxidant therapy could reduce death or cardiovascular disease in human patients with CKD.[211] The study did suggest that antioxidant therapy may lead to reduced serum creatinine and may therefore reduce the risk of progression to end-stage renal disease, and there was no evidence that supplementing with antioxidants was harmful. However, the review was based on few studies and overall a low event rate. The conclusion of this *Cochrane Review* was therefore insufficient evidence to support routine use of antioxidant therapy at this time, although there was sufficient evidence to support that further studies should be performed to explore the potentially beneficial effects of antioxidant therapy.[211]

There have been few studies to date that have explored oxidative stress in relation to feline CKD.[212] Two studies have attempted to evaluate oxidative stress in cats with CKD using different methods. A study by Keegan and colleagues[213] evaluated superoxide dismutase, antioxidant capacity, GSH:GSSG ratio, neutrophil phagocytosis, and oxidative burst in cats with CKD and age-matched control cats. Results from this study indicated that cats with CKD had significantly higher GSH:GSSG ratios and significantly reduced antioxidant capacity. There was no significant difference in superoxide dismutase activity between groups, whereas neutrophil burst was significantly higher in the CKD cats.[213] Together, these results were interpreted as evidence that antioxidant mechanisms are activated in cats with CKD. Krofič Žel and colleagues[214] measured selenium concentrations, plasma and erythrocyte glutathione peroxidase activity, and total plasma antioxidant capacity. Selenium concentrations were investigated because selenium is an integral component of glutathione peroxidase. This study identified that IRIS stage 4 cats had significantly higher plasma glutathione peroxidase activity but that there was no significant difference in the other markers either among IRIS stage or between CKD and control cats.[214] These results suggest that at stage 4 CKD cats may still be able to induce antioxidant mechanism and that selenium deficiency does not seem to be a factor in cats with IRIS stage 1 to 4 CKD and a non-age-matched control group.[214]

To date, only one study has evaluated antioxidant supplementation in cats. This study evaluated dietary supplementation with vitamin C and E in a group of 10 elderly cats with CKD compared with healthy non-age-matched controls.[215] They used 8-hydroxy-2'-deoxyguanosine, a product of DNA oxidation and a comet assay, which is a gel electrophoresis–based method for measuring DNA breaks in eukaryotic cells. Supplementation significantly decreased DNA damage markers in this study, providing preliminary support for antioxidants in cats with CKD.[215]

Overall the results of these studies only begin to touch the surface in terms of the role of oxidative stress in cats with CKD and whether any form of antioxidant supplementation would be of benefit. Further work is required in this area before routine antioxidant supplementation in cats can be advocated.

SUMMARY

Given the similarities in mammalian physiology, it seems likely that many of the pathophysiologic mechanisms implicated in the development and progression of kidney disease from experimental and human studies are likely to be common and important in the cat. However, further studies are required that will help demonstrate the links between environmental and individual factors that predispose cats to CKD, perhaps optimizing the way that health care is provided for cats in the earlier stages of their life. An improved understanding of the factors associated with progression of disease and the key mediators of these changes may allow the adaption of treatment strategies for cats diagnosed with CKD. Particularly in relation to proteinuria, RAAS activation, and hypoxia, further clinical evidence that modulating these parameters improves outcome is required.

REFERENCES

1. Chakrabarti S, Syme HM, Brown CA, et al. Histomorphometry of feline chronic kidney disease and correlation with markers of renal dysfunction. Vet Pathol 2012;50(1):147–55.
2. McLeland SM, Cianciolo RE, Duncan CG, et al. A comparison of biochemical and histopathologic staging in cats with chronic kidney disease. Vet Pathol 2014;52(3):524–34.
3. Dibartola SP, Rutgers HC, Zack PM, et al. Clinicopathologic findings associated with chronic renal disease in cats: 74 cases (1973-1984). J Am Vet Med Assoc 1987;190:1196–202.
4. Minkus G, Reusch C, Hörauf A, et al. Evaluation of renal biopsies in cats and dogs—histopathology in comparison with clinical data. J Small Anim Pract 1994;35:465–72.
5. Lulich JP, Osborne CA, O'Brien TD, et al. Feline renal failure: questions, answers, questions. Compend Cont Ed Pract Vet 1992;14:127–52.
6. Marino CL, Lascelles BDX, Vaden SL, et al. Prevalence and classification of chronic kidney disease in cats randomly selected from four age groups and in cats recruited for degenerative joint disease studies. J Feline Med Surg 2014;16:465–72.
7. Lindeman RD, Tobin J, Shock NW. Longitudinal studies on the rate of decline in renal function with age. J Am Geriatr Soc 1985;33:278–85.
8. Garg AX, Papaioannou A, Ferko N, et al. Estimating the prevalence of renal insufficiency in seniors requiring long-term care. Kidney Int 2004;65:649–53.
9. Glassock RJ, Winearls C. Ageing and the glomerular filtration rate: truths and consequences. Trans Am Clin Climatol Assoc 2009;120:419–28.
10. Perico N, Remuzzi G, Benigni A. Aging and the kidney. Curr Opin Nephrol Hypertens 2011;20:312–7.
11. Yang H, Fogo AB. Cell senescence in the aging kidney. J Am Soc Nephrol 2010; 21:1436–9.
12. Denic A, Glassock RJ, Rule AD. Structural and functional changes with the aging kidney. Adv Chronic Kidney Dis 2016;23:19–28.
13. Stenvinkel P, Larsson TE. Chronic kidney disease: a clinical model of premature aging. Am J Kidney Dis 2013;62:339–51.
14. Lawler DF, Evans RH, Chase K, et al. The aging feline kidney: a model mortality antagonist? J Feline Med Surg 2006;8:363–71.
15. Hao C-M, Haase VH. Sirtuins and their relevance to the kidney. J Am Soc Nephrol 2010;21:1620–7.
16. Kuro-o M, Matsumura Y, Aizawa H, et al. Mutation of the mouse klotho gene leads to a syndrome resembling ageing. Nature 1997;390:45–51.
17. John GB, Cheng C-Y, Kuro-o M. Role of klotho in aging, phosphate metabolism, and CKD. Am J Kidney Dis 2011;58:127–34.
18. Kuro-o M. A potential link between phosphate and aging–lessons from Klotho-deficient mice. Mech Ageing Dev 2010;131:270–5.

19. Melk A, Kittikowit W, Sandhu I, et al. Cell senescence in rat kidneys in vivo increases with growth and age despite lack of telomere shortening. Kidney Int 2003;63:2134–43.
20. Melk A, Ramassar V, Helms LMH, et al. Telomere shortening in kidneys with age. J Am Soc Nephrol 2000;11:444–53.
21. Melk A, Schmidt BMW, Takeuchi O, et al. Expression of p16INK4a and other cell cycle regulator and senescence associated genes in aging human kidney. Kidney Int 2004;65:510–20.
22. Quimby JM, Maranon DG, Battaglia CL, et al. Feline chronic kidney disease is associated with shortened telomeres and increased cellular senescence. Am J Physiol Renal Physiol 2013;305:F295–303.
23. Greene JP, Lefebvre SL, Wang M, et al. Risk factors associated with the development of chronic kidney disease in cats evaluated at primary care veterinary hospitals. J Am Vet Med Assoc 2014;244:320–7.
24. Boyd LM, Langston C, Thompson K, et al. Survival in cats with naturally occurring chronic kidney disease (2000–2002). J Vet Intern Med 2008;22:1111–7.
25. Paepe D, Saunders JH, Bavegems V, et al. Screening of ragdoll cats for kidney disease: a retrospective evaluation. J Small Anim Pract 2012;53:572–7.
26. Dibartola SP, Buffington CA, Chew DJ, et al. Developement of chronic renal failure in cats fed a commercial diet. J Am Vet Med Assoc 1993;202:744–51.
27. Reynolds BS, Chetboul V, Nguyen P, et al. Effects of dietary salt intake on renal function: a 2-year study in healthy aged cats. J Vet Intern Med 2013;27:507–15.
28. Hughes KL, Slater MR, Geller S, et al. Diet and lifestyle variables as risk factors for chronic renal failure in pet cats. Prev Vet Med 2002;55:1–15.
29. Lappin MR, Jensen WA, Jensen TD, et al. Investigation of the induction of antibodies against Crandell-Rees feline kidney cell lysates and feline renal cell lysates after parenteral administration of vaccines against feline viral rhinotracheitis, calicivirus, and panleukopenia in cats. Am J Vet Res 2005;66:506–11.
30. Lappin MR, Basaraba RJ, Jensen WA. Interstitial nephritis in cats inoculated with Crandell Rees feline kidney cell lysates. J Feline Med Surg 2006;8:353–6.
31. Whittemore JC, Hawley JR, Jensen WA, et al. Antibodies against Crandell Rees feline kidney (CRFK) cell line antigens, α-enolase, and annexin A2 in vaccinated and CRFK hyperinoculated cats. J Vet Intern Med 2010;24:306–13.
32. Ronco C, Haapio M, House AA, et al. Cardiorenal syndrome. J Am Coll Cardiol 2008;52:1527–39.
33. Pouchelon JL, Atkins CE, Bussadori C, et al. Cardiovascular–renal axis disorders in the domestic dog and cat: a veterinary consensus statement. J Small Anim Pract 2015;56:537–52.
34. Schmiedt CW, Brainard BM, Hinson W, et al. Unilateral renal ischemia as a model of acute kidney injury and renal fibrosis in cats. Vet Pathol 2016;53:87–101.
35. Syme HM, Barber PJ, Markwell PJ, et al. Prevalence of systolic hypertension in cats with chronic renal failure at initial evaluation. J Am Vet Med Assoc 2002;220:1799–804.
36. Jepson RE, Elliott J, Brodbelt D, et al. Effect of control of systolic blood pressure on survival in cats with systemic hypertension. J Vet Intern Med 2007;21:402–9.
37. Bijsmans ES, Jepson RE, Chang YM, et al. Changes in systolic blood pressure over time in healthy cats and cats with chronic kidney disease. J Vet Intern Med 2015;29(3):855–61.

38. Syme HM, Markwell PJ, Pfeiffer D, et al. Survival of cats with naturally occurring chronic renal failure is related to severity of proteinuria. J Vet Intern Med 2006; 20:528–35.

39. Jepson RE, Brodbelt D, Vallance C, et al. Evaluation of predictors of the development of azotemia in cats. J Vet Intern Med 2009;23:806–13.

40. Chakrabarti S, Syme HM, Elliott J. Clinicopathological variables predicting progression of azotemia in cats with chronic kidney disease. J Vet Intern Med 2012; 26:275–81.

41. Zini E, Benali S, Coppola L, et al. Renal morphology in cats with diabetes mellitus. Vet Pathol 2014;51:1143–50.

42. Syme HM. Cardiovascular and renal manifestations of hyperthyroidism. Vet Clin North Am Small Anim Pract 2007;37:723–43, vi.

43. DiBartola SP, Broome MR, Stein BS, et al. Effect of treatment of hyperthyroidism on renal function in cats. J Am Vet Med Assoc 1996;208:875–8.

44. Graves TK, Olivier NB, Nachreiner RF, et al. Changes in renal function associated with treatment of hyperthyroidism in cats. Am J Vet Res 1994;55:1745–9.

45. van Hoek I, Lefebvre HP, Peremans K, et al. Short- and long-term follow-up of glomerular and tubular renal markers of kidney function in hyperthyroid cats after treatment with radioiodine. Domest Anim Endocrinol 2009;36:45–56.

46. Williams TL, Elliott J, Syme HM. Association of iatrogenic hypothyroidism with azotemia and reduced survival time in cats treated for hyperthyroidism. J Vet Intern Med 2010;24:1086–92.

47. Williams TL, Elliott J, Syme HM. Calcium and phosphate homeostasis in hyperthyroid cats–associations with development of azotaemia and survival time. J Small Anim Pract 2012;53:561–71.

48. Palm CA, Westropp JL. Cats and calcium oxalate: strategies for managing lower and upper tract stone disease. J Feline Med Surg 2011;13:651–60.

49. Adams LG. Nephroliths and ureteroliths: a new stone age. N Z Vet J 2013;61: 212–6.

50. Kyles AE, Hardie EM, Wooden BG, et al. Clinical, clinicopathologic, radiographic, and ultrasonographic abnormalities in cats with ureteral calculi: 163 cases (1984-2002). J Am Vet Med Assoc 2005;226:932–6.

51. Ross SJ, Osborne CA, Lekcharoensuk C, et al. A case control study of the effects of nephrolithiasis in cats with chronic kidney disease. J Am Vet Med Assoc 2007;230:1854–9.

52. White JD, Stevenson M, Malik R, et al. Urinary tract infections in cats with chronic kidney disease. J Feline Med Surg 2012;15(6):459–65.

53. Mayer-Roenne B, Goldstein RE, Erb HN. Urinary tract infections in cats with hyperthyroidism, diabetes mellitus and chronic kidney disease. J Feline Med Surg 2007;9:124–32.

54. Bailiff NL, Westropp JL, Nelson RW, et al. Evaluation of urine specific gravity and urine sediment as risk factors for urinary tract infections in cats. Vet Clin Pathol 2008;37:317–22.

55. Weese JS, Blondeau JM, Boothe D, et al. Antimicrobial use guidelines for treatment of urinary tract disease in dogs and cats: Antimicrobial Guidelines Working Group of the International Society for Companion Animal Infectious Diseases. Vet Med Int 2011;2011:9.

56. Medapalli RK, He JC, Klotman PE. HIV-associated nephropathy: pathogenesis. Curr Opin Nephrol Hypertens 2011;20:306–11.

57. Poli A, Tozon N, Guidi G, et al. Renal alterations in feline immunodeficiency virus (FIV)-infected cats: a natural model of lentivirus-induced renal disease changes. Viruses 2012;4:1372–89.
58. Baxter KJ, Levy JK, Edinboro CH, et al. Renal disease in cats infected with feline immunodeficiency virus. J Vet Intern Med 2012;26:238–43.
59. White JD, Malik R, Norris JM, et al. Association between naturally occurring chronic kidney disease and feline immunodeficiency virus infection status in cats. J Am Vet Med Assoc 2010;236:424–9.
60. Sieg M, Heenemann K, Rückner A, et al. Discovery of new feline paramyxoviruses in domestic cats with chronic kidney disease. Virus Genes 2015;51:294–7.
61. Sakaguchi S, Koide R, Miyazawa T. In vitro host range of feline morbillivirus. J Vet Med Sci 2015;77:1485–7.
62. Sakaguchi S, Nakagawa S, Yoshikawa R, et al. Genetic diversity of feline morbilliviruses isolated in Japan. J Gen Virol 2014;95:1464–8.
63. Woo PCY, Lau SKP, Wong BHL, et al. Feline morbillivirus, a previously undescribed paramyxovirus associated with tubulointerstitial nephritis in domestic cats. Proc Natl Acad Sci U S A 2012;109:5435–40.
64. Koide R, Sakaguchi S, Miyazawa T. Basic biological characterization of feline morbillivirus. J Vet Med Sci 2015;77:565–9.
65. Furuya T, Sassa Y, Omatsu T, et al. Existence of feline morbillivirus infection in Japanese cat populations. Arch Virol 2013;159:371–3.
66. Furuya T, Wachi A, Sassa Y, et al. Quantitative PCR detection of feline morbillivirus in cat urine samples. J Vet Med Sci 2015;77:1701–3.
67. Lapointe C, Plamondon I, Dunn M. Feline leptospirosis serosurvey from a Quebec referral hospital. Can Vet J 2013;54:497–9.
68. Schuller S, Francey T, Hartmann K, et al. European consensus statement on leptospirosis in dogs and cats. J Small Anim Pract 2015;56:159–79.
69. Rodriguez J, Blais MC, Lapointe C, et al. Serologic and urinary PCR survey of leptospirosis in healthy cats and in cats with kidney disease. J Vet Intern Med 2014;28:284–93.
70. Markovich JE, Ross L, McCobb E. The prevalence of leptospiral antibodies in free roaming cats in Worcester County, Massachusetts. J Vet Intern Med 2012;26:688–9.
71. Arbour J, Blais M-C, Carioto L, et al. Clinical leptospirosis in three cats (2001–2009). J Am Anim Hosp Assoc 2012;48:256–60.
72. Shropshire SB, Veir JK, Morris AK, et al. Evaluation of the Leptospira species microscopic agglutination test in experimentally vaccinated cats and Leptospira species seropositivity in aged azotemic client-owned cats. J Feline Med Surg 2015. [Epub ahead of print].
73. Sykes JE, Westropp JL, Kasten RW, et al. Association between Bartonella species infection and disease in pet cats as determined using serology and culture. J Feline Med Surg 2010;12:631–6.
74. Prunotto M, Ghiggeri G, Bruschi M, et al. Renal fibrosis and proteomics: current knowledge and still key open questions for proteomic investigation. J Proteomics 2011;74:1855–70.
75. Mack M, Yanagita M. Origin of myofibroblasts and cellular events triggering fibrosis. Kidney Int 2015;87:297–307.
76. Sun DF, Fujigaki Y, Fujimoto T, et al. Possible involvement of myofibroblasts in cellular recovery of uranyl acetate-induced acute renal failure in rats. Am J Pathol 2000;157:1321–35.

77. Fujigaki Y, Muranaka Y, Sun D, et al. Transient myofibroblast differentiation of interstitial fibroblastic cells relevant to tubular dilatation in uranyl acetate-induced acute renal failure in rats. Virchows Arch 2004;446:164–76.

78. Kramann R, Dirocco DP, Maarouf OH, et al. Matrix producing cells in chronic kidney disease: origin, regulation, and activation. Curr Pathobiol Rep 2013;1: 301–11.

79. Eddy AA. Overview of the cellular and molecular basis of kidney fibrosis. Kidney Int Suppl (2011) 2014;4:2–8.

80. Eddy AA. The origin of scar-forming kidney myofibroblasts. Nat Med 2013;19: 964–6.

81. LeBleu VS, Taduri G, O'Connell J, et al. Origin and function of myofibroblasts in kidney fibrosis. Nat Med 2013;19:1047–53.

82. Kramann R, Humphreys BD. Kidney pericytes: roles in regeneration and fibrosis. Semin Nephrol 2014;34:374–83.

83. Pallone TL, Silldorff EP. Pericyte regulation of renal medullary blood flow. Nephron Exp Nephrol 2001;9:165–70.

84. Ohashi R, Shimizu A, Masuda Y, et al. Peritubular capillary regression during the progression of experimental obstructive nephropathy. J Am Soc Nephrol 2002; 13:1795–805.

85. Humphreys BD, Lin S-L, Kobayashi A, et al. Fate tracing reveals the pericyte and not epithelial origin of myofibroblasts in kidney fibrosis. Am J Pathol 2010;176:85–97.

86. Strutz F, Okada H, Lo CW, et al. Identification and characterization of a fibroblast marker: FSP1. J Cell Biol 1995;130:393–405.

87. Iwano M, Plieth D, Danoff TM, et al. Evidence that fibroblasts derive from epithelium during tissue fibrosis. J Clin Invest 2002;110:341–50.

88. Piera-Velazquez S, Li Z, Jimenez SA. Role of Endothelial-Mesenchymal Transition (EndoMT) in the pathogenesis of fibrotic disorders. Am J Pathol 2011; 179:1074–80.

89. Zeisberg EM, Potenta SE, Sugimoto H, et al. Fibroblasts in kidney fibrosis emerge via endothelial-to-mesenchymal transition. J Am Soc Nephrol 2008; 19:2282–7.

90. Shin D-M, Jeon J-H, Kim C-W, et al. TGFβ mediates activation of transglutaminase 2 in response to oxidative stress that leads to protein aggregation. FASEB J 2008;22:2498–507.

91. Rohatgi R, Flores D. Intra-tubular hydrodynamic forces influence tubulo-interstitial fibrosis in the kidney. Curr Opin Nephrol Hypertens 2010;19:65–71.

92. Farris AB, Colvin RB. Renal interstitial fibrosis: mechanisms and evaluation. Curr Opin Nephrol Hypertens 2012;21:289–300.

93. Wolf G. Renal injury due to renin–angiotensin–aldosterone system activation of the transforming growth factor-β pathway. Kidney Int 2006;70:1914–9.

94. Liu Y. Renal fibrosis: new insights into the pathogenesis and therapeutics. Kidney Int 2006;69:213–7.

95. Pilling D, Gomer RH. Differentiation of circulating monocytes into fibroblast-like cells. Methods Mol Biol 2012;904:191–206.

96. Reich B, Schmidbauer K, Rodriguez Gomez M, et al. Fibrocytes develop outside the kidney but contribute to renal fibrosis in a mouse model. Kidney Int 2013;84: 78–89.

97. Mimura I, Nangaku M. The suffocating kidney: tubulointerstitial hypoxia in end-stage renal disease. Nat Rev Nephrol 2010;6:667–78.

98. Serón D, Alexopoulos E, Raftery MJ, et al. Number of interstitial capillary cross-sections assessed by monoclonal antibodies: relation to interstitial damage. Nephrol Dial Transplant 1990;5:889–93.
99. Choi Y-J, Chakraborty S, Nguyen V, et al. Peritubular capillary loss is associated with chronic tubulointerstitial injury in human kidney: altered expression of vascular endothelial growth factor. Hum Pathol 2000;31:1491–7.
100. Kawakami T, Mimura I, Shoji K, et al. Hypoxia and fibrosis in chronic kidney disease: crossing at pericytes. Kidney Int Suppl (2011) 2014;4:107–12.
101. Tanaka S, Tanaka T, Nangaku M. Hypoxia as a key player in the AKI-to-CKD transition. Am J Physiol Renal Physiol 2014;307:F1187–95.
102. Yamaguchi I, Tchao BN, Burger ML, et al. Vascular endothelial cadherin modulates renal interstitial fibrosis. Nephron Exp Nephrol 2012;120:e20–31.
103. Zeisberg M, Neilson EG. Mechanisms of tubulointerstitial fibrosis. J Am Soc Nephrol 2010;21:1819–34.
104. Yang L, Besschetnova TY, Brooks CR, et al. Epithelial cell cycle arrest in G2/M mediates kidney fibrosis after injury. Nat Med 2010;16:535–43, 1p following 143.
105. Abbate M, Zoja C, Remuzzi G. How does proteinuria cause progressive renal damage? J Am Soc Nephrol 2006;17:2974–84.
106. Sawashima K, Mizuno S, Mizuno-Horikawa Y, et al. Expression of alpha-smooth muscle actin and fibronectin in tubulointerstitial lesions of cats with chronic renal failure. Am J Vet Res 2000;61:1080–6.
107. Yabuki A, Mitani S, Fujiki M, et al. Comparative study of chronic kidney disease in dogs and cats: induction of myofibroblasts. Res Vet Sci 2010;88:294–9.
108. Habenicht LM, Webb TL, Clauss LA, et al. Urinary cytokine levels in apparently healthy cats and cats with chronic kidney disease. J Feline Med Surg 2012;15(2):99–104.
109. Arata S, Ohmi A, Mizukoshi F, et al. Urinary transforming growth factor-beta1 in feline chronic renal failure. J Vet Med Sci 2005;67:1253–5.
110. Lawson J, Wheeler-Jones C, Syme H, et al. Urinary active TGF-beta 1 in feline chronic kidney disease #NU4. J Vet Intern Med 2015;29:1122–256.
111. Bobkova IN, Chebotareva NV, Kozlovskaia LV, et al. Urine excretion of a monocytic chemotaxic protein-1 and a transforming growth factor beta1 as an indicator of chronic glomerulonephritis progression. Ter Arkh 2006;78:9–14 [in Russian].
112. Johnson TS, Skill NJ, El Nahas AM, et al. Transglutaminase transcription and antigen translocation in experimental renal scarring. J Am Soc Nephrol 1999;10:2146–57.
113. Johnson TS, El-Koraie AF, Skill NJ, et al. Tissue transglutaminase and the progression of human renal scarring. J Am Soc Nephrol 2003;14:2052–62.
114. Sánchez-Lara AC, Elliott J, Syme HM, et al. Feline chronic kidney disease is associated with upregulation of transglutaminase 2: a collagen cross-linking enzyme. Vet Pathol 2015;52(3):513–23.
115. Elliott J, Rawlings JM, Markwell PJ, et al. Survival of cats with naturally occurring chronic renal failure: effect of dietary management. J Small Anim Pract 2000;41:235–42.
116. Finch NC, Geddes RF, Syme HM, et al. Fibroblast growth factor 23 (FGF-23) concentrations in cats with early nonazotemic chronic kidney disease (CKD) and in healthy geriatric cats. J Vet Intern Med 2013;27:227–33.
117. Finch NC, Syme HM, Elliott J. Parathyroid hormone concentration in geriatric cats with various degrees of renal function. J Am Vet Med Assoc 2012;241:1326–35.

118. Geddes RF, Elliott J, Syme HM. Relationship between plasma fibroblast growth factor-23 concentration and survival time in cats with chronic kidney disease. J Vet Intern Med 2015;29(6):1494–501.
119. Brenner BM. Nephron adaptation to renal injury or ablation. Am J Physiol 1985; 249:F324–37.
120. Hostetter TH, Olson JL, Rennke HG, et al. Hyperfiltration in remnant nephrons: a potentially adverse response to renal ablation. Am J Physiol 1981;241:F85–92.
121. Brown SA, Brown CA. Single-nephron adaptations to partial renal ablation in cats. Am J Physiol 1995;269:R1002–8.
122. Brown SA, Crowell WA, Brown CA, et al. Pathophysiology and management of progressive renal disease. Vet J 1997;154:93–109.
123. Ross LA, Finco DR, Crowell WA. Effects of dietary phosphorus restriction on the kidneys of cats with reduced renal mass. Am J Vet Res 1982;43:1023–6.
124. Adams LG, Polzin DJ, Osborne CA, et al. Influence of dietary protein/calorie intake on renal morphology and function in cats with 5/6 nephrectomy. Lab Invest 1994;70:347–57.
125. Siragy HM, Carey RM. Role of the intrarenal renin-angiotensin-aldosterone system in chronic kidney disease. Am J Nephrol 2010;31:541–50.
126. Navar LG, Prieto MC, Satou R, et al. Intrarenal angiotensin II and its contribution to the genesis of chronic hypertension. Curr Opin Pharmacol 2011;11:180–6.
127. Kobori H, Nangaku M, Navar LG, et al. The intrarenal renin-angiotensin system: from physiology to the pathobiology of hypertension and kidney disease. Pharmacol Rev 2007;59:251–87.
128. Ferrão FM, Lara LS, Lowe J. Renin-angiotensin system in the kidney: what is new? World J Nephrol 2014;3:64–76.
129. Lv L-L, Liu B-C. Role of non-classical renin-angiotensin system axis in renal fibrosis. Front Physiol 2015;6:117.
130. Benigni A, Gagliardini E, Remuzzi A. Changes in glomerular perm-selectivity induced by angiotensin II imply podocyte dysfunction and slit diaphragm protein rearrangement. Semin Nephrol 2004;24:131–40.
131. Bohrer MP, Deen WM, Robertson CR, et al. Mechanism of angiotensin II-induced proteinuria in the rat. Am J Physiol 1977;233:F13–21.
132. Durvasula RV, Petermann AT, Hiromura K, et al. Activation of a local tissue angiotensin system in podocytes by mechanical strain1. Kidney Int 2004;65:30–9.
133. Macconi D, Remuzzi G, Benigni A. Key fibrogenic mediators: old players. Renin–angiotensin system. Kidney Int Suppl (2011) 2014;4:58–64.
134. Wolf G, Wenzel U, Burns KD, et al. Angiotensin II activates nuclear transcription factor-kappaB through AT1 and AT2 receptors1. Kidney Int 2002;61:1986–95.
135. Yokoi H, Sugawara A, Mukoyama M, et al. Role of connective tissue growth factor in profibrotic action of transforming growth factor-β: a potential target for preventing renal fibrosis. Am J Kidney Dis 2001;38:S134–8.
136. Nangaku M, Fujita T. Activation of the renin-angiotensin system and chronic hypoxia of the kidney. Hypertens Res 2008;31:175–84.
137. Wang Z, Tang L, Zhu Q, et al. Hypoxia-inducible factor-1[alpha] contributes to the profibrotic action of angiotensin II in renal medullary interstitial cells. Kidney Int 2011;79:300–10.
138. Hollenberg NK. Aldosterone in the development and progression of renal injury. Kidney Int 2004;66:1–9.
139. Remuzzi G, Cattaneo D, Perico N. The aggravating mechanisms of aldosterone on kidney fibrosis. J Am Soc Nephrol 2008;19:1459–62.

140. Lai L, Chen J, Hao C-M, et al. Aldosterone promotes fibronectin production through a Smad2-dependent TGF-β1 pathway in mesangial cells. Biochem Biophys Res Commun 2006;348:70–5.
141. Juknevicius I, Segal Y, Kren S, et al. Effect of aldosterone on renal transforming growth factor-β. Am J Physiol Renal Physiol 2004;286:F1059–62.
142. Sun Y, Zhang J, Zhang JQ, et al. Local angiotensin II and transforming growth factor-β1 in renal fibrosis of rats. Hypertension 2000;35:1078–84.
143. Nishiyama A, Yao L, Nagai Y, et al. Possible contributions of reactive oxygen species and mitogen-activated protein kinase to renal injury in aldosterone/salt-induced hypertensive rats. Hypertension 2004;43:841–8.
144. Han KH, Kang YS, Han SY, et al. Spironolactone ameliorates renal injury and connective tissue growth factor expression in type II diabetic rats. Kidney Int 2006;70:111–20.
145. Ruggenenti P, Cravedi P, Remuzzi G. Mechanisms and treatment of CKD. J Am Soc Nephrol 2012;23(12):1917–28.
146. Ruggenenti P, Perticucci E, Cravedi P, et al. Role of remission clinics in the longitudinal treatment of CKD. J Am Soc Nephrol 2008;19:1213–24.
147. Mann JFE, Schmieder RE, McQueen M, et al. Renal outcomes with telmisartan, ramipril, or both, in people at high vascular risk (the ONTARGET study): a multicentre, randomised, double-blind, controlled trial. Lancet 2008;372:547–53.
148. Persson F, Rossing P, Parving H-H. Direct renin inhibition in chronic kidney disease. Br J Clin Pharmacol 2013;76:580–6.
149. Gentile G, Remuzzi G, Ruggenenti P. Dual renin-angiotensin system blockade for nephroprotection: still under scrutiny. Nephron 2015;129:39–41.
150. Watanabe T, Mishina M. Effects of benazepril hydrochloride in cats with experimentally induced or spontaneously occurring chronic renal failure. J Vet Med Sci 2007;69:1015–23.
151. Mathur S, Brown CA, Dietrich UM, et al. Evaluation of a technique of inducing hypertensive renal insufficiency in cats. Am J Vet Res 2004;65:1006–13.
152. Lefebvre HP, Toutain PL. Angiotensin-converting enzyme inhibitors in the therapy of renal diseases. J Vet Pharmacol Ther 2004;27:265–81.
153. Tauger F, Baatz G, Nobiling R. The renin-angiotensin system in cats with chronic renal failure. J Comp Pathol 1996;115:239–52.
154. Mitani S, Yabuki A, Taniguchi K, et al. Association between the intrarenal renin-angiotensin system and renal injury in chronic kidney disease of dogs and cats. J Vet Med Sci 2013;75:127–33.
155. Mitani S, Yabuki A, Sawa M, et al. Intrarenal distributions and changes of angiotensin-converting enzyme and angiotensin-converting enzyme 2 in feline and canine chronic kidney disease. J Vet Med Sci 2014;76:45–50.
156. Steele J, Henik R, Stepien R. Effects of angiotensin-converting enzyme inhibition on plasma aldosterone concentration, plasma renin activity, and blood pressure in spontaneously hypertensive cats with chronic renal disease. Vet Ther 2002;3:157–66.
157. Jepson RE, Syme HM, Elliott J. Plasma renin activity and aldosterone concentrations in hypertensive cats with and without azotemia and in response to treatment with amlodipine besylate. J Vet Intern Med 2014;28:144–53.
158. Jensen J, Henik RA, Brownfield M, et al. Plasma renin activity and angiotensin I and aldosterone concentrations in cats with hypertension associated with chronic renal disease. Am J Vet Res 1997;58:535–40.
159. King JN, Gunn-Moore DA, Tasker S, et al. Tolerability and efficacy of benazepril in cats with chronic kidney disease. J Vet Intern Med 2006;20:1054–64.

160. Brown SA, Brown CA, Jacobs G, et al. Effects of the angiotensin converting enzyme inhibitor benazepril in cats with induced renal insufficiency. Am J Vet Res 2001;62:375–83.
161. Mizutani H, Koyama H, Watanabe T, et al. Evaluation of the clinical efficacy of benazepril in the treatment of chronic renal insufficiency in cats. J Vet Intern Med 2006;20:1074–9.
162. Sent U, Gössl R, Elliott J, et al. Comparison of efficacy of long-term oral treatment with telmisartan and benazepril in cats with chronic kidney disease. J Vet Intern Med 2015;29:1479–87.
163. Jamerson KA, Townsend RR. The attributable burden of hypertension: focus on CKD. Adv Chronic Kidney Dis 2011;18:6–10.
164. Klag MJ, Whelton PK, Randall BL, et al. Blood pressure and end stage renal disease in men. N Engl J Med 1996;334:13–8.
165. Klahr S, Levey AS, Beck GJ, et al. The effects of dietary protein restriction and blood-pressure control on the progression of chronic renal disease. N Engl J Med 1994;330:877–84.
166. Griffin K, Pothugunta K, Polichnowski AJ, et al. The role of systemic blood pressure in the progression of chronic kidney disease. Curr Cardiovasc Risk Rep 2015;9:1–9.
167. Weir MR, Townsend RR, Fink JC, et al. Hemodynamic correlates of proteinuria in chronic kidney disease. Clin J Am Soc Nephrol 2011;6:2403–10.
168. Zoja C, Abbate M, Remuzzi G. Progression of renal injury toward interstitial inflammation and glomerular sclerosis is dependent on abnormal protein filtration. Nephrol Dial Transplant 2015;30:706–12.
169. Verroust PJ, Christensen EI. Megalin and cubulin—the story of two multipurpose receptors unfolds. Nephrol Dial Transplant 2002;17:1867–71.
170. Gómez-Garre D, Largo R, Tejera N, et al. Activation of NF-κB in tubular epithelial cells of rats with intense proteinuria: role of angiotensin II and endothelin-1. Hypertension 2001;37:1171–8.
171. Eddy AA, Giachelli CM. Renal expression of genes that promote interstitial inflammation and fibrosis in rats with protein-overload proteinuria. Kidney Int 1995;47:1546–57.
172. Donadelli R, Abbate M, Zanchi C, et al. Protein traffic activates NF-kB gene signaling and promotes MCP-1–dependent interstitial inflammation. Am J Kidney Dis 2000;36:1226–41.
173. Kramer AB, Ricardo SD, Kelly DJ, et al. Modulation of osteopontin in proteinuria-induced renal interstitial fibrosis. J Pathol 2005;207:483–92.
174. Nangaku M. Complement regulatory proteins in glomerular diseases. Kidney Int 1998;54:1419–28.
175. David S, Biancone L, Caserta C, et al. Alternative pathway complement activation induces proinflammatory activity in human proximal tubular epithelial cells. Nephrol Dial Transplant 1997;12:51–6.
176. Abbate M, Zoja C, Corna D, et al. Complement-mediated dysfunction of glomerular filtration barrier accelerates progressive renal injury. J Am Soc Nephrol 2008;19:1158–67.
177. Cao W, Zhou QG, Nie J, et al. Albumin overload activates intrarenal renin–angiotensin system through protein kinase C and NADPH oxidase-dependent pathway. J Hypertens 2011;29:1411–21.
178. Caruso-Neves C, Pinheiro AAS, Cai H, et al. PKB and megalin determine the survival or death of renal proximal tubule cells. Proc Natl Acad Sci U S A 2006;103:18810–5.

179. Koral K, Erkan E. PKB/Akt partners with Dab2 in albumin endocytosis. Am J Physiol Renal Physiol 2012;302:F1013-24.
180. Benigni A, Gagliardini E, Remuzzi A, et al. Angiotensin-converting enzyme inhibition prevents glomerular-tubule disconnection and atrophy in passive Heymann nephritis, an effect not observed with a calcium antagonist. Am J Pathol 2001;159:1743-50.
181. Erkan E, Garcia CD, Patterson LT, et al. Induction of renal tubular cell apoptosis in focal segmental glomerulosclerosis: roles of proteinuria and Fas-dependent pathways. J Am Soc Nephrol 2005;16:398-407.
182. Zoccali C, Ruggenenti P, Perna A, et al. Phosphate may promote CKD progression and attenuate renoprotective effect of ACE inhibition. J Am Soc Nephrol 2011;22:1923-30.
183. Haut LL, ALfrey AC, Guggenheim S, et al. Renal toxicity of phosphate in rats. Kidney Int 1980;17:722-31.
184. Craig JM. Observations on the kidney after phosphate loading in the rat. Arch Pathol 1959;68:306-15.
185. Koizumi T, Murakami K, Nakayama H, et al. Role of dietary phosphorus in the progression of renal failure. Biochem Biophys Res Commun 2002;295:917-21.
186. Finco DR, Brown SA, Crowell WA, et al. Effects of dietary phosphorus and protein in dogs with chronic renal failure. Am J Vet Res 1992;53:2264-71.
187. Kendrick J, Chonchol M. The role of phosphorus in the development and progression of vascular calcification. Am J Kidney Dis 2011;58:826-34.
188. Shuto E, Taketani Y, Tanaka R, et al. Dietary phosphorus acutely impairs endothelial function. J Am Soc Nephrol 2009;20:1504-12.
189. Kang D-H, Kanellis J, Hugo C, et al. Role of the microvascular endothelium in progressive renal disease. J Am Soc Nephrol 2002;13:806-16.
190. Cozzolino M, Brancaccio D, Gallieni M, et al. Pathogenesis of vascular calcification in chronic kidney disease. Kidney Int 2005;68:429-36.
191. Ohnishi M, Razzaque MS. Dietary and genetic evidence for phosphate toxicity accelerating mammalian aging. FASEB J 2010;24:3562-71.
192. Di Marco GS, Hausberg M, Hillebrand U, et al. Increased inorganic phosphate induces human endothelial cell apoptosis in vitro. Am J Physiol Renal Physiol 2008;294:F1381-7.
193. Chen Z, Chen D, McCarthy TL, et al. Inorganic phosphate stimulates fibronectin expression in renal fibroblasts. Cell Physiol Biochem 2012;30:151-9.
194. Beck GR, Zerler B, Moran E. Phosphate is a specific signal for induction of osteopontin gene expression. Proc Natl Acad Sci U S A 2000;97:8352-7.
195. Eräranta A, Riutta A, Fan M, et al. Dietary phosphate binding and loading alter kidney angiotensin-converting enzyme mRNA and protein content in 5/6 nephrectomized rats. Am J Nephrol 2012;35:401-8.
196. Geddes RF, Elliott J, Syme HM. The effect of feeding a renal diet on plasma fibroblast growth factor 23 concentrations in cats with stable azotemic chronic kidney disease. J Vet Intern Med 2013;27(6):1354-61.
197. Ross SJ, Osborne CA, Kirk CA, et al. Clinical evaluation of dietary modification for the treatment of spontaneous chronic kidney disease in cats. J Am Vet Med Assoc 2006;229:949-57.
198. Nangaku M. Chronic hypoxia and tubulointerstitial injury: a final common pathway to end-stage renal failure. J Am Soc Nephrol 2006;17:17-25.
199. Nangaku M, Eckardt K-U. Hypoxia and the HIF system in kidney disease. J Mol Med 2007;85:1325-30.

200. Semenza GL, Wang GL. A nuclear factor induced by hypoxia via de novo protein synthesis binds to the human erythropoietin gene enhancer at a site required for transcriptional activation. Mol Cell Biol 1992;12:5447–54.
201. Leonard MO, Cottell DC, Godson C, et al. The role of HIF-1α in transcriptional regulation of the proximal tubular epithelial cell response to hypoxia. J Biol Chem 2003;278:40296–304.
202. Norman JT, Clark IM, Garcia PL. Hypoxia promotes fibrogenesis in human renal fibroblasts. Kidney Int 2000;58:2351–66.
203. Norman JT, Orphanides C, Garcia P, et al. Hypoxia-induced changes in extracellular matrix metabolism in renal cells. Nephron Exp Nephrol 1999;7:463–9.
204. Manotham K, Tanaka T, Matsumoto M, et al. Transdifferentiation of cultured tubular cells induced by hypoxia. Kidney Int 2004;65:871–80.
205. King JN, Tasker S, Gunn-Moore DA, et al. Prognostic factors in cats with chronic kidney disease. J Vet Intern Med 2007;21:906–16.
206. Small DM, Coombes JS, Bennett N, et al. Oxidative stress, anti-oxidant therapies and chronic kidney disease. Nephrology (Carlton) 2012;17:311–21.
207. Cadenas E, Davies KJA. Mitochondrial free radical generation, oxidative stress, and aging1. Free Radic Biol Med 2000;29:222–30.
208. Brune B, Zhou J, Von Knethien A. Nitric oxide, oxidative stress and apoptosis. Kidney Int 2003;63:S22–4.
209. Vlassara H, Torreggiani M, Post JB, et al. Role of oxidants/inflammation in declining renal function in chronic kidney disease and normal aging. Kidney Int Suppl 2009;(114):S3–11.
210. Dounousi E, Papavasiliou E, Makedou A, et al. Oxidative stress is progressively enhanced with advancing stages of CKD. Am J Kidney Dis 2006;48:752–60.
211. Jun M. Antioxidants for chronic kidney disease. Nephrology (Carlton) 2013;18: 576–8.
212. Brown SA. Oxidative stress and chronic kidney disease. Vet Clin North Am 2008; 38:157–66.
213. Keegan RF, Webb CB. Oxidative stress and neutrophil function in cats with chronic renal failure. J Vet Intern Med 2010;24:514–9.
214. Krofič Žel M, Tozon N, Nemec Svete A. Plasma and erythrocyte glutathione peroxidase activity, serum selenium concentration, and plasma total antioxidant capacity in cats with IRIS stages I–IV chronic kidney disease. J Vet Intern Med 2014;28:130–6.
215. Yu S, Paetau-Robinson I. Dietary supplements of vitamins E and C and beta-carotene reduce oxidative stress in cats with renal insufficiency. Vet Res Commun 2006;30:403–13.

Controversies in Veterinary Nephrology: Renal Diets Are Indicated for Cats with International Renal Interest Society Chronic Kidney Disease Stages 2 to 4: The Pro View

David J. Polzin, DVM, PhD*, Julie A. Churchill, DVM, PhD

KEYWORDS

• Chronic kidney disease • Cats • Nutrition • Renal diets

KEY POINTS

• Veterinarians should closely monitor nutritional status (including at least body weight and body condition and muscle mass scores) in cats with CKD and (1) take steps as needed to assure adequate renal diet is consumed, (2) identify and mitigate factors promoting catabolism, and (3) modify diets judicially as needed to meet the needs of individual cats.
• Clinical trials have confirmed that cats with chronic kidney disease (CKD) fed renal diets survive significantly longer than cats with CKD fed typical feline diets.
• Cats consuming renal diets in amounts adequate to meet their daily energy requirements have been shown to maintain stable, adequate nutrition, as measured by body weight and body condition scores, for at least 2 years.

THE EFFECTS OF IMPAIRED KIDNEY FUNCTION ON FOOD AND WATER INTAKE

Perhaps the most important function of the kidneys is maintaining the internal milieu by eliminating metabolic wastes and excesses and deficits of ingested foodstuffs and water because a normal internal milieu is essential for normal cell metabolism and function. In order to achieve this, substances entering the body in excess must be excreted (with or without metabolic modification), whereas essential substances must be retained in appropriate quantities (ie, not too much, not too little). Healthy kidneys are able to achieve this goal over a great range of intakes of foodstuffs and water. However, when kidney function declines, the kidney's ability to adapt

The authors have nothing to disclose.
Department of Veterinary Clinical Sciences, College of Veterinary Medicine, University of Minnesota, 1352 Boyd Avenue, St Paul, MN 55108, USA
* Corresponding author.
E-mail address: polzi001@umn.edu

appropriately to various ranges of intakes of foodstuffs becomes challenged. Essentially the tolerable ranges of intake for most nutrients and water narrow as kidney function declines.

The impact of declining kidney function on retention and excretion of specific substances varies depending on how the substances are handled by the nephrons and whether or not active compensatory mechanisms mitigate changes in concentrations. For example, creatinine is essentially all excreted by glomerular filtration with no secretion, reabsorption, or renal metabolism. As a consequence, serum creatinine concentration increases progressively as glomerular filtration rate (GFR) declines. In contrast, serum phosphorus concentration typically does not begin to increase until GFR declines by about 75% or more. The kidneys manage phosphorus by glomerular filtration and renal tubular reabsorption; however, multiple factors, such as fibroblast growth factor-23 (FGF-23), parathyroid hormone, calcitriol, and ionized calcium, act to mitigate elevation in serum phosphorus concentration until the adaptive processes can no longer prevent progressive hyperphosphatemia. Although these adaptive processes delay the onset of hyperphosphatemia, there are significant adverse trade-offs, such as chronic kidney disease (CKD) mineral and bone disorder and progression of CKD. Thus, failing to adjust dietary intake of phosphorus according to loss of kidney function ultimately harms the kidneys and patients.

When a cat with impaired kidney function consumes a food substance in excess of the kidneys' ability to excrete it, the substance, or its metabolites, will be retained in the body. An example of this principle is the azotemia that develops when protein intake is not reduced in advanced CKD. In turn, when an individual with impaired kidney function consumes a substance in a quantity less than the kidney's ability to conserve it, a deficiency of that substance will develop. A common example of this principle is dehydration developing in cats with CKD because of inadequate water consumption concurrent with polyuria due to impaired urine concentration.

Many of the tools we use to manage cats with CKD are based on these physiologic principals. The trade-off for failing to adequately modify intakes of dietary elements and water in CKD include excesses and deficits of dietary elements and water, and at least some of these imbalances promote uremia and/or progression of CKD. When specific dietary elements are managed actively, compensatory adaptations may be deleterious to the kidneys and/or patients, as is true of mitigating phosphorus retention.

No doubt, there are limits to the extent to which the intake of any given dietary element may be therapeutically modified; nutritional requirements likely do impact these limits. However, it may be necessary to balance therapeutic dietary modifications with the challenge of impaired kidney function in order to optimize the overall health of patients. Ultimately the best way to assess this balance will be regular careful assessment of the patients' response to therapeutic modifications considering overall health.

FELINE RENAL DIETS AND NUTRITION IN CHRONIC KIDNEY DISEASE

Renal diets (RDs) are diets specifically formulated for the purpose of clinical management of cats with CKD.[1] They are generally accepted to be useful in cats with moderate to advanced CKD.[1–5] They are not solely modified based on the impact of declining kidney function but also supplemented with nutrients thought to ameliorate complications of CKD, such as omega-3 polyunsaturated fatty acids and antioxidants.[1] They have been considered standard therapy for managing cats with CKD for many years and are supported by evidence from clinical studies in cats.[1–5] For the purpose of this discussion, the term *RDs* shall include commercially produced diets specifically designed for cats with CKD and similar diets formulated for cats with CKD by boarded veterinary nutritionists.

The use of RDs in treating cats with CKD has become a topic of controversy, weighing the potential benefits of RDs mitigating the clinical consequences of CKD versus the purported potential risk of protein malnutrition consequent to the high protein requirements of cats. As a result of this controversy, some veterinarians have recommended feeding diets containing high levels of dietary protein instead of RDs. This divergence in therapeutic opinion has evolved from recent studies suggesting that senior cats may require more protein than younger cats and the observation that, at least in some cats with CKD, body weight, body condition score, and/or muscle mass may decline over time.[6] The specific point of disagreement between these two schools of thought is focused on how much protein should be fed to cats with CKD. More specifically, those advocating feeding higher-protein diets to cats with CKD have generally recommended feeding commercial or nonrenal therapeutic diets containing more protein instead of feeding the currently available RDs specifically designed for cats with CKD.

Veterinarians use therapeutic diets in much the same way as they use pharmaceuticals to manage many medical conditions. When they prescribe feeding a RD for cats with CKD, they expect the diet to achieve 4 specific goals. These goals are (1) to ameliorate or prevent clinical consequences of CKD and uremia; (2) to slow progression of CKD and/or prolong survival; (3) to minimize derangements of electrolyte, mineral, and acid-base balance; and (4) to maintain adequate nutrition.[7]

To achieve these multifaceted goals, modifications beyond just reducing protein content is incorporated in the formulating of RD for cats, including reduced phosphate and sodium content; increased omega-3-polyunsaturated fatty acids, antioxidants, fiber, vitamin D, and potassium content; and a neutral effect on systemic pH.[7] Most of these dietary formulations are extrapolated from studies examining one or occasionally 2 diet modifications. However, clinical trials of RDs have been performed to evaluate the overall effectiveness of the sum of dietary modifications.[2–4]

EVIDENCE SUPPORTING RENAL DIETS AS EFFECTIVE IN CATS WITH CHRONIC KIDNEY DISEASE

Three studies address the effectiveness of feline RDs in mitigating uremic crises and extending suvival.[2–4] The first study (study 1) compared a manufactured protein- and phosphorus-restricted RD with making no diet change from the cat's (nonrenal) previous diet.[2] The design of this study was neither randomized nor masked; cats that chose not to eat the RD continued on their usual diet. Cats that consumed the RD (mean survival time = 633 days) survived significantly longer than the cats that continued to consume their regular diet (mean survival time = 264 days). In addition, the serum urea nitrogen and serum phosphorus concentrations declined; the increase parathyroid hormone concentrations were prevented in cats consuming the RD.

The second study (study 2) was a randomized, masked clinical trial with 22 cats randomized to a manufactured RD and 23 cats or feline maintenance diet (MD). The principal dietary modifications in the RD in this study included reduced protein, phosphorus, sodium, and supplementation with polyunsaturated fatty acids; the MD was formulated using the average nutrient contents of the 10 most popular dry maintenance foods for cats.[3] Cats in this study had serum creatinine values ranging from 2.0 mg/dL to 4.5 mg/dL (International Renal Interest Society [IRIS] CKD stages 2 and 3). Risks of uremic crises and renal deaths were significantly reduced among cats that consumed the RD. Among the 22 cats fed RD, there were no uremic crises or renal deaths over 2 years of study. In contrast, among the 23 cats consuming MD, 6 developed clinical and biochemical evidence of uremia and 5 died of renal causes. Mean serum phosphorus concentrations were significantly lower among cats consuming the RD diet compared with cats consuming the RD at 12 months (RD = 3.8 mg/dL vs MD = 4.2 mg/dL; $P<.04$) and 24 months (RD = 3.8 mg/dL vs MD = 50.8 mg/dL; $P<.001$).[3] Mean serum urea nitrogen concentrations were also significantly lower among cats consuming the RD diet compared with cats consuming the RD at 12 months (RD = 40.1 mg/dL vs MD = 52.2 mg/dL; $P<.001$) and 24 months (RD = 3.8 mg/dL vs MD = 4.4 mg/dL; $P<.02$).

The third study was a retrospective study performed in 31 first-opinion veterinary practices in The Netherlands and compared survival times for cats with IRIS CKD Stages 2, 3, and 4 fed one or more of 7 commercial feline RDs with cats not fed a RD.[4] Median survival time for cats fed a RD was 16 months compared with 7 months for cats fed their usual diet.

The consistent findings in these 3 studies using different diets and methodologies and performed in 3 different countries by 3 independent groups of researchers strongly support the conclusion that RDs favor better clinical outcomes (longer survival and reduced uremic crises). Further, a randomized, masked clinical trial performed in dogs also demonstrated canine RDs, which are formulated similar to feline RDs, reduce the risk of developing uremia and early death due to CKD in dogs. Although each of these studies have limitations in their methodology and size, the fact that findings in these diverse studies are all supportive of the clinical impact of RDs is meaningful because taken together they support the generalization that diet therapy with RD is effective in favorably influencing clinical outcomes in CKD.

Studies have also shown that feline RDs are effective in minimizing derangements of electrolyte, mineral, and acid-base balance.[2,3,8,9] Although debate continues regarding the optimal nutrient profile, there is less controversy about the detrimental effects of phosphorus in cats with CKD. Clinical studies have confirmed feeding RDs lowers plasma phosphorus concentrations compared with cats with CKD consuming their usual diet. One of these studies demonstrated further that an RD can reduce FGF-23 compared with cats consuming their usual diet.[8] The phosphatonin, FGF-23, enhances urinary excretion of excess phosphorus very early in the course of CKD. The elevated FGF-23 concentration in CKD represents a response to retention of dietary phosphorus in the body. Phosphorus is perhaps the single most important metabolite recognized for managing cats with CKD because elevated serum phosphorus concentrations and FGF-23 concentrations have been implicated in promoting progression of CKD.[9]

The available clinical studies provide evidence that RDs fed to cats with CKD do sustain them for extended periods, thereby belying claims that RDs promote weight loss when presented properly and adequate intake is assured.[2,3] In the nonrandomized clinical trial (referenced earlier), body weight remained stable through midsurvival in both cats fed the RD as well as cats fed the MD.[2] In the randomized, masked clinical trial, both body condition score and body weight did not change significantly after 12 and 24 months on the RD.[3] In addition, cats fed the RD and those fed the MD did not differ significantly in body condition score or body weight at baseline and 12 and 24 months. For the duration of this study, (2+ years) cats did not have clinical signs of malnutrition.

WHAT IS THE RATIONAL FOR PROTEIN RESTRICTION IN RENAL DIETS?

It has been known for more than a century that protein restriction reduces the clinical signs of uremia.[10,11] Indeed, most clinical signs of uremia are caused by accumulation of products of protein metabolism.[a] Although limiting protein intake to ameliorate clinical signs of uremia has been standard practice for decades, the decision as to when protein restriction should be initiated remains controversial. There are 2 schools of thought on this question. The first is that initiating protein restriction should be delayed until the cat begins to display clinical signs of uremia, typically during late IRIS CKD stage 3 or IRIS CKD stage 4. The alternative position is that dietary protein restriction should begin early in IRIS CKD stages 2 or 3 because it may slow progression of CKD, delay onset of uremic signs, and facilitate better acceptance of diet change. Delaying diet therapy until the owner recognizes that the cat is beginning to manifest clinical signs of uremia significantly risks the cat developing an overt uremic crisis before diet treatment can be started, an expensive, unnecessary, and potentially fatal adventure.[3] Further, evidence that RDs reduce uremic crises and mortality in cats in IRIS CKD stage 3,[2–4] and initiating diet therapy this late in the course of CKD, may make the diet change more difficult. On the other hand, although initiating diet therapy in cats with IRIS CKD stage 2 may be effective in slowing progression of CKD, the evidence supporting RDs in this CKD stage is less compelling than evidence supporting efficacy of RDs in IRIS CKD stage 3, although this is in large part due to IRIS CKD stage 3 being the focus of the studies rather than earlier stages of kidney disease. One possible concern regarding RDs in some cats with IRIS CKD stage 2 is that initiating protein restriction with a calorically dense food may contribute to body fat gain with lean mass loss if protein requirements are not met with a RD.

Studies in rodents and humans provide evidence that limiting protein intake may slow progression and extend survival in CKD. Studies in rodent models of CKD have shown that feeding a high-protein diet is associated with development of glomerular sclerosis, proteinuria, and progressive decline in kidney function, whereas feeding low-protein diets prevented these effects.[12] From these observations in rats, studies were performed to determine whether reducing protein intake slowed progression in humans.[13] Although the interpretation of these studies has been controversial, recent meta-analysis studies have suggested that protein intake does delay progression and reduce renal mortality in humans with CKD. A meta-analysis performed by the Cochrane Collaboration concluded that reducing protein intake in patients with CKD (Kidney Disease Outcomes Quality Initiative [KDOQI] stages 3–5) reduced the occurrence of renal death by 32% compared with unrestricted protein intake.[14] Although evidence that protein restriction per se reduces renal mortality in cats with CKD is lacking, it is unknown whether it contributes to the effectiveness of feline RDs in reducing renal mortality and warrants further study.

Although not the only source of phosphorus in feline diets, protein is a significant source of phosphorus; excessive dietary intake of phosphorus has been linked to progression of CKD in cats and other species.[8,15,16] Thus, limiting dietary protein is a strategy for limiting dietary phosphorus intake. Feeding RDs to cats with CKD has been shown to reduce serum phosphorus concentrations and FGF-23 levels.[2,3] Not all dietary proteins provide the same amount of phosphorus, so the amount of phosphorus linked to protein depends on the type and amount of protein. For example, plant-source proteins generally provide lower amounts of phosphorus compared with animal-source protein.[17] Thus, it is possible to provide higher protein diets, yet limit dietary phosphorus intake by using greater proportion of vegetable protein or other proteins that contain lower available phosphorus content. **Table 1** compares

---

[a] The toxins responsible for the uremic syndrome are not completely known. It is assumed that uremia is due to multiple retained toxins (supported by the effectiveness of dialysis therapy), although urea and creatinine do not seem to be substantial contributors to the toxicity.

Table 1
Protein, phosphorus, and sodium levels of the most commonly used therapeutic diets for managing cats with chronic kidney disease

Product Name Feline Formulations	Calories: Cup or Can	Protein (g/100 kcal)	Phosphorus (mg/100 kcal)
ProPlan Veterinary Diet Feline NF Kidney Function canned	193 kcal/5.5-oz can	7.23	120
ProPlan Veterinary Diet Feline Kidney Function dry	398 per cup	6.61	110
Hill's Prescription Diet k/d Feline Renal Health dry	499 kcal per cup	6.4	108
Hill's Prescription Diet k/d Feline canned with chicken	183 kcal/5.5-oz can	6.5	85
Hill's Prescription Diet k/d Feline chicken and vegetable stew	78 kcal/2.9-oz can	6.5	105
Hill's Prescription Diet k/d Feline canned vegetable and tuna stew	77 kcal/2.9-oz can	6.7	107
Hill's Prescription Diet k/d Feline canned with ocean white fish	187 kcal/5.5-oz can	6.6	117
Hill's Prescription Diet g/d Feline dry	297 kcal per cup	7.9	135
Hill's Prescription Diet g/d Feline canned	165 kcal/5.5-oz can	8.2	123
Iams VF Renal Plus Feline dry	514 kcal per cup	7.1	93
Iams VF Renal Plus Feline canned	199 kcal/6-oz can	7.2	128
Royal Canin Veterinary Diet Feline Renal Support A	345 kcal per cup	5.8	110
Royal Canin Veterinary Diet Feline Renal Support F	373 kcal per cup	6.5	110
Royal Canin Veterinary Diet Feline Renal Support S	398 kcal per cup	5.8	100
Royal Canin Veterinary Diet Feline Renal Support D	97 kcal/3-oz can	6.2	80
Royal Canin Veterinary Diet Feline Renal Support E	171 kcal/5.8-oz can	6.6	90
Royal Canin Veterinary Diet Feline Renal Support T	82 kcal/3-oz can	6.2	100
Royal Canin Veterinary Diet Feline Multifunction Renal + Hydrolyzed dry	400 kcal per cup	6.1	110

the protein, phosphorus, and sodium levels of the most commonly used therapeutic diets for managing feline patients with CKD.

The goal of limiting dietary phosphorus intake may influence the maximum amount of protein that can be fed. Although the amount of phosphorus in diets can be mitigated somewhat by administration of intestinal phosphorus binders, the ability of intestinal phosphorus binders to limit phosphorus uptake from diets containing high levels of phosphorus is finite. This limitation, combined with the fact many cats resist administration of medications, increases owner frustration and reduces quality of life for cats having to receive unpalatable medications with every feeding. This limitation lowers adherence and makes the strategy of supplementing high-protein foods with phosphorus binders of questionable efficacy. Administering phosphorus binders at dosages greater than the recommended dose range can lead to adverse drug effects: toxic effects due to absorption of cations associated with the binders (eg, aluminum, calcium, lanthanum, and so forth).[18]

In order to be effective in slowing progressive kidney disease, it is recommended that intestinal phosphate binders be dosed to achieve specific serum phosphorus targets (**Table 2**). Clearly no single dose will be appropriate for all cats. As described earlier, RDs significantly reduce serum phosphorus concentration and they are associated with better long-term survival. However, in one study, cats fed both the RD and MD were found to be within recommended targets for phosphorus; but RD was associated with both a significantly lower serum phosphorus concentration and significantly better survival outcomes compared with the MD diet. Thus, dietary restriction of phosphorus seems to be clinically important even when cats with CKD have serum phosphorus concentrations within the recommended guidelines for phosphorus. Because phosphorus content is not the sole dietary difference between RD and MD, these findings cannot prove that the favorable outcomes with RD are due solely to phosphorus alone.

THE INTERNATIONAL RENAL INTEREST SOCIETY'S GUIDELINES FOR DIETARY THERAPY IN CHRONIC KIDNEY DISEASE

The IRIS provides guidelines on when RDs should be fed to cats with CKD.[5] These guidelines are based on the cat's IRIS CKD stage and magnitude of proteinuria. RDs are not currently recommended for cats in IRIS CKD stage 1. The IRIS' guidelines for cats in IRIS CKD stage 2 do not recommend RDs; however, they suggest considering feeding a RD in this stage because cats may be more likely to accept a RD than in later stages of CKD. Studies supporting clinical benefits of feeding RDs have included cats with serum creatinine concentrations from 2.1 mg/dL to 2.8 mg/dL, suggesting that diet therapy may extend survival in at least in the latter half of IRIS CKD stage 2.[2,3] Cats with early IRIS CKD stage 2 has not specifically been evaluated. In addition, RDs are recommended for cats in IRIS CKD stage 2 when needed to achieve serum phosphorus goals.[5] However, because elevated FGF-23 concentrations are elevated in IRIS CKD stage 2 and have been linked to progression of CKD in cats, and RDs have been shown to reduce FGF-23 concentrations in cats with CKD, it may be appropriate to recommend RDs for IRIS CKD stage 2 cats from these findings.[8,19] In addition, has been shown to predict IRIS guidelines recommend feeding RDs to cats in IRIS CKD

Table 2		
Serum phosphate targets according to IRIS chronic kidney disease stage		
Recommended Treatment Goals for Serum Phosphorus Concentrations		
IRIS Stage	Target Serum Phosphorus Concentration	
Stage	(mg/dL)	(mmol/dL)
1	2.5–4.5	0.81–1.45
2	2.5–4.5	0.81–1.45
3	2.5–5.0	0.81–1.61
4	2.5–6.0	0.81–1.94

stages 3 and 4 and for all cats with persistent urine protein/creation ratio (UPC) values exceeding 0.4.

Cats in IRIS CKD stages 1 and 2 are unlikely to require protein restriction for the purpose of preventing or ameliorating clinical signs of uremia. The exception to this generality would be when substantial loss of lean muscle mass artifactually lowers serum creatinine values thereby underestimating the cat's true IRIS CKD stage. There seems to be no renal advantage of feeding high-protein diets in these stages (meaning diets that exceed minimum protein requirements for the cat's life stage). Although high-protein diets may increase GFR, studies have indicated that high-protein diets promote proteinuria and development of glomerular lesions.[20] Although high-protein intake has not been convincingly proven to promote progression of CKD in cats, proteinuria has been shown to be associated with CKD.[15,21,22] In addition, most high-protein diets contain high-phosphorus content that is likely to promote progressive decline in kidney function.[9]

The IRIS' guidelines recommend that cats with IRIS CKD stages 3 and 4 should be fed RDs. The justification for this recommendation is based on studies that confirm RDs are associated with longer survival and reduced risk of uremic signs.[2–4] In contrast to cats in IRIS CKD stages 1 and 2, cats in IRIS CKD stages 3 and 4 are likely to develop clinical and biochemical abnormalities (consequences) when fed diets unrestricted in protein content and/or absent other characteristic of RDs. In these stages, the trade-off for increasing protein intake is an increasing risk of uremic toxicity and its various consequences.[10] Because cats in IRIS CKD stages 3 and 4 are at risk of uremic crisis and death due to consequences of CKD, feeding excessive protein would be predicted to shorten survival and clinically healthy interval, as has been shown in clinical trials in cats with CKD.[3] In addition, studies in rodents and humans suggest that the uremic environment is likely to promote protein and calorie wasting.[23–26] This topic warrants further investigation in uremic cats with CKD.

MUSCLE WASTING AND THE UREMIC ENVIRONMENT

It is being proposed that feeding RDs to cats with CKD causes moderate to severe loss of lean muscle mass. From this hypothesis, it has been recommended that cats with CKD should be fed diets containing higher- and, in some instances, high-protein diets. Because feeding excessive protein to cats with CKD may promote uremia in cats with IRIS CKD stages 3 and 4, it is worthwhile to ask whether protein restriction, CKD, or both lead to muscle wasting in these cats. If uremia alone or in concert with dietary protein restriction is the cause for the loss of lean mass in cats, then markedly increasing dietary protein intake may be the wrong response to the problem of sarcopenia in cats with CKD. Unfortunately, there are no studies that directly address the effect of uremia on protein requirements in cats with CKD. To attempt to answer this question, it is necessary to look beyond just feline evidence to the human and rodent studies on this question.

It is common for cats with CKD to lose weight and body condition and develop sarcopenia. This decline in nutritional status may develop before or after initiation of a RD, suggesting that feeding a MD alone does not always prevent development of sarcopenia. There is great variation in the clinical presentation of cats with CKD. In some cats, declining body weight and body condition scores and muscle wasting may be among the earliest clinical signs leading to a diagnosis of CKD. In some cats with CKD, the decline in nutrition status seems to be associated with concurrent diseases and complications of CKD. For example, urinary tract infections (UTIs) are a common complication in CKD cats. Cats with CKD and concurrent UTI often develop substantial loss of body weight and muscle mass associated with UTI. Treatment of the UTI may slow or stop weight loss; but restoring the previous body weight often improves very slowly or not at all, particularly in geriatric cats.

As in cats, muscle wasting is an important and common complication in humans with CKD. It is associated with increased mortality and has often been attributed to malnutrition associated with impaired appetite and prescribed dietary restrictions (primarily protein).[27,28] Malnutrition is defined as faulty nutrition due to inadequate or unbalanced intake of nutrients or their impaired assimilation or utilization.[26] However, malnutrition does not seem to be the sole mechanism leading to sarcopenia in most humans with CKD.[24,26]

The evidence that dietary protein restriction in humans with CKD is usually not the sole cause for sarcopenia includes several studies indicating that low-protein diets do not typically lead to malnutrition in patients with CKD. In a study of body composition as assessed by dual-energy x-ray absorptiometry (DEXA) in human patients with severe CKD, 2 years of a very-low-protein diet (0.3 g/kg/d protein) was determined to be safe for a "long period."[29] Lean body mass decreased over the first 6 months but thereafter increased progressively over 6 to 24 months in this study. A systematic literature review examining the effects of low-protein diets on body composition in humans with CKD concluded there was no strong evidence low-protein diets impaired body condition in patients with moderate to severe CKD.[30] Body condition in these studies was determined by DEXA, bioelectrical impedance analysis, and anthropometry. Another literature-based study examined the impact of low-protein and very-low-protein diets in patients with KDOQI CKD stages 3–5. They found that both diets were capable of sustaining mean and body cell mass for extended periods in CKD.[31] However, these investigators reported intercurrent diseases and periods of spontaneous reduction in calorie and protein intake markedly reduced the risk for malnutrition. It has been suggested that even small changes in protein metabolism may lead to marked loss of protein stores in patients with CKD.[26] Cats have a 4-fold greater protein requirement compared with humans and would clearly develop malnutrition on the protein intakes described in these studies. However, these studies indicate that uremia itself can contribute to sarcopenia; therefore, feeding excess protein may also promote sarcopenia.

Evidence supports that sarcopenia of CKD in humans and rodents is due, at least in part, to activation of complex mechanisms that stimulate loss of skeletal muscle involving activation of mediators that stimulate the ATP-dependent ubiquitin-proteasome system (UPS).[24,32] Studies in humans and rodents have identified the UPS as the major pathway degrading protein in skeletal muscle.[33] The UPS also has been shown to be a probable mediator of lean muscle mass loss in cats with feline immunodeficiency virus infections.[34] Mediators that have been identified in promoting muscle protein breakdown in CKD include inflammation, metabolic acidosis, angiotensin II, and neural and hormonal factors that cause defects in insulin/insulinlike growth factor intracellular signaling processes.[24,35,36]

It is likely changes in body composition involve many factors beyond diet formulation. Protein-energy wasting (PEW) is a state of nutritional and metabolic derangements occurring in human patients with CKD and characterized by simultaneous loss of systemic body protein and energy stores, leading ultimately to loss of muscle and fat mass and cachexia.[28,37] Uremic sarcopenia, characterized by muscle weakness and progressive muscle wasting, is one of the principal clinical outcomes of PEW.[25] The cause of PEW is proposed to include hypercatabolism, uremic toxins, malnutrition, and inflammation. Persistent low-grade inflammation recognized by elevated levels of biomarkers, such as C-reactive protein, has been reported to be a common finding in humans with end-stage renal disease.[38] A consensus statement by the International Society of Renal Nutrition and Metabolism on the cause of PEW concluded that, although insufficient food intake due to poor appetite and dietary restrictions may contribute to PEW, other factors are required for the full syndrome to develop.[23] These factors include uremia-induced alterations, such as increased energy expenditure, persistent inflammation, acidosis, and multiple endocrine disorders that render a state of hypermetabolism leading to excess catabolism of muscle and fat. PEW should be discriminated from malnutrition because CKD-related factors may contribute to the development of PEW, which are in addition to or independent of inadequate nutrient intake due to anorexia and/or dietary restrictions.[28] Factors that may contribute to PEW include decreased protein and energy intake, hypermetabolism, metabolic acidosis, decreased physical activity, decreased anabolism, comorbidities, lifestyle, and, when relevant, dialysis.[28] Similarly, cats with CKD are often seniors and may have concurrent reductions in protein and fat digestibility, along with reduced food intake.

It is likely that cats with CKD develop pathophysiologic derangements similar to PEW and uremic sarcopenia such as humans with CKD do. Further, the currently available evidence indicates that feline RDs do not consistently lead to reduced body weight and condition scores. Taken together, the available evidence provides reasonable doubt concerning the proposal that simply increasing protein intake is likely to prevent or ameliorate the changes in body composition.

FEEDING HIGHER-PROTEIN DIETS TO CATS WITH CHRONIC KIDNEY DISEASE

Current evidence does not support a recommendation to feed MDs or any diets other than RDs to cats with IRIS CKD stages 3 and 4. Based on the clinical trial data, feeding cats MDs or other diets that do not incorporate the modifications found in RDs would be expected to result in higher mortality and earlier onset signs of uremia compared with cats fed RDs.[2–4] Although some of the cats in these clinical trials were in IRIS CKD stage 2, the entire range of stage 2 was not included in these studies and the number of stage 2 cats studied was insufficient to establish the impact of diet. Although clinical studies indicate that modifications included in RDs have a favorable impact on survival and delaying onset of uremia, at least in IRIS CKD stages 3 and 4, the specific contribution of each modification has not been fully established. Thus, the beneficial effects of RDs are viewed as a diet effect. The specific therapeutic impact of altering or eliminating any one or more of the modifications in RDs is also largely unknown. However, based on the recognized association between protein intake and uremic signs, it is likely that excessive protein intake would promote premature onset of uremic signs and may promote sarcopenia associated with PEW. Based on the established role of dietary phosphorus content in slowing the progression of CKD, diets containing excessive phosphorus content would be predicted to accelerate progressive decline in kidney function. Because of these potentially adverse effects, clinical studies comparing RDs with higher-protein diets, with or without other dietary modifications found in RDs, should be performed before recommending higher-protein diets for cats with IRIS CKD stages 3 and 4.

Although there is no effective therapy short of dialysis or renal transplantation that will mitigate the increase in uremic toxins associated with increased protein intake, angiotensin-converting enzyme inhibitors (ACEi) and intestinal phosphorus binders have been suggested to mitigate some of the consequences of feeding diets other than RDs to cats with CKD. Specifically, ACEi are recommended to reduce proteinuria associated with higher protein intake, and intestinal phosphorus intestinal binders are recommended to mitigate phosphorus retention associated with higher-phosphorus diets.[39–41]

High-protein intake promotes proteinuria, which in turn has been linked to poor outcomes in cats with CKD.[20,39–41] However, providing standard dosing of 0.25 to 0.5 mg/kg of enalapril or benazepril has yet to be shown to alter progression or reduce mortality in cats with spontaneous CKD.[40] It is likely ACEi therapy must substantially reduce the magnitude of proteinuria in order to be effective in slowing progression or reducing mortality in CKD.[42] Thus, dosing of ACEi should be adjusted such that proteinuria does in fact decline, ideally to less than a UPC of less than 0.4. If the UPC cannot be reduced to less than 0.4, an alternate goal might be to reduce UPC from the pretreatment baseline UPC by 50%.[40] Similarly, dosing intestinal phosphorus binders should be adjusted to target serum phosphorus concentration according to IRIS CKD stage.

RENAL DIETS: WHERE DO WE GO FROM HERE?

The RDs tested in clinical trials were formulated by several pet food companies using what was interpreted as the best evidence on dietary protein requirements in cats (see **Table 1**). The shortfall of these studies is that diet intake was not evaluated, so no information is known about actual protein or phosphorus intake, only the concentration of nutrients in the foods provided. Although some of these diets have subsequently had modest modifications in their protein content, more recent studies suggest that dietary protein requirements for cats may be greater than previously thought, particularly for senior cats, which are overrepresented among cats with CKD.

Unfortunately, the recent suggestion that cats may require more protein in their diets has led to a variety of dietary recommendations that are untested and potentially harmful for cats with IRIS CKD stage 3 or higher. Reassessment of feline protein requirements should not be taken to justify feeding cats with CKD high-protein diets that exceed their protein requirements (5.2 g protein per kilogram of body weight). At least in IRIS CKD stages 3 and 4, such diets are likely to harm rather than benefit cats with CKD by increasing the risk of uremic signs and failing to provide any of the other modifications RDs provide. They are usually high in phosphorus, typically too high to adequately mitigate by supplementing intestinal phosphate binders.

Clinical recommendations that are based on opinion and/or extrapolation from normal cats to cats with CKD should not be state of the art. Nutritional studies performed in normal senior cats are a basis for a hypothesis as to what level of protein might be optimum for cats with CKD; however, it is inadequate for a recommendation for treatment. The authors think the optimum level of protein for feline RDs should be established by properly performed randomized controlled clinical trials in cats with spontaneous CKD. Because only limited studies have examined the role of RDs in IRIS CKD stage 2, studies including cats with the entire range of IRIS CKD stage 2 should be performed to determine the clinical effects of RDs in these cats and better determine the optimal time to implement dietary modification. Until studies of the type described earlier are performed, the authors think the current recommendation to feed RDs to cats with IRIS CKD stages 3 and 4 should stand because current data supports this recommendation. Cats in earlier stages should be evaluated regularly while supporting hydration and meeting but not exceeding nutritional requirements.

CLINICAL DECISION PROCESS FOR FEEDING CATS WITH CHRONIC KIDNEY DISEASE

Ideally recommendations for any specific nutritional therapy should be based on evidence-based nutrition. An evidence-based decision for determining patient care is defined as the integration of the best research evidence with clinical expertise and patient preferences.[43] *Best research evidence* means clinically relevant research, especially from patient-centered clinical studies. *Clinical expertise* refers to the use of clinical skills to identify each patient's unique health state, establish a diagnosis, and determine the risks and benefits of potential interventions. For veterinary practice, the concept of patient preferences must include the unique expectations of each owner (**Fig. 1**). In addition, if a therapeutic intervention is not readily available, then it is unlikely to benefit patients.

This concern is a true concern when trying to balance the unique nutritional needs of a cat while balancing the modifications considered beneficial in managing CKD. There are a finite number of therapeutic renal products that have similar levels of protein and phosphorus (see **Table 1**). Pet foods are formulated to provide complete nutrition. Supplementation of other foods that do not provide complete nutrition can imbalance the overall diet. For cats with CKD, it is recommended that no more than 10% of daily calories be provided as foodstuffs that are not nutritionally balanced for cats.

The first approach is to assess patients with a thorough diet history, physical examination (including body and muscle condition scoring, body weight, and weight history), and relevant diagnostics to determine the IRIS CKD stage. In IRIS CKD stages 3 and 4, there is stronger research evidence for the use of RDs and assuring cats meets their water and energy requirement to maintain a stable healthy body weight, condition, and hydration.

In cats with IRIS CKD stage 2, the clinical research is less clear and the clinical expertise and cat preferences may have slightly greater weight in the decision-making process. Ideally, the authors would evaluate the cat for any other comorbidities (including overweight/underweight status) or nutritional risk factors so that they

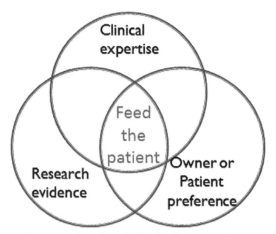

Fig. 1. Venn diagram demonstrating the relationship between clinical experiences, research evidence, and owner preference in developing clinical recommendations. The relative emphasis on each circle varies according to the quantity and volume of input from each area. These circles may change over time as needed information becomes available.

can be addressed.[44] The food would be evaluated to assure it meets nutritional and quality standards recommended by the American Animal Hospital Association and the World Small Animal Association.[44,45] In the absence of strong clinical evidence, the authors recommend prioritizing these nutritional goals: (1) promote and increase water intake, transitioning to all or part canned food if necessary; (2) meet individual calorie needs to maintain healthy stable weight; (3) in the context of caloric needs, select a product that provides high-quality protein to meet but not exceed the needs; (4) reduce dietary phosphorus; and (5) align nutritional balance if necessary (assuring treats and medication vehicles do not exceed 10% of the daily caloric intake).

Once a diet plan is made, a vigilant monitoring plan is an equally important part of managing early stages of CKD in order to detect any signs of progressive changes. Reassess patients 4 to 6 weeks after transitioning to a new diet and then every 3 to 4 months. Each follow-up evaluation should include an assessment of patients' food intake, the body weight, body condition score and muscle condition score to monitor nutritional status and any signs of progression of CKD (hypertension, proteinuria, increasing renal values [serum creatinine and urea nitrogen concentrations, symmetric dimethylarginine]) that would signal an indication for further nutritional intervention with a RD.

SUPPORTING NUTRITION BY PROMOTING ADEQUATE FOOD CONSUMPTION

To achieve the proposed benefits of RDs, cats must consume an adequate amount of diet daily. Some cats (with or without CKD) are especially selective in their food preferences. It is the responsibility of the veterinary team and the client to assure that nutritional targets are met by selecting an appropriate diet prescription, providing an ideal recommendation for calorie intake and daily food consumption, regularly monitoring body weight and body condition score, and communicating regular progress reports, including phone contact and clinic visits. The dietary transition phase can range from easy to demanding depending on the cat and the pet owner; but in any case, it essential for successful long-term treatment. Although it is true that some clients may not be sufficiently motivated to engage in this process, many committed pet owners will largely commit to these efforts. Educate the pet owner about the process and the need to sustain adequate nutrition will help promote the owner to become a partner in achieving the treatment goals.

Although many cats readily accept a gradual change to RDs, some cats do not. Often the reason for poor acceptance of RDs is inappropriate introduction of the diets. Cats often poorly accept abrupt changes in diet. The authors generally recommend a gradual introduction to the new diet over several days to weeks by progressively increasing the proportion of the RD. Progressive introduction of the diet may be achieved by gradually mixing more RD in with the old diet (starting with ~10%–20% RD) or by concurrently providing separate bowls of the old and RDs, then gradually reducing the amount of the old diet.

It also is important to not introduce the RD in inappropriate settings. Force-feeding of cats while in the veterinary hospital or when uremic/nauseated is likely to promote a dietary aversion. Long-term RDs should be introduced when the cat is feeling well and at home in a comfortable environment that is most likely to facilitate an appetite.

Impaired appetite, nausea, and vomiting are among the most common signs of CKD and uremia. If nausea or vomiting is present, it should be corrected using antiemetic therapy before exposing the cat to the new diet. Recent studies in cats have indicated that H_2-blockers (eg, famotidine, ranitidine), proton pump inhibitors (omeprazole, pantoprazole, esomeprazole), and sucralfate are unlikely to be useful in managing gastrointestinal signs of uremia in cats.[46] In contrast, antiemetic therapy is useful in managing uremic nausea and vomiting.[47] Although antiemetic drugs generally do not directly enhance appetite, they may minimize loss of food and fluids via emesis. Maropitant acts on the chemoreceptor trigger zone as well as in the gut. It has been documented in a masked placebo-controlled clinical trial to be effective in suppressing vomiting in cats with IRIS CKD stages 2 and 3.[45]

Hyporexia and anorexia are common in cats with IRIS CKD stages 3 and 4. Mirtazapine (1.87 mg per cat by mouth every 48 hours; 3.75–30 mg per dog by mouth every 24 hours) has been shown in a masked placebo-controlled crossover clinical trial to be an effective appetite stimulant in cats with CKD.[48] It significantly increased appetite, activity, and body weight in cats with CKD. In addition, it was associated with a significant decrease in vomiting.

Failure to stabilize patients at an acceptable body condition score and body weight is likely to adversely affect long-term outcomes. Placing an esophagostomy tube is indicated for cats with progressively declining body condition score and body weight despite all dietary management and pharmacologic efforts to achieve adequate nutrition. Tube feeding is a very effective and convenient way to provide food, water, and medications to cats with CKD. It is useful to stabilize or improve nutrition, clinical signs, and longevity as well as owner satisfaction. In general, tube placement is less likely to be effective when the decision to proceed is delayed until severe reduction in body condition score and body weight are present and advanced uremia and malnutrition have developed.

Owners often express a wide range of feelings about placing feeding tubes, and they may need a period of time to become comfortable with the concept. The discussion that placing a feeding tube in their cat may ultimately become necessary should generally arise early in the course of treatment of CKD. Propose that the veterinarian and pet owner shall jointly make every reasonable effort to meet the pet's nutrition needs by the methods described earlier before agreeing to place a feeding tube. This bargain with the pet owner will incentivizes them to make a determined effort to meet the cat's nutritional needs. Should they fail to meet nutritional needs after a serious effort, they are more likely to be convinced of the need to place a feeding tube.

In most patients, nutritional status can be stabilized using tube-feeding RDs. However, if a cat that has been nutritionally stable suddenly begins to lose weight and/or body condition score, a diagnostic search should be initiated for possible causes for loss of body mass, including progression of kidney disease, inflammatory conditions, and UTIs and other infections. Because loss of body mass resulting from these conditions is often difficult or impossible to restore, early recognition, diagnosis, and treatment is essential.

REFERENCES

1. Roudebush P, Polzin DJ, Ross SJ, et al. Therapies for feline chronic kidney disease. What is the evidence? J Feline Med Surg 2009;11:195–210.
2. Elliott J, Rawlings JM, Markwell PJ, et al. Survival of cats with naturally occurring chronic renal failure: effect of dietary management. J Small Anim Pract 2000;41: 235–42.
3. Ross SJ, Osborne CA, Kirk CA, et al. Clinical evaluation of dietary modification for treatment of spontaneous chronic kidney disease in cats. J Am Vet Med Assoc 2006;229:949–57.
4. Plantinga EA, Everts H, Kastelein AMC, et al. Retrospective study of the survival of cats with acquired chronic renal insufficiency offered different commercial diets. Vet Rec 2005;157:185–7.

5. Available at: www.iris-kidney.com. Accessed April 23, 2016.
6. Cupp CJ, Kerr WW. Effect of diet and body composition on life span in aging cats. Proc Nestle Purina Companion Animal Nutrition Summit: focus on gerontology. Clearwater Beach (FL), March 26–7, 2010. p. 36–42.
7. Polzin D. Chronic kidney disease. In: Ettinger S, Feldman E, editors. Textbook of veterinary internal medicine. Philadelphia: Saunders; 2010. p. 2036–67.
8. Geddes RF, Elliott J, Syme HM. The effects of feeding a renal diet on plasma fibroblast growth factor 23 concentrations in cats with stable azotemic chronic kidney disease. J Vet Intern Med 2013;27:1354–61.
9. Geddes RF, Finch NC, Syme HM, et al. The role of phosphorus in the pathology of chronic kidney disease. J Vet Emerg Crit Care 2013;23:122–33.
10. Walser M, Mitch W, Maroni DJ, et al. Should protein intake be restricted in predialysis patients? Kidney Int 1999;55:771–7.
11. Meyers T, Hostetter T. Pathophysiology of uremia. In: Brenner BM, editor. The kidney. Philadelphia: WB Saunders; 2008. p. 1681–96.
12. Brenner BM, Meyer TW, Hostetter TH. Dietary protein intake and the progressive nature of kidney disease: the role of hemodynamically mediated glomerular injury in the pathogenesis of progressive glomerular sclerosis in aging, renal ablation, and intrinsic renal disease. N Engl J Med 1982;307(11):652–9.
13. Klahr S, Levey AS, Beck GJ, et al. The effects of dietary protein restriction and blood-pressure control on the progression of chronic renal disease. N Engl J Med 1994;330:877–84.
14. Fouque D, Laville M. Low protein diets for chronic kidney disease in non-diabetic adults [review]. Cochrane Database Syst Rev 2009;(3):CD001892.
15. King JN, Tasker S, Gunn-Moore DA. Prognostic factors in cats with chronic kidney disease. J Vet Intern Med 2007;21:906–16.
16. Alfrey AC. Effect of dietary phosphate restriction on renal function and deterioration. Am J Clin Nutr 1988;47:146–52.
17. Chen X, Wei G, Jalili T, et al. The associations of plant protein intake with all-cause mortality in CKD. Am J Kidney Dis 2015;67:423–30.
18. Segev G, Bandt C, Francey T, et al. Aluminum toxicity following administration of aluminum-based phosphate binders in 2 dogs with renal failure. J Vet Intern Med 2008;22:1432–5.
19. Finch NC, Geddes RF, Syme HM. Fibroblast growth factor 23 (FGF-23) concentrations in cats with early nonazotemic chronic kidney disease (CKD) and in healthy geriatric cats. J Vet Intern Med 2013;27:227–33.
20. Adams LG, Polzin DJ, Osborne CA, et al. Influence of dietary protein/calorie intake on renal morphology and function in cats with 5/6 nephrectomy. Lab Invest 1994;70:347–57.
21. Syme HM, Markwell PJ, Pfeiffer D, et al. Survival of cats with naturally occurring chronic renal failure is related to severity of proteinuria. J Vet Intern Med 2008;20:528–35.
22. Jepson RE, Brodbelt D, Vallance C, et al. Evaluation of predictors of the development azotemia in cats. J Vet Intern Med 2009;23:806–13.
23. Carrero JJ, Stenvinkel S, Cuppari L. Etiology of the protein-energy wasting syndrome in chronic kidney disease: a consensus statement from the International Society of Renal Nutrition and Metabolism (ISRNM). J Ren Nutr 2013;23:77–90.
24. Workeneh BT, Mitch WE. Review of muscle wasting associated with chronic kidney disease. Am J Clin Nutr 2010;91(Suppl):1128S–32S.
25. Fahal IH. Uaremic sarcopenia: aetiology and implications. Nephrol Dial Transplant 2014;29:1655–65.

26. Mitch WE. Malnutrition is an unusual cause of decreased muscle mass in chronic kidney disease. J Ren Nutr 2007;17:66–9.

27. Laflamme D, Gunn-Moore D. Nutrition of ageing cats. Vet Clin Small Anim 2014; 44:761–74.

28. Obi Y, Qader H, Kovesdy C, et al. Latest consensus and update on protein-energy wasting in chronic kidney disease. Curr Opin Clin Nutr Metab Care 2015;18:254–62.

29. Chauveau P, Vendrely B, Haggan WE, et al. Body composition of patients on a very low-protein diet: a two-year survey with DEXA. J Ren Nutr 2003;13:282–7.

30. Eyre S, Attman P. Protein restriction and body composition in renal disease. J Ren Nutr 2008;18:167–86.

31. Dumler F. Body composition modifications in patients under low protein diets. J Ren Nutr 2011;21:76–81.

32. Mitch WE. Proteolytic mechanisms, not malnutrition, cause loss of muscle mass in kidney failure. J Ren Nutr 2006;16:208–11.

33. Mitch WE, Goldberg AL. Mechanisms of muscle wasting. The role of ubiquitin-proteasome pathway. N Engl J Med 1996;335:1897–905.

34. Piedimonte G, Crinelli R, Salda LD, et al. Protein degradation and apoptotic death in lymphocytes during FIV infection: activation of the ubiquitin-proteasome proteolytic system. Exp Cell Res 1999;248:381–90.

35. Deger SM, Sundell MB, Siew ED, et al. Insulin resistance and protein metabolism in chronic hemodialysis patients. J Ren Nutr 2013;23:e59–66.

36. Price SR, Gooch JL, Donaldson SK, et al. Muscle atrophy in chronic kidney disease results from abnormalities in insulin signaling. J Ren Nutr 2010;20(5S): S24–8.

37. Guarnieri G, Antonione R, Biolo G. Mechanisms of malnutrition in uremia. J Ren Nutr 2003;13:153–7.

38. Miyamoto T, Carrero JJ, Stenvinkel P. Inflammation as a risk factor and target for therapy in chronic kidney disease. Curr Opin Nephrol Hypertens 2011;20:662–8.

39. King JN, Gunn-Moore DA, Tasker S, et al. Tolerability and efficacy of benazepril in cats with chronic kidney disease. J Vet Intern Med 2006;20:1054–64.

40. Mizutani H, Koyama H, Watanabe H, et al. Evaluation of the clinical efficacy of benazepril in the treatment of chronic renal insufficiency in cats. J Vet Intern Med 2006;20:1074–9.

41. Kidder AC, Chew D. Treatment options for hyperphosphatemia in feline CKD: what's out there? J Feline Med Surg 2009;11:913–24.

42. Brown SA, Francey T, Polzin DJ, et al. The IRIS canine GN study group standard therapy subgroup: consensus recommendations for standard therapy of glomerular disease in dogs. J Vet Intern Med 2013;27(Suppl 1):S27–43.

43. Sackett DL, Stauss SE, Richardson WS. Introduction. In: Sackett DL, Stauss SE, Richardson WS, editors. Evidence-based medicine: how to practice and teach EBM. 2nd edition. Philadelphia: Churchill-Livingstone; 2005. p. 1–12.

44. Baldwin K, Bartges J, Buffington T, et al. AAHA nutritional assessment guidelines for dogs and cats. J Am Anim Hosp Assoc 2010;46(4):285–96.

45. Available at: http://www.wsava.org/sites/default/files/Recommendations%20on% 20Selecting%20Pet%20Foods.pdf.

46. McLeland SM, Lunn KF, Duncan CG, et al. Relationship among serum creatinine, serum gastrin, calcium-phosphorus product, and uremic gastropathy in cats with chronic kidney disease. J Vet Intern Med 2014;28(3):827–37.

47. Quimby JM, Brock WT, Moses K, et al. Chronic use of maropitant for the management of vomiting and inappetence in cats with chronic kidney disease: a masked placebo-controlled clinical trial. J Feline Med Surg 2015;17:692–7.
48. Quimby JM, Lunn KF. Mirtazapine as an appetite stimulant and anti-emetic in cats with chronic kidney disease: a masked placebo-controlled crossover clinical trial. Vet J 2013;197:651–5.

Controversies in Veterinary Nephrology: Renal Diets Are Indicated for Cats with International Renal Interest Society Chronic Kidney Disease Stages 2 to 4: The Con View

CrossMark

Margie A. Scherk, DVM[a],*, Dottie P. Laflamme, DVM, PhD[b]

KEYWORDS

- Feline • Chronic kidney disease • Therapeutic nutrition • Protein • Potassium
- Phosphorus • Diet • Malnutrition

KEY POINTS

- The ideal dietary nutrient composition to optimize the health of cats with chronic kidney disease (CKD) remains unclear.
- Limited research has been published regarding dietary management for cats with CKD; although some benefits were documented, there is inadequate evidence to support protein restriction.
- Phosphorus restriction seems to be of value in CKD, but inadequate data are available to determine the degree of restriction needed.
- Adequate studies have not been performed comparing the value of dietary modification with appropriate pharmaceutical interventions.
- Hypokalemia should be avoided and corrected and caloric intake to support ideal body and muscle condition should be maintained.

INTRODUCTION: PATHOPHYSIOLOGY OF FELINE CHRONIC KIDNEY DISEASES AND GOALS OF DIETARY MANAGEMENT

Three important principles to consider regarding dietary management of cats with chronic kidney disease (CKD) include (1) abnormalities in normal homeostasis produced by renal insufficiency are influenced by dietary intake, (2) the kidney is

Dr D.P. Laflamme is a consultant for Nestle Purina PetCare Company. Dr M.A. Scherk has nothing to disclose.
[a] CatsINK 4381 Gladstone Street, Vancouver, British Columbia V5N 4Z4, Canada; [b] Scientific Communications, 473 Grandma's Place, Floyd, VA 24091, USA
* Corresponding author.
E-mail address: hypurr@aol.com

Vet Clin Small Anim 46 (2016) 1067–1094
http://dx.doi.org/10.1016/j.cvsm.2016.06.007
0195-5616/16/$ – see front matter

susceptible to self-perpetuating injury, which may be influenced by dietary modification, and (3) the responses of cats with CKD to dietary or pharmaceutical management will vary dramatically and individualized therapy with appropriate follow-up are required.[1] This article considers these principles and the available evidence regarding dietary management of cats with CKD.

To understand the abnormalities in homeostasis, one must consider normal kidney functions and the impact of renal disease on those functions. The primary function of the kidney is to serve as a filter, retaining important substances and releasing toxic and unnecessary excess of metabolism into the urine. These functions can be disrupted in CKD. Etiologies of CKD include hypoxia, pyelonephritis, toxins, ureterolithiasis and nephrolithiasis, retroviral infection, morbillivirus infection, leptospirosis, glomerulonephritis, renal neoplasia, amyloidosis, and hypokalemic nephropathy, as well as congenital conditions. Unlike humans and dogs, primary glomerular disease is rare in cats; however, glomerular dysfunction may occur secondary to inflammatory conditions, (eg, immune-mediated, pancreatitis, triaditis), or lymphoma.

It is generally accepted that the ultimate/common histomorphologic endpoint in feline CKD is interstitial fibrosis.[2–4] There seem to be multiple paths to this outcome as well as wide variations in the degree of expression. It is hypothesized that chronic renal injury results in inflammation and infiltration by inflammatory cells (most commonly lymphocytes and plasma cells). This inflammation stimulates the production of profibrotic mediators (including transforming growth factor-beta, upregulation of the renin-angiotensin-aldosterone system [RAAS], transglutaminase 2, and endothelin 1), which activate matrix-producing cells and initiate fibrogenesis. Newly formed myofibroblasts and transformed tubular epithelial cells perpetuate the process. Chronic hypoxia and oxidative stress also contribute to the process.[4–6] Activation of the RAAS results in increased angiotensin II levels that result in efferent arteriolar vasoconstriction and glomerular hypertension. Excess protein in the glomerular filtrate is believed to be toxic to tubules, although it may not cause fibrosis directly; proteinuria may instead reflect decreased tubular uptake in affected kidneys.[4] Taken together, and likely with elegant processes we do not yet understand, a self-perpetuating process occurs. However, renal pathology in cats seems to follow a different trajectory compared with that in dogs.[7] Clinically, we see this as cats living much longer after a diagnosis of CKD compared with dogs; cats with CKD can live for several years.[8]

Despite potential species differences and regardless of underlying etiology, it seems that progression of CKD is inevitable, although the rate of progression varies widely between cats, occurring over months to years. Identified risk factors contributing to decreased survival time include renal azotemia,[9–11] hyperphosphatemia,[8,10,11] urine protein:creatinine ratio of greater than 0.4[10,11] or greater than 0.2,[9] decreased hemoglobin and hematocrit,[9–11] and leukocytosis.[10] Left untreated, systemic hypertension affects quality of life,[12] increases risk of target organ damage,[13] may contribute to endothelial dysfunction and arterial structural changes resulting in hypoxia,[14] and may induce glomerular hypertension and proteinuria. When appropriately treated, however, it does not seem to contribute to progression of CKD.[9,11] Similarly, urinary tract infections, despite potentially initiating the inflammatory process, are not recognized to contribute to progression.[11] Plasma calcium, bicarbonate, and potassium levels may play a role in clinical disease, but are not recognized to affect progression.

By altering the load of dietary and metabolic metabolites reaching the kidney, it is thought to be possible to alter the trajectory of the ongoing damage. Thus, the current standard of care is to feed patients with CKD protein restricted diets that are further modified to be restricted in phosphorus and sodium, and supplemented with potassium, B vitamins, antioxidants, and long-chain omega-3 fatty acids. Assuming this is appropriate for other species, does this dictum suit cats—obligatory carnivores—as well?

What is the significance of being an obligatory carnivore? Cats certainly require more protein than dogs, humans, or other omnivores do and, similar to mink, have been identified as being hypercarnivorous.[15] Cats have adapted to metabolize a native diet that is extremely high in protein (~52% of calories) and low in carbohydrate without developing ketonemia.[16–18] They readily use protein and amino acids to generate the glucose needed by their brains and cells. Yet, healthy cats are capable of dealing with a wide range of protein and carbohydrate intakes, and can metabolize carbohydrates to spare protein to a great extent, so long as their minimum protein needs are met.[19] However, like other species when protein needs are not met, cats undergo a gradual loss of lean body mass (LBM), catabolizing muscle and other lean tissues to meet the needs for protein turnover and ongoing metabolic needs. This effect may be worsened in cats with CKD, because protein catabolism is increased and synthesis decreased in other species with CKD.[20] Unknown is whether or not cats' kidneys deal with the amino acids and nitrogen metabolites derived from catabolism of LBM differently than those derived from dietary protein.

Independent of protein, does the available evidence support the need for all of the recommended nutrient modifications found in commercial "renal" diets, or would a different nutrient profile be more appropriate for cats with CKD? Is restricting phosphorus and sodium, increasing the pH, adding potassium, B vitamins, antioxidants, and essential fatty acids warranted in this species? This article attempts to address these questions nutrient, by nutrient.

DIETARY MANAGEMENT IN CHRONIC KIDNEY DISEASE
Protein

Protein restriction has been recommended for patients with kidney disease for decades.[21,22] This section explores the research evaluating protein restriction for cats with CKD, and also the implications of protein restriction in aging cats since most cats with CKD are elderly.

Much of the evidence to support the practice of protein restriction comes from rodent or canine studies, and many of these studies used diets that differed in multiple nutrients, such as phosphorus, in addition to protein. There are few studies in cats, and even fewer not confounded by multiple nutrient differences among diets tested.

Two studies have been performed in cats with induced CKD, both using a five-sixths nephrectomy model.[23–25] The Adams study evaluated diets containing either 27.6% or 51.7% protein (dry matter basis) fed over the course of 1 year. They reported that the group fed the higher protein diet had significantly higher inulin clearance, lower serum creatinine, and maintained body weight better than cats fed the lower protein diet. However, cats fed the higher protein diet developed greater renal pathology and had greater serum urea nitrogen concentrations compared with those fed the lower protein diet. Critically, however, the higher protein diet was deficient in potassium, as evidenced by more than one-half of the cats fed this diet developing clinical manifestations of hypokalemia. Hypokalemia is recognized to cause or contribute to renal dysfunction in cats.[26] Potassium was supplemented after the first 3 months of the study, but markers of renal dysfunction including urine protein excretion were notably worse in this group by this time. Other differences between diet groups included calorie intake, with cats fed the lower protein diet consuming fewer calories. Reduced calorie intake has been suggested to have a protective effect regarding kidney function.[27] Because of these confounding factors, it cannot be clearly determined if the renal pathology assessed at the end of the study was due to protein or due to other factors. A second study was conducted in cats to attempt to address this issue.[25] Using the same five-sixths nephrectomy model in cats, the study was designed to control for both protein and calorie intake. Potassium intake was adequate in all cats in this study. Cats with CKD fed the high protein, high calorie diet maintained body weight, whereas those fed the low protein diet lost weight. Markers of renal function, including glomerular filtration rate (GFR) and serum creatinine, were better in cats fed the higher protein diets although these effects did not achieve statistical significance. There were no effects from diet on urine protein/creatinine ratios. Renal histopathology showed no effects from protein intake on tubular lesions, fibrosis or cellular infiltrate, and a mild, nonsignificant increase in mesangial matrix accumulation. However, greater calorie intake was associated with significantly greater cellular infiltrate and tubular lesions, with a nonsignificant trend toward increased fibrosis. Overall, the results of this study showed no association between higher protein intake and renal lesions, proteinuria, or decreased GFR, which tended to refute the findings of the Adams study. Given this, and because the diet model and study design were similar, one must wonder if the differences in results were due to some differences in the diets. Between the 2 studies, differences included protein sources, fat content, and changes in cats' body weight, but the most obvious difference was the inadequate potassium intake and resulting hypokalemia in the Adams study.

No clinical studies in cats with naturally occurring CKD have been conducted where only dietary protein levels were compared although several studies evaluated protein restricted "renal" diets in cats with spontaneous CKD (**Table 1**). Two of these were either retrospective studies or nonrandomized studies. In the first of these, 50 cats with CKD were entered into the study.[28] Among these, 29 cats were offered dry or canned commercial protein-restricted, phosphorus-restricted renal diets. For the other 21 cats, the renal diet was not fed either because the cat refused the diet or the owner refused the diet. This group was kept on commercial maintenance diets. Phosphorus binders were used as needed to control hyperphosphatemia in cats fed the renal diet, with 34% using a phosphorus binder, but were not offered for cats fed the maintenance diets. The combination of renal diet with phosphorus binders resulted in this group living longer and having lower phosphate and parathyroid hormone (PTH) concentrations. A retrospective study compared results in cats with CKD fed either commercial protein and phosphorus-restricted diets from several manufacturers, or other diets including commercial maintenance diets.[29] Cats fed the renal diets survived longer compared with those fed maintenance diets.

Two randomized, controlled prospective clinical evaluating diets for cats with spontaneous CKD also have been published. The first of these included 35 cats randomly divided into uneven groups so that 25 cats were offered a low-protein renal diet and 10 cats received a control maintenance diet for 24 weeks.[30] Cats fed the maintenance diet lost weight, showed increases in serum urea nitrogen and creatinine, and greater clinical deterioration compared with those fed the renal diet. In a subsequent study, 45 cats with International Renal Interest Society (IRIS) stage 2 or 3 were randomly assigned to a renal or maintenance diet and followed for 2 years.[31] As in previous studies, cats fed the renal diet showed greater survival. Unfortunately, none of these studies specifically evaluated protein. Therefore, although these studies are often used to support the feeding of protein-restricted diets, one must consider the many differences among the diets. At this time, there is inadequate evidence to support the need to restrict protein in cats with CKD.

Table 1
Summary of interventional studies evaluating dietary effects on chronic kidney disease in cats

Reference	Type of Study	Type of Subjects	Number Enrolled	Nutrients vs Control	Duration	Key Dietary Effects	Comments
Adams et al,[23] 1993; Adams et al,[24] 1994	Randomized, controlled	5/6 Nephrectomy-induced CKD	22	Protein	12 mo	High protein led to hypokalemia, increased GFR, proteinuria, and renal injury	Reduced calorie intake with low protein and potassium depletion in high protein group confounded study
Finco et al,[25] 1998	Randomized, controlled	5/6 Nephrectomy-induced CKD	28	Protein, calories	12 mo	No effect from protein; high calorie intake led to increased renal tubular injury	Minimal effects from any dietary treatment in this study
Ross et al,[47] 1982	Randomized, controlled	5/6 Nephrectomy-induced CKD	16	Phosphorus	≤343 d	High phos led to increased serum [phos] PTH and renal pathology	No diet effects on mean serum urea N or creatinine
Buranakarl et al,[65] 2004	Sequential cross-over	Healthy cats + 2 models of induced CKD	21	Sodium	7 d per diet	Low Na activated RAAS and induced hypokalemia; High Na increased GFR in CKD cats	Short-term study
Theisen et al,[82] 1997	Randomized, controlled clinical	Natural stable CKD	11	Potassium supplement	6 mo	Increased muscle potassium, improved acid-base status with potassium gluconate vs sodium gluconate	Supplement given on top of potassium adequate diet in normokalemic cats had no effect on markers of renal function

(continued on next page)

Table 1
(continued)

Reference	Type of Study	Type of Subjects	Number Enrolled	Nutrients vs Control	Duration	Key Dietary Effects	Comments
Barber et al,[53] 1999	Nonrandomized clinical	Natural stable CKD	23	Renal diet with multiple nutrient modifications ± Phos binder vs maintenance diet	≤147 d	Untreated group showed increased serum creatinine, urea nitrogen, phosphate and PTH	Unable to assess nutrient effect because study compared renal diet + Phos binders as needed vs maintenance diet; control diet high protein but low calorie
Elliott et al,[28] 2000	Nonrandomized clinical	Natural stable CKD	50	Renal diet with multiple nutrient modifications ± Phos binder vs various diets	5 y	Treated cats had reduced serum phosphate, PTH and longer survival	Biased by design: owners could choose renal diet or not; clinical improvement with renal diet and Phos binders, but unable to determine which components are important
Harte et al,[30] 1994	Randomized, controlled clinical	Natural stable CKD	35	Renal diet with multiple nutrient modifications vs maintenance diet	24 wk	Renal diet reduced serum urea nitrogen, creatinine, phosphate	Clinical improvement with renal diet, but unable to determine which components are important

Study	Study type	Population	N	Comparison	Duration	Results	Comments
Ross et al,[31] 2006	Randomized, controlled clinical	Natural stable CKD, IRIS stage 2, 3	45	Renal diet with multiple nutrient modifications vs maintenance diet	2 y	More uremic episodes and renal-related death in maintenance group. Serum urea N and creatinine higher for maintenance group from beginning, no change over time	Clinical improvement with renal diet, but unable to determine which components are important
Geddes et al,[54] 2013	Nonrandomized, retrospective	Natural stable CKD, IRIS stage 2, 3	44	Renal diet with multiple nutrient modifications vs various diets	28–56 d	Renal diet reduced phosphate, PTH, FGF-23 in CKD cats with hyperphosphatemia	No effect of either diet on creatinine; effect on renal diet greater in cats with existing hyperphosphatemia
Plantinga et al,[29] 2005	Retrospective, nonrandomized	Natural stable CKD	321	Renal diets with multiple nutrient modifications vs various diets	NA	All renal diets resulted in prolonged median survival vs various diets	Compared multiple commercial renal diets vs various diets; suggested that diet highest in long chain fatty acids associated with best response

Abbreviations: CKD, chronic kidney disease; FGF-23, fibroblast growth factor-23; GFR, glomerular filtration rage; IRIS, International Renal Interest Society; NA, not applicable; phos, phosphorus; PTH, parathyroid hormone; RAAS, renin-angiotensin-aldosterone system.

It has been suggested that protein restriction will reduce proteinuria in patients with CKD. This is based on pathophysiologic reasoning that proteinuria damages tubules and results in interstitial inflammation.[4,32,33] Because proteinuria is a recognized negative prognostic factor in cats with CKD, this could be important. Studies have evaluated reduction in proteinuria and impact on quality of life in naturally occurring feline CKD using pharmacologic agents: angiotensin-converting enzyme inhibitors[10,12] and angiotensin receptor blocker.[34] However, there is very limited evidence to support a benefit from restriction of dietary protein. There are 2 studies in dogs with X-linked hereditary nephropathies showing a reduction in proteinuria with dietary protein restriction,[35,36] but no studies evaluating protein restriction on quality of life or survival in dogs with glomerular disease. In cats with surgically induced CKD fed protein restricted diets that caused hypokalemia, proteinuria was significantly greater than in cats fed a low-protein diet.[24] However, once potassium supplementation was initiated, proteinuria began to decrease, returning to near baseline levels after several months. In another study using the same experimental model of CKD, a high protein, potassium-replete diet was not associated with an increase in proteinuria.[25] Likewise, when cats with naturally occurring stage 2 and 3 CKD were fed a protein-restricted renal diet or maintenance diet, there was no difference in proteinuria.[31] Thus, the evidence does not support a role for dietary protein restriction for the management of proteinuria in CKD cats.

The goal of dietary management in any disease condition is to provide balanced nutritional support for the patient while also addressing the clinical signs or reducing ongoing pathology from the disease. Given this, one must consider also the potential detrimental effects from protein-restricted diets in aging cats. Cats are obligate carnivores and have a basal protein requirement that is considerably greater than many other species, including dogs. In healthy subjects, even marginally inadequate protein intake contributes to reduced protein turnover and loss of LBM over time, whereas increased protein intake can result in increased LBM.[37,38] Loss of LBM as a result of aging or catabolic diseases increases the risks of morbidity and mortality. In other species with CKD, endogenous protein synthesis is decreased and catabolism increased, and mortality in CKD patients is related to loss of muscle mass.[20]

It is common for aging cats and cats with CKD to experience a loss of body weight and LBM.[39–42] In cats with CKD, lower body weight is associated with increased mortality[8,42]; thus prevention or reversal of loss may be a reasonable goal as part of patient management. To date, there are no controlled studies showing that prevention of loss of body weight or LBM extends survival in CKD cats. However, in healthy aging cats, preservation of body weight and LBM was associated with reduced risk for mortality.[41] Other research showed that increased dietary protein intake helps to slow or reduce the age-associated loss of LBM in cats.[43] In that study, research cats (aged 7–17 years) fed lower protein diets (7.5–10.4 g protein/100 Kcal metabolizable energy) lost weight over the 12 month study, whereas those fed 12.75 g protein/100 Kcal metabolizable energy were better able to maintain body weight. Further, although initial age had a significant impact on the amount of protein intake needed to maintain LBM, cats fed more protein lost less LBM over time.[43] Given that most cats with CKD are older cats, this questions the relative value of protein restriction in these patients. Other factors in patients with CKD that can influence loss of LBM include energy intake and metabolic acidosis. These issues are addressed in separate sections within this paper.

Based on the available evidence, protein restriction per se is not warranted in cats with CKD. If a commercial renal diet is fed for its other benefits, it is recommended to select a higher protein option. It is important to monitor for adequate intake and for loss of body weight and LBM. A muscle mass score, such as that recommended by the World Small Animal Veterinary Association (www.wsava.org/guidelines/global-nutrition-guidelines) should be used to monitor changes. Should a decline be apparent, consideration should be given to feeding a higher protein diet and addressing other renal pathologies through use of available medications.

Phosphorus

Phosphorus retention and secondary hyperparathyroidism are common complications of feline CKD.[44] In healthy animals, phosphorus balance is controlled predominantly via the kidneys. In CKD, phosphorus excretion is compromised, leading to an increase in PTH concentrations, decreased production of active 1,25-dihydroxyvitamin D, and increased fibroblast growth factor 23 (FGF-23), all of which help to increase phosphorus excretion. These mechanisms result in normalization of serum phosphorus concentrations in early CKD. As CKD progresses, serum phosphorus concentrations increase, despite continued increases in PTH and FGF-23. In cats with CKD, serum phosphorus concentrations are inversely associated with survival.[8,10,11,45] Several experimental studies have documented that controlling the increases in serum phosphorus, PTH and FGF-23 resulted in reduced renal pathology, morbidity and mortality in remnant kidney models of CKD (in rats,[46] cats[47–50]).

Dietary phosphate restriction was evaluated in cats with induced CKD.[47] In that study, cats were fed diets with either 0.42% (dry basis) or 1.56% (dry basis) phosphorus for 65 to 343 days. Serum phosphorus and PTH concentrations were increased in cats fed the higher phosphorus diet, but neither diet had a measureable impact on progression of renal function during the study. However, kidneys from cats fed the higher phosphorus diet showed mineralization, fibrosis, and mononuclear cell infiltration, whereas those from cats fed the restricted phosphorus diet showed none of these changes[47] Subsequent studies in experimental models have shown similarly that renal injury is reduced with phosphorus restriction independent of dietary protein content.[48,51,52]

No clinical studies have been performed in cats with spontaneous CKD to evaluate dietary phosphorus restriction alone, although several studies evaluated phosphorus-restricted "renal" diets in cats with spontaneous CKD. These studies were reviewed previously in the protein section, and showed that cats fed the phosphorus-restricted diets had lower serum phosphorus and PTH concentrations, and lived longer compared with cats fed maintenance diets without phosphate binders or restriction.[28,29,31] An additional short-term, nonrandomized study evaluated a renal diet and phosphate binders (as needed) to control plasma phosphate and PTH concentrations in cats with CKD.[53] Plasma phosphate, creatinine, and urea nitrogen all increased over time in untreated cats and were reduced significantly in cats receiving the renal diet and phosphate binders. Another small, short (4–8 weeks), nonrandomized, retrospective study that also evaluated renal diets showed that hyperphosphatemic CKD cats fed a renal diet showed significant reductions in plasma phosphate, PTH, and FGF-23.[54] In CKD cats with normal serum phosphorus, the renal diet resulted in a reduction in FGF-23, but no change in phosphate or PTH. In neither group was a significant change in creatinine seen. Unfortunately, none of these studies evaluated differences in phosphorus alone. Therefore, although these studies are often used to support the feeding of phosphorus-restricted diets, one must consider the many differences among the diets.

In addition to the studies on dietary phosphorus restriction, 1 study evaluated the use of a phosphate binder in cats with CKD, using a remnant kidney model.[44] In this study, cats with stage 1 or 2 CKD fed a maintenance diet with a phosphorus binder had significantly lower serum phosphorus and PTH compared with those fed the same diet but without the phosphorus binder. The beneficial effects on serum phosphorus and PTH persisted throughout the 9-month study. There were no differences in serum creatinine, blood urea nitrogen, or GFR by time or treatment during the study.

The evidence supports a real benefit to controlling phosphorus, but many questions remain. Is there an optimum dietary concentration for renal diets? This question is further complicated by the fact that phosphorus availability can differ greatly based on the composition of the diet. For example, phosphorus from vegetarian diets is less bioavailable compared with meat-based diets, and phosphates from inorganic sources are more bioavailable compared with those from organic or meat sources.[55,56] Is restriction of dietary phosphorus superior, in terms of cat well-being and progression of disease, compared with phosphate binders? Do these differ based on stage of CKD progression? Because it seems that PTH and FGF-23 are increased before serum phosphorus increases, should these substances be used as the markers advising the use of phosphate binding or restriction? If so, what would be the appropriate reference value? Given the numerous unanswered questions, at this time, no specific guidelines can be provided for optimum dietary phosphorus content. Dietary phosphate restriction or phosphate binders should be tailored to the individual patient to achieve a serum phosphorus concentration within the low normal range, as recommended by IRIS (http://iris-kidney.com/guidelines/recommendations.aspx).

Sodium

The main rationale for dietary sodium restriction is to manage hypertension. Hypertension is a common finding in cats with CKD and may contribute to the progression of renal disease.[13,57] Hypertension seems to cause proteinuria, with a direct association between degrees of hypertension, proteinuria, and progression of renal lesions in dogs with experimentally induced renal failure.[58] Although similar data are not available in cats, proteinuria is a negative prognostic factor in cats with CKD.[9,59]

Limited evidence addresses the link, if any, between dietary sodium and blood pressure in cats. A single case report indicated that a cat with idiopathic hypertension had been fed a high sodium diet and that sodium restriction, along with pharmaceutical management, was used to manage the case successfully.[60] However, no attempt was made to isolate any effects of sodium in that case. Multiple studies in cats have since shown no impact of dietary sodium ranging between 0.3% and 1.3% of diet dry matter on systemic blood pressure.[61–64] On the contrary, restriction of sodium has been shown to activate the RAAS and may actually lead to progression of vascular, renal and cardiac lesions.[13,65] Further, low sodium intake (50 mg/kg body weight) increased urinary potassium loss,[65] which can contribute to renal injury.

High sodium intake has been suggested to cause renal damage independent of effects on blood pressure.[62] In a study that included various groups of cats including 6 with mild renal insufficiency, a diet providing 1.2% sodium was associated with increases in serum creatinine and urea nitrogen during a 12-week trial.[62] Other studies did not confirm this and, instead, showed no adverse effects from sodium at similar dietary amounts in studies lasting 6 months to 2 years.[63,64] In a 6-month study that included 9 cats with mild renal insufficiency, there was no impact from dietary sodium (0.55% vs 1.1% diet dry matter).[63] None of these studies reported adverse effects from high sodium intake on urine protein/creatinine ratios. On the contrary, the data showed numerical but nonsignificant decreases in urine protein/creatinine ratios with the higher sodium intakes.[63,65]

Activation of the RAAS and increases in plasma aldosterone concentrations are recognized as a contributing factor to ongoing renal damage.[66–68] This may be associated with the increase in oxidative stress and increased secretion of inflamma-tory mediators recognized to occur in response to elevations in aldosterone and RAAS.[69,70] Although species-specific differences do exist regarding the link between RAAS and renal injury, aldosterone is increased in cats with CKD and activation of the RAAS does promote ongoing renal injury in cats with CKD.[65,67,68,71] In cats with exper-imentally induced CKD, plasma aldosterone was increased over healthy cats regard-less of dietary sodium intake and was greatest in cats fed the lowest sodium diet.[65] Further, low dietary sodium was recognized as a risk factor for the development of CKD in cats.[72] Therefore, excessive restriction of dietary sodium, which stimulates the RAAS, should be avoided in cats with CKD.

What constitutes "excessive restriction" is, unfortunately, poorly defined. Among the studies cited, dietary sodium ranged from approximately 0.33% to approximately 1.3% sodium on a dry matter basis. All of these are in excess of the suggested min-imum requirements for normal adult cats,[73] yet the lower intakes were associated with inappropriate kaliuresis, reduced the GFR, and increased aldosterone concentrations in CKD cats.[65] Whereas 1 report suggests possible detrimental effects from sodium at 1.2% of the diet in cats with existing CKD, other studies refute this finding. Therefore, we conclude that the evidence does not support feeding sodium-restricted diets to cats with CKD.

Fatty acids

Prostaglandins (PG) play an important role in renal function and sodium and water bal-ance. By altering vascular tone in the kidneys, PG affect renal blood flow and GFR[74,75] Specific PG production can be influenced by alterations in dietary fatty acids. Diets rich in long-chain omega-3 fatty acids will yield less PGE2 and thromboxane A-2, compared with diets rich omega-6 fatty acids. PGE2 helps to maintain renal blood flow and is generally considered to be beneficial. However, thromboxane A-2 de-creases renal blood flow and GFR, a potentially detrimental effect. In humans, mice, and dogs, PG production is increased in CKD, although this has not been documented in cats.

In remnant kidney model dogs, omega-3 supplementation, (specifically eicosapen-taenoic acid [EPA] and docosahexaenoic acid) at 15% of the diet, resulted in decreased intraglomerular hypertension, decreased proteinuria, maintenance of GFR, and increased survival.[76,77] Also, the dogs fed the EPA and docosahexaenoic acid–enhanced diet had decreased renal lesions relative to those fed omega-6 poly-unsaturated fatty acid–enhanced diet. Similar data are not available for cats; however, these researchers did evaluate the impact of omega-3 and omega-6 fatty acids on renal function in healthy cats. Both renal blood flow and GFR were increased in cats fed the diet rich in omega-3 fatty acids.[78]

The amount of omega-3 polyunsaturated fatty acid that is most effective for reducing inflammation is unknown in different species and may also depend on the degree and type of disease. Although omega-6 fatty acids are essential, excessive di-etary omega-6 levels and a very high omega-6:omega-3 is suggested to contribute to or promote cardiovascular disease, cancer, autoimmune, and inflammatory diseases in humans.[79] Brown[5] reported benefits of supplementing both omega-6:omega-3 polyunsaturated fatty acids at 5:1 and antioxidants (vitamin E, carotenoids, and lutein) on reducing the rate of decline of GFR in a remnant kidney model with older Beagles.

One retrospective study compared survival of cats with CKD eating maintenance di-ets with those eating 1 of 7 commercially available renal diets. The renal diet associ-ated with longest survival had the highest EPA concentration.[29] However, owing to the retrospective nature of the study, lack of consistency in management between participating practitioners and clients, and other differences in the diets, causality could not be established.

Recent evidence has been presented[80] prospectively evaluating serum fatty acids in cats with IRIS stages 2 to 4 CKD. Cats were fed either a renal diet or a maintenance diet and were compared with age-matched healthy cats fed the maintenance diet. No differences were found in serum EPA or docosahexaenoic acid levels between any of the 3 groups, suggesting in this small study that feeding a renal diet does not provide benefit through increased blood omega-3 concentrations.

To date all evidence is circumstantial for benefit of fatty acids in feline CKD. Given that cats typically do not develop glomerular disease, they may not benefit from omega-3 fatty acids. On the other hand, because proteinuria seems to be a significant risk factor in cats with CKD, and omega-3 fatty acids may reduce proteinuria in other species, additional research is warranted to determine if cats would benefit from omega-3 fatty acids.

Potassium

Hypokalemia occurs in 20% to 30% of cats with CKD. However, clinical hypokalemia develops only after there is depletion of body stores of potassium or when extracellular potassium is redistributed into cells, such as with metabolic alkalosis.[81] Because CKD is often associated with metabolic acidosis, which causes potassium to be shifted out of the cells and into the plasma, developing hypokalemia may be masked until body stores are depleted. In 1 study of cats with CKD and normal serum potassium, muscle potassium content was low.[82] Therefore, the incidence of subclinical potassium depletion in cats with CKD is not known.

The gain or loss of potassium is influenced by diet, but also by the RAAS, and by alterations in renal tubular resorption. Experimentally induced chronic metabolic acidosis can cause potassium depletion and hypokalemia.[81,83] Multiple studies in cats fed acidifying diets showed that these lower serum potassium concentrations and increase the risk for development of hypokalemia.[26,81,84–86] Further, acidifying diets that were also low in potassium reduced GRF by 20% in healthy cats,[84] and induced renal failure in 3 of 9 previously healthy young cats.[26,85] The low potassium, acidifying diets also resulted in a reduction in plasma renin activity and increase in aldosterone, which tended to return to normal with potassium supplementation.[84] Supplementation of potassium reduced serum creatinine in 1 group of hypokalemic cats with increased creatinine concentrations, and restored GFR in a different study, confirming a link with renal function.[81,84] It was suggested that the effects of acidosis and potassium depletion might be additive in their adverse effects on the kidneys.[84] Independent of acid–base balance, another study that was designed to evaluate the impact of protein restriction in cats with induced CKD identified worsened renal function in cats fed a potassium-depleting diet.[23] Four of the 7 cats fed this diet developed hypokalemia.

Clinical studies evaluating potassium supplementation in cats with naturally occurring CKD are lacking. The only published study in cats with CKD recruited only cats with normal serum potassium and fed all cats a diet with abundant potassium.[82] They found no benefit to additional potassium supplementation in this very small study. However, among all 7 cats provided with supplemental potassium gluconate, GRF increased or remained stable during the 6-month study compared with only 3 of the 4 treated with sodium gluconate. Likewise, serum creatinine remained stable and serum urea nitrogen decreased 8.3% in the potassium treated group, whereas creatinine increased by 8.3% and serum urea nitrogen increased by 17.5% in the other group.[82]

Based on the available evidence, provision of adequate potassium in a nonacidifying diet is important for renal function. However, because hyperkalemia occasionally occurs in cats with CKD, each patient must be assessed individually and there are insufficient data upon which to make a specific recommendation regarding potassium supplementation for cats with CKD. As potassium will shift in or out of cells based on changes in acid–base, in is critical to address acid–base status before assessing potassium status.

Acid–Base Balance

Metabolic acidosis is a common complication from CKD. In healthy animals, kidneys serve as the major homeostatic control point for maintaining acid–base balance. In response to acidosis, healthy kidneys increase net reabsorption of bicarbonate and increase secretion of hydrogen ions. In CKD, these homeostatic mechanisms fail, resulting in pronounced acidosis in 53% to 80% of cats with CKD.[22,87] In addition, acidosis may cause or contribute to decreased renal function or progression of CKD either directly, or through potassium wasting.[84,88] Healthy cats fed a low potassium, acidifying diet developed negative potassium balance, metabolic acidosis and decreased renal function.[84] Whether this was due to the potassium depletion or the acidosis could not be determined from that study.

Among the important adverse effects caused by acidosis are anorexia, nausea, vomiting, lethargy, weakness, and weight loss as well as increased protein catabolism, decreased protein synthesis, and loss of LBM, most of which may be improved by correction of acid–base balance.[22,89,90] In human CKD patients, loss of muscle mass is linked with greater mortality.[20] Glucocorticoids, insulin, insulinlike growth factor 1, and PTH all play important roles in the body's response to acidosis, as reviewed by Franch.[90] Release of calcium carbonate from bone to buffer the acid results in an increase in renal calcium excretion and negative calcium balance. Acidosis-induced activation of the ubiquitin–proteosome proteolytic system and branched-chain ketoacid dehydrogenase in muscle are part of the homeostatic mechanism that contribute to negative nitrogen balance and loss of muscle mass. Acidosis also seems to impair insulin signaling functions through its effect on phosphoinositide 3-kinase, resulting in increased protein degradation and loss of LBM.[91] In healthy rats, induced acidosis resulted in at 70% increase in proteolysis and a 145% increase in amino acid oxidation.[92] These changes would not only result in loss of LBM, but could generate more byproducts of protein oxidation including urea nitrogen and potential uremic toxins.

Increased intake of meat and animal proteins can contribute to acidosis, unless the diet has buffering agents added to counteract this. Commercial renal diets for cats and dogs typically are both protein restricted and have appropriate buffering agents as well as other nutrient modifications. This again raises the question as to whether protein restriction per se is actually beneficial in feline CKD, or if benefits attributed to protein restriction are actually due to other dietary factors including pH buffering.

Can simply correcting acid–base imbalance reduce or prevent the loss of LBM or slow the progression of CKD? Experimental evidence in rats suggests this to be true, but results vary depending on the experimental model.[20] In human patients, retrospective studies have shown clear associations between acidosis and increased mortality in CKD.[20] As cited in de Brito-Ashurst,[93] several short-term trials in CKD patients receiving dialysis showed that correction of acidosis resulted in normalized protein catabolism and improved markers of nutritional status. A 2-year prospective, controlled clinical trial was conducted in nondialysis human CKD patients with both groups receiving the same standard care but 1 group also receiving bicarbonate supplementation.[93] Of the 67 patients in the control group, 17 progressed to end-stage renal failure within the first year compared with none in the treatment group. During the second year, creatinine clearance progressively deteriorated in the remaining patients in the control group but not in the treatment group. Additionally, the bicarbonate-treated group was able to consume more protein, showed an increase in normalized protein nitrogen appearance (a marker of nitrogen balance), and increased LBM as assessed by mid-arm muscle circumference.[93] Even subtle differences in acid–base balance can influence protein balance. In a small cross-over study in human CKD patients undergoing peritoneal dialysis, adjusting the arterial pH to either the high normal (pH 7.44) or low normal (7.37) had a significant impact on net nitrogen balance, serum urea nitrogen, and total body protein synthesis.[94]

At this time, no data in cats address the potential benefit of independently controlling acidosis on LBM, protein metabolism, or progression of CKD. However, clinical studies with "renal" diets designed with an alkalinizing effect as well as other nutrient modifications have shown positive benefits when fed to cats with CKD.[29,31] It has been suggested that the need to provide therapy to maintain normal acid–base balance may increase if cats with CKD are fed protein-restricted diets,[22] yet a comparative evaluation showed no incremental benefit of higher dietary base excess among commercial renal diets.[29] Further research is needed to better define both the role of alkalinization and the optimum amount to address acid–base imbalance in CKD.

Although the evidence supports the need to correct metabolic acidosis in CKD cats, data on which to create specific treatment and monitoring parameters are lacking. Current IRIS guidelines suggest that blood bicarbonate or TCO_2 should be maintained in the range of 16 to 24 mmol/L once the patient is stabilized and hydrated. If needed, potassium citrate or sodium bicarbonate should be supplemented to effect.

Energy Intake, Loss of Body Weight, and Body Condition

Studies of healthy aging cats, identify a decline in feline digestive capability with increasing age.[39,95,96] Both fat digestion and protein digestion tend to decrease in cats more than 12 years of age.[39] Many otherwise healthy geriatric cats have increased requirements for calories and protein owing to digestive and metabolic inefficiencies.[39,97–99] Maintaining weight and body condition in nonobese cats prolongs lifespan.[41] Cats diagnosed with CKD may live for many years.[8,10] Because most cats with CKS are older, these observations in healthy aging cats must be considered when considering dietary management for CKD patients.

Weight loss, with loss of muscle and LBM, is common among healthy aging cats.[98] Sarcopenia, the age-associated loss of LBM, occurs slowly over many years. Insufficient dietary protein intake can exacerbate LBM loss, especially in aging cats.[43] Loss of body weight also tends to occur slowly in geriatric cats unless associated with disease. Loss of body fat tends to occur much later in life, and is a predictor of mortality. Maintaining body weight and LBM seems to reduce the risk for morbidity and mortality in aging cats. Cachexia is the more aggressive loss of LBM and body mass that occurs secondary to disease, especially neoplasia, heart failure and kidney failure. Although dietary management alone cannot prevent or reverse sarcopenia or cachexia, inadequate calorie or protein intake can worsen it.[43,100] In healthy adult cats, 32% to 34% of calories from protein seems to be adequate to maintain LBM.[38,99] Limited research suggests that apparently healthy geriatric cats may need more than this, although no published studies have addressed this question in cats with CKD.[43]

Thin body condition, as well as poor muscle condition and weight loss, are common in cats with CKD with 2 of the most consistent findings among cats with CKD being inappetance and weight loss.[42,101–103] Weight loss usually begins before a diagnosis of CKD is made.[39,102,104] Retrospective evaluation of the medical records of IRIS staged CKD cats showed a weight loss of 8.9% in the 12 months before diagnosis of CKD but also showed that this weight loss began up to 3 years earlier.[42] and increased in severity after diagnosis and initiation of treatment.[42] This is similar to the data reported by Perez-Camargo[39] in colony cats. Among cats dying from CKD, median body weight loss began about 2.5 years before death, accelerating as the disease progressed.[39] How much of that weight loss was related to the condition and how much related to diet composition or preference, nausea, inappetence, and other factors, is unknown and would be difficult to parse out. In 1 retrospective study, cats with body weights below the median (4.2 kg) at time of diagnosis of CKD had a significantly shorter survival time after diagnosis.[42] In a different study, sustained weight loss occurred in at least 67% of cats with CKD. Those that lost weight had a median survival time of 401 days compared with 771 days for all cats.[8] These data suggest that preventing or minimizing weight loss in CKD cats by improving palatability and ensuring adequate consumption of calories and protein might prolong lifespans.

In other species, loss of LBM in CKD patients is associated with increased morbidity and mortality. This loss seems to be due, at least in part, to inappropriately increased muscle protein catabolism coupled with reduced protein synthesis.[20] Compared with healthy human patients, those with CKD had a 27% to 37% reduction in synthesis of muscle proteins.[20] Even small but persistent imbalances between protein synthesis and degradation cause substantial protein loss over time. Although simply providing more dietary protein will not eliminate the CKD-stimulated protein loss, reducing protein intake may accelerate the loss.

Another important factor that may increase the loss of LBM is metabolic acidosis.[20,92,105] Metabolic acidosis secondary to CKD results in loss of muscle protein predominantly through stimulation of catabolism. Buffering the diet to correct acidosis decreases the protein degradation, stimulates protein synthesis, and decreased loss of LBM.[20,88,90,105] Increasing dietary protein intake may also aid in acid–base balance because protein provides the ammonia that allows for renal excretion of acidic hydrogen ions via ammonium.[106] Finally, a critical factor influencing loss of body weight and LBM is calorie intake. Regardless of the macronutrient balance in the diet, inadequate calorie intake will contribute to loss of weight, LBM, and fat mass. Poor intake is a common finding reported in cats with CKD.

Exact energy requirements for patients with CKD cannot be calculated owing to considerable individual variability. The average geriatric cat requires more calories per unit body weight compared with middle aged cats, primarily owing to difficulties with digestion and metabolism. Approximately 33% of apparently healthy cats older than 12 have a reduced ability to digest fat and about 20% of cats older than 14 have trouble digesting protein.[39] Cats with illness that may influence their metabolic efficiency, such as diabetes mellitus, hyperthyroidism, or CKD, will likely have further increases in needs. The most appropriate way to determine if an individual patient is consuming adequate calories is to track actual intake and weight changes: cats that are losing weight are not consuming enough calories.

Getting adequate calories into cats with reduced appetites can be difficult. This can be particularly difficult when attempting to feed a reduced protein food, because cats generally prefer higher protein diets. Several feeding management approaches to consider are listed in **Table 2**. To reduce the risk of development of a diet aversion, it is always preferred to stabilize and hydrate patients before introducing them to a new diet and to introduce it to them in a familiar environment, rather than in the hospital setting. If it is deemed appropriate to introduce a commercial renal diet, 1 option is to provide samples from several manufacturers, including both dry and wet foods, and allow the cat to select what it finds most palatable. Because most cats with CKD

Table 2	
Feeding management recommendations to increase calorie intake in cats with CKD	
Stabilize patient before introducing a new diet.	Introducing a new diet while the patient is feeling ill or is stressed from being hospitalized, there is a greater likelihood that an aversion to the food will form and the food will be rejected.
Introduce any new food gradually	Each day, provide the cat with the new food in its old bowl and the old food in a new bowl. Once the new food is being at least partly consumed, gradually decrease the amount of the old food and increase the amount of the new food offered. Transitions can occur in as little as 1 wk, or take up to a month.
Provide a choice of wet and dry foods	Some cats have an aversion to either dry or wet food, so should receive the type of food they prefer.
Provide a choice of foods from different manufacturers	Although all pet food companies strive to make their foods palatable, individual cats may choose those from 1 maker over another. This is also an approach to consider if a patient stops eating 1 brand and seeks variety.
Consider access to the bowl	Many cats with chronic kidney disease have concurrent osteoarthritis. Raising the food and water bowls several inches can make eating and drinking less painful. If food bowls are on raised surfaces, consider providing ramps or other access aids. Wider lower bowls that don't interfere with whiskers may also be considered
Offer palatable foods	If a patient refuses all options of the veterinary preferred diet, offer foods that the cat prefers and manage the disease via pharmaceutical options
Appetite stimulants and feeding tubes	Appetite stimulants (eg, cyproheptadine 1 mg orally every 12 h, mirtazapine 2 mg orally every 48 h) can be used very short term, but should not be relied on for long-term management. If voluntary intake is inadequate, placement of a permanent, large-bore feeding tube should be strongly considered.

are geriatric, many tips on feeding geriatric cats and providing an appropriate environment also would apply to CKD cats and may help with food intake.[98,107,108] Appetite stimulants (eg, mirtazapine 2 mg orally every 48 hours) can be used as a short-term adjunct to feeding management.[109] As with all cats, it is important to monitor food intake and changes in body weight so that necessary adjustments can be made. If intake remains poor, feeding tubes should be strongly considered.

Water

In healthy cats with access to water, drinking increases or decreases as needed to maintain hydration. Drinking water intake ranges from about 100 to 150 mL per cat per day when cats eat dry food to as little as 5 mL/kg per day[110] or even no water at all with very high moisture diets.[111–113] Cats with CKD will often consume considerably more water than healthy cats but, owing to excess losses, may become dehydrated.

Water is essential to perfuse tissues with oxygen and nutrient carrying and waste scavenging mechanisms. Dehydration may contribute to renal ischemia and deterioration of kidney function by compromising renal blood flow. The clinical consequences of dehydration include all of the manifestations of uremia owing to concentration of uremic toxins, as well as constipation. Rehydration aids in acid–base and electrolyte homeostasis and dilutes uremic toxins. The most physiologic route to maintain hydration is through increasing water ingestion. Adding water to the food, offering flavored liquids, installing a pet fountain, and ensuring that the water is fresh may make other methods unnecessary. Dividing the daily energy requirement into multiple small meals was shown to result in increased water intake in healthy cats in 1 study,[114] and ad libitum feeding was associated with significantly greater water intake in a different study.[115] Feeding canned foods may aid with hydration. Cats eating 100% wet food consumed twice as much water than when they ate dry only, retained more water suggesting improved hydration, and had larger volumes and less concentrated urine.[111–113,116] Therefore, when acceptable to both owner and cat, feeding canned food may be preferred for cats with CKD.

Controlled, randomized studies assessing the efficacy of fluid therapy in the treatment and ongoing management of CKD in cats are lacking. However, with an impaired ability to concentrate urine, despite polydipsia, exogenous fluids are required both to correct dehydration as well as to maintain hydration and euvolemia in IRIS stages 3 and 4 as well as in acute on chronic crises. Discussion of types of fluids, routes, amounts, and frequency of administration is beyond the scope of this nutrition article.

Other Nutrients

Consistent with studies in human patients, several studies have identified increased oxidative stress in cats with CKD.[6,117–119] Recent evidence suggests that oxidative stress may play a key role in fibrosis development,[120] a very common finding in feline CKD. The finding of oxidative stress is not unto itself a surprising finding, but does raise the question of how, and if, it should be addressed. In a small nonrandomized, controlled study, cats with IRIS stage 2 or greater were fed a dry diet supplemented with vitamins E and C and beta-carotene. Markers for DNA damage were reduced compared with the preceding period during which they were fed a nonsupplemented diet, suggesting that the antioxidants reduced oxidative stress in these cats.[117] Unfortunately, the study was not designed to identify specific antioxidants or dosages of antioxidants that might be effective in controlling oxidative stress in CKD, so additional research is warranted.

COMMENTARY: FUTURE DIRECTIONS

Dietary protein is not toxic to kidneys. Creatinine and urea, whether generated through the catabolism of exogenous or endogenous protein, are 2 of a long list of purported uremic toxins (**Table 3**). A review of the effects of uremic toxins on multiple organ systems in humans with CKD and acute kidney injury concludes that neither creatinine nor urea concentrations reflect GFR or toxicity owing to the presence and interactions of many other endogenous metabolites.[121] No single uremic toxin accounts for the clinical spectrum of uremia. Instead, uremia results from the interactions of inflammation, malnutrition, hypoalbuminemia, increased concentrations of protein-bound solutes as well as generation of nonnutritional toxins.[122–124]

Although uremic toxins can result in malnutrition, malnutrition itself results in inflammation, morbidity, and mortality in human patients with CKD.[123] Possible explanations include that (a) not all protein and nutritional degradation metabolites are toxic, (b) hypoalbuminemia enhances protein-bound toxin availability, (c) tissue catabolism results in generation of more toxic solutes than those from protein metabolism, (d) compounds unrelated to protein degradation contribute to inflammation and malnutrition, and (e) renal clearance is required for removal of nonprotein derived toxins.

Table 3		
List of purported uremic toxins		
Small Water Soluble Solutes	**Protein-bound Solutes**	**Middle Molecules**
Asymmetric dimethylarginine	3-Deoxyglucosone	Adrenomedullin
Benzylalcohol	CMPF	Atrial natriuretic peptide
β-Guanidinopropionic acid	Fructoselysine	β2-Microglobulin
β-Lipotropin	Glyoxal	β-Endorphin
Creatinine	Hippuric acid	Cholecystokinin
Cytidine	Homocysteine	Clara cell protein
Guanidine	Hydroquinone	Complement factor D
Guanidinoacetic acid	Indole-3-acetic acid	Cystatin C
Guanidinosuccinic acid	Indoxyl sulfate	Degranulation inhibiting protein I
Hypoxanthine	Kinurenine	Delta-sleep–inducing peptide
Malondialdehyde	Kynurenic acid	Endothelin
Methylguanidine	Methylglyoxal	Hyaluronic acid
Myoinositol	N-carboxymethyllysine	Interleukin 1β
Orotic acid	P-cresol	Interleukin 6
Orotidine	Pentosidine	Kappa-Ig light chain
Oxalate	Phenol	Lambda-Ig light chain
Pseudouridine	P-OH hippuric acid	Leptin
Symmetric dimethylarginine	Quinolinic acid	Methionine-enkepahlin
Urea	Spermidine	Neuropeptide Y
Uric acid	Spermine	Parathyroid hormone
Xanthine		Retinol binding protein
		Tumor necrosis factor alpha

Abbreviation: CMPF, carboxy-methyl-propyl-furanpropionic acid.
From Vanholder R, Glorieux G, De Smet R, et al. New insights in uremeic toxins. Kidney Int 2003;63:S7; with permission.

Despite numerous experimental studies and clinical trials having been performed, questions about feeding and managing the cat with CKD remain. Some of these include the following.

1. Do we rely too much on diet? Are there other approaches we could use to reduce uremic toxin production or absorption? Renal diets were developed at a time when there were no effective medications for CKD. Now, the availability of phosphorus binders, potassium gluconate or citrate, omega-3 fatty acids, angiotensin-converting enzyme inhibitors, angiotensin receptor blockers, and amlodipine provide greater ability to address the specific needs of the individual patient without inducing malnutrition.

2. Do different types of kidney disease require different dietary therapies? Fibrosis associated with interstitial changes is the endpoint for most cats; however, what etiology initiates the process is generally unknown in an individual cat.

3. At what point in disease progression should dietary therapy be implemented, if at all? In theory, would it be better to address acid–base balance initially, and then phosphorus binding, or vice versa?

4. What is the optimal amount of protein for cats with CKD? How much restriction, if any, is necessary? Interestingly, the benefits of protein restriction in human CKD remains an area of controversy with metaanalyses failing to show clear advantages.[125–127] Similar to cats, protein malnutrition, sarcopenia, and iron deficiency are clinical problems in human CKD patients following low protein regimes. A prospective study in human CKD patients contrasting protein and phosphorus restriction concluded that the risks associated with protein restriction may

outweigh the benefits from phosphorus restriction, and suggested that protein restriction as a means to control phosphorus intake is not justified.[128] Kasiske and associates[129] conclude that the relatively weak effect on progression of renal disease provided by dietary protein restriction in human CKD suggests that better therapies are needed.

5. Does the type of protein, or the amino acid composition of the protein, make a difference in cats? There is evidence in humans and rats that types of protein can differentially influence the effect of protein on GFR, acid–base and other effects.[130–132] This effect was not observed in dogs,[133] and no data are available for cats.

6. Will a cat in IRIS stage 3 or 4 benefit adequately if phosphorus is restricted by means other than diet? No controlled clinical trials address this question. One study using a remnant kidney model demonstrated persistent benefit of a chitosan calcium carbonate phosphorus binder when stage 1 and 2 cats were fed a maintenance diet.[44]

7. Might some cats with advanced disease benefit from increased dietary protein levels? As discussed, regular reassessment of the patient enables evaluation of muscle and body condition, which is helpful in changing dietary treatment recommendations if warranted. As loss of LBM is detrimental as well as predictive of progression, increasing dietary protein and using alternate methods to restrict phosphorus or uremic toxins should be considered. When patients fail to eat adequate calories (protein, fat, or carbohydrate), then feeding support is required. Would a more palatable diet help? Evidence-based guidelines for type of assistance and timing would be helpful.

8. Do we rely too heavily on creatinine as a measure of azotemia? What are the actual uremic toxins that cause adverse effects in cats and what can we do about them? This remains an area of potential research.

9. Should we be investigating phosphatonins (eg, FGF-23) and their role in phosphate homeostasis in cats and potentially seeking ways to block or correct FGF-23 as GFR declines? Finch and colleagues[134] reported an inverse relationship between FGF-23 concentrations and GFR and demonstrated that FGF-23 is increased in cats that go on to become azotaemic before phosphate concentrations increase. PTH also changes before serum phosphorus. Would these be better markers of progression of renal dysfunction?

10. Progression of renal fibrosis is thought to be related to the ongoing production of proinflammatory and profibrotic cytokines. Proteinuria, hypoxia, hyperphosphatemia, ageing, and chronic inflammation have been investigated and are believed to maintain this state.[4] Should the focus of early identification (eg, symmetric dimethylarginine) and treatment be modification of the inflammatory mediators?

11. Is it appropriate to restrict protein in cats with proteinuria? Although protein in the urine may initiate an inflammatory response that ultimately progresses to interstitial fibrosis,[4] muscle wasting and a perceived decreased quality of life may result in an earlier death, either owing to general decline in health or earlier requested euthanasia. Would this be better addressed pharmacologically rather than risking malnutrition? Malnutrition also results in inflammation and mortality; therefore, preventing malnutrition (as well as sarcopenia), is critically important when managing the feline CKD patient.

SUMMARY

As stated, we agree that (1) abnormalities in normal homeostasis produced by renal insufficiency are influenced by dietary intake, (2) the kidney is susceptible to

Table 4
Summary of evidence supporting nutrient modification in cats with chronic kidney disease

Nutrient	Documentation for Benefit to Change	Evidence-based Target for Dietary Intake	Comments
Protein	Conflicting results in remnant kidney model; no data testing protein restriction independent of other nutrients in spontaneous CKD cats	Restriction not supported; recommended target: 30%–40% of calories from protein	Commercial renal diets provide as little as 20% of calories from protein.
Phosphorus	0.42% superior to 1.56% (dry basis) in remnant kidney cats; no data testing phosphorus restriction independent of other nutrients in spontaneous CKD cats	Some restriction is supported, but inadequate data on which to base a dietary target	IRIS guidelines suggest maintaining serum phosphorus in the low normal range. PTH and FGF-23 may be elevated even with normal serum phosphorus
Sodium	Conflicting data on adverse effects at 1.2% dietary sodium (dry basis); adverse effects from too little sodium noted in remnant kidney models at about 0.33% sodium, dry basis	Restriction is contraindicated; avoid sodium levels >1.0% of diet dry matter	Commercial renal diets may contain insufficient sodium and stimulate the RAAS system; if low-sodium diet is fed, consider potassium supplementation
Potassium	Hypokalemia is associated with renal dysfunction but no benefit documented in eukalemic CKD cats	Treat hypokalemic cats as needed to maintain serum potassium within the normal range	Correct acid–base imbalance before testing potassium
Omega-3 fatty acids	15% dietary omega-3 fatty acids affect GFR and renal blood flow; no data to support long-term benefit from supplementation	No data in cats with CKD	Long-chain n-3 fatty acids, especially EPA, reduce inflammation, blood pressure and proteinuria in other species
Alkalinization	No studies in cats have evaluated bicarbonate supplementation alone	No data in cats with CKD	IRIS guidelines suggest maintaining normal TCO2 levels
Calories	No studies in cats have evaluated calorie supplementation alone	Maintain calorie intake sufficient to support ideal body condition	Individual calorie needs vary greatly but are typically increased in aged cats
Water	No studies in cats have evaluated hydration alone	No data in cats with CKD; healthy cats need about 50 mL water/kg body weight	Rehydration as needed aids in acid–base and electrolyte homeostasis and dilutes uremic toxins

Abbreviations: CKD, chronic kidney disease; FGF-23, fibroblast growth factor-23; GFR, glomerular filtration rage; IRIS, International Renal Interest Society; PTH, parathyroid hormone; RAAS, renin-angiotensin-aldosterone system.

Given the smaller number and size of the studies in veterinary medicine, we are unable to perform metaanalysis, thus it seems prudent to make the following recommendation: when prescribing restricted protein renal diets practitioners must carefully monitor their patients' protein and energy intake and nutritional status, as evidenced by body and muscle condition as well as enjoyment of meals/quality of life. If deterioration in any of these is noted with no other apparent reason, alternate diets or means to reduce phosphorus should be considered.

self-perpetuating injury, which may be influenced by dietary modification, and (3) the responses of cats with CKD to dietary or pharmaceutical management will vary dramatically, making individualized therapy with appropriate follow-up necessary.[76] Although clinical studies have shown a benefit from feeding commercial renal diets compared with maintenance diets for cats with CKD, numerous nutrients differed in each study and it is not clear that all nutrient modifications are necessary. As is the case throughout veterinary medical research, we lack statistical power owing to small studies, small numbers of studies, and lack of confirming or refuting studies, and are therefore left to draw conclusions based on very limited data. The sum of the evidence (**Table 4**) suggests that addressing the dysregulation of phosphorus that occurs in CKD is of value. Whether this is best done through phosphorus-restricted diets or the addition of phosphate binders remains to be determined. Evidence regarding a beneficial effect in CKD from dietary protein restriction is lacking, as is evidence to support sodium restriction. Evidence in other species suggests a benefit for addressing acid–base imbalances and there is evidence to support potassium supplementation when potassium depletion is detected. Limited evidence suggests a potential benefit from long-chain omega-3 fatty acid supplementation. Finally, it should be noted that dietary management of CKD is no longer the only option. Appropriate medical management, for example, phosphate binders, alkalinizing agents, angiotensin-converting enzyme inhibitors, and so on, may preclude the need for special diets.

REFERENCES

1. Brown SA. Evaluation of chronic renal disease: a staged approach. Compend Contin Educ Pract Vet 1999;21(8):752–63.
2. DiBartola SP, Rutgers HC, Zack PM, et al. Clinicopathologic findings associated with chronic renal disease in cats: 74 cases (1973-1984). J Am Vet Med Assoc 1987;190(9):1196–202.
3. Chakrabarti S, Syme HM, Brown CA, et al. Histomorphometry of feline chronic kidney disease and correlation with markers of renal dysfunction. Vet Pathol 2013;50(1):147–55.
4. Lawson J, Elliott J, Wheeler-Jones C, et al. Renal fibrosis in feline chronic kidney disease: known mediators and mechanisms of injury. Vet J 2015;203:18–26.
5. Brown SA. Oxidative stress and chronic kidney disease. Vet Clin North Am Small Anim Pract 2008;38:157–66.
6. Keegan RF, Webb CB. Oxidative stress and neutrophil function in cats with chronic renal failure. J Vet Intern Med 2010;24:514–9.
7. Lawler DF, Evans RH, Chase K, et al. The aging feline kidney: a model mortality antagonist? J Feline Med Surg 2006;8:363–71.
8. Boyd LM, Langston C, Thompson K, et al. Survival in cats with naturally occurring chronic kidney disease (2000-2002). J Vet Intern Med 2008;22:1111–7.
9. Syme HM, Markwell PJ, Pfeiffer D, et al. Survival of cats with naturally occurring chronic renal failure is related to severity of proteinuria. J Vet Intern Med 2006; 20:528–35.
10. King JN, Tasker S, Gunn-Moore DA, et al, BENRiC (Benazepril in Renal insufficiency in Cats) Study Group. Prognostic factors in cats with chronic kidney disease. J Vet Intern Med 2007;21:906–16.
11. Chakrabarti S, Syme HM, Elliott J. Clinicopathological variables predicting progression of azotemia in cats with chronic kidney disease. J Vet Intern Med 2012; 26:275–81.

12. King JN, Gunn-Moore DA, Tasker S, et al, Benazepril in Renal insufficiency in Cats Study Group. Tolerability and efficacy of benazepril in cats with chronic kidney disease. J Vet Intern Med 2006;20:1054–64.

13. Brown S, Atkins C, Bagley R, et al. Guidelines for the identification, evaluation, and management of systemic hypertension in dogs and cats. J Vet Intern Med 2007;21:542–58.

14. Jepson RE. Feline systemic hypertension: classification and pathogenesis. J Feline Med Surg 2011;13:25–34.

15. Eisert R. Hypercarnivory and the brain: protein requirements of cats reconsidered. J Comp Physiol B 2011;181:1–17.

16. Plantinga EA, Bosch G, Hendriks WH. Estimation of the dietary nutrient profile of free-roaming feral cats: possible implications for nutrition of domestic cats. Br J Nutr 2011;106:S35–48.

17. Hewson-Hughes AK, Hewson-Hughes VL, Miller AT, et al. Geometric analysis of macronutrient selection in the adult domestic cat, Felis catus. J Exp Biol 2011; 214:1039–51.

18. Hewson-Hughes AK, Hewson-Hughes VL, Colye A, et al. Consistent proportional macronutrient intake selected by adult domestic cats (Felis catus) despite variations in macronutrient and moisture content of foods offered. J Comp Physiol B 2013;183:525–36.

19. Green AS, Ramsey JJ, Villaverde C, et al. Cats are able to adapt protein oxidation to protein intake provided their requirement for dietary protein is met. J Nutr 2008;138:1053–60.

20. Wang XH, Mitch WE. Mechanisms of muscle wasting in chronic kidney disease. Nat Rev Nephrol 2014;10:504–16.

21. Polzin DJ, Osborne CA, Adams LG. Effect of modified protein diets in dogs and cats with chronic renal failure: current status. J Nutr 1991;121:S140–4.

22. Polzin DJ, Osborne CA, Ross S, et al. Dietary management of feline chronic renal failure: where are we now? In what direction are we headed? J Feline Med Surg 2000;2:75–82.

23. Adams LG, Polzin DJ, Osborne CA, et al. Effects of dietary protein and calorie restriction in clinically normal cats and cats with surgically induced chronic renal failure. Am J Vet Res 1993;54:1653–62.

24. Adams LG, Polzin DJ, Osborne CA, et al. Influence of dietary protein/calorie intake on renal morphology and function in cats with 5/6 nephrectomy. Lab Invest 1994;70:347–57.

25. Finco DR, Brown SA, Brown CA, et al. Protein and calorie effects on progression of induced chronic renal failure in cats. Am J Vet Res 1998;59:575–82.

26. DiBartola SP, Buffington CA, Chew DJ, et al. Development of chronic renal disease in cats fed a commercial diet. J Am Vet Med Assoc 1993;202:744–51.

27. Tapp DC, Kobayashi S, Fernandes G, et al. Protein restriction or calorie restriction? A critical assessment of the influence of selective calorie restriction in the progression of experimental renal disease. Semin Nephrol 1989;9:343–53.

28. Elliott J, Rawlings JM, Markwell PJ, et al. Survival of cats with naturally occurring chronic renal failure: effect of dietary management. J Small Anim Pract 2000;41: 235–42.

29. Plantinga EA, Everts H, Kastelein AMC, et al. Retrospective study of the survival of cats with acquired chronic renal insufficiency offered different commercial diets. Vet Rec 2005;157:185–7.

30. Harte JG, Markwell PJ, Moraillon RM, et al. Dietary management of naturally occurring chronic renal failure in cats. J Nutr 1994;124:26660S–2S.

31. Ross SJ, Osborne CA, Kirk CA, et al. Clinical evaluation of dietary modification for treatment of spontaneous chronic kidney disease in cats. J Am Vet Med Assoc 2006;229:949–57.

32. Lees GE, Brown SA, Elliott J, et al. Assessment and management of proteinuria in dogs and cats: 2004 ACVIM Forum Consensus Statement (small animal). J Vet Intern Med 2005;19:377–85.

33. Littman MP. Protein-losing nephropathy in small animals. Vet Clin Small Anim 2011;41:31–62.

34. Sent U, Gössl R, Elliott J, et al. Comparison of efficacy of long-term oral treatment with telmisartan and benazepril in cats with chronic kidney disease. J Vet Intern Med 2015;29:1479–87.

35. Burkholder WJ, Lees GE, LeBlanc AK, et al. Diet modulates proteinuria in heterozygous female dogs with X-linked hereditary nephropathy. J Vet Intern Med 2004;18:165–75.

36. Valli VE, Baumal R, Thorner P, et al. Dietary modification reduces splitting of glomerular basement membranes and delays death due to renal failure in canine X-linked hereditary nephritis. Lab Invest 1991;65:67–73.

37. Nguyen P, Leray V, Dumon H, et al. High protein intake affects lean body mass but not energy expenditure in nonobese neutered cats. J Nutr 2004;134: 2084S–6S.

38. Laflamme DP, Hannah SS. Discrepancy between use of lean body mass or nitrogen balance to determine protein requirements for adult cats. J Feline Med Surg 2013;15:691–7.

39. Perez-Camargo G. Cat nutrition: what's new in the old? Comp Cont Edu Small Anim Pract 2004;26(Suppl 2A):5–10.

40. Cupp CJ, Kerr WW, Jean-Philippe C, et al. The role of nutritional interventions in the longevity and maintenance of long-term health in aging cats intern. J Appl Res Vet Med 2008;6:69–81.

41. Cupp CJ, Kerr WW. Effect of diet and body composition on life span in aging cats. In: Proceedings of the nestle Purina companion animal nutrition summit: focus on gerontology. St. Louis (MO): Nestlé Purina PetCare; 2010. p. 36–42.

42. Freeman LM, Lachaud MP, Matthews S, et al. Evaluation of weight loss over time in cats with chronic kidney disease [Research report] [abstract]. J Vet Intern Med 2015;29:935.

43. Laflamme DP, Hannah SS. The effect of protein intake on changes in lean body mass in aging cats. J Fel Med Surg 2016, in press.

44. Brown SA, Rickertson M, Sheldon S. Effects of an intestinal phosphorus binder on serum phosphorus and parathyroid hormone concentration in cats with reduced renal function. Intern J Appl Res Vet Med 2008;6(3):155–60.

45. Kuwahara Y, Ohba Y, Kitoh K, et al. Association of laboratory data and death within one month in cats with chronic renal failure. J Small Anim Pract 2006; 47:446–50.

46. Ibels LS, Alfrey AC, Haut L, et al. Preservation of function in experimental renal disease by dietary restriction of phosphate. N Engl J Med 1976;298:122–6.

47. Ross LA, Finco DR, Crowell WA. Effect of dietary phosphorus restriction on the kidneys of cats with reduced renal mass. Am J Vet Res 1982;43:1023–6.

48. Finco DR, Brown SA, Crowell WA, et al. Effects of phosphorus/calcium-restricted and phosphorus/calcium-replete 32% protein diets in dogs with chronic renal failure. Am J Vet Res 1992;53:157–63.

49. Koizumi M, Komaba H, Fukagawa M. Parathyroid function in chronic kidney disease: role of FGF23-Klotho axis. Contrib Nephrol 2013;180:110–23.

50. Bohnert BN, Daniel C, Amann K, et al. Impact of phosphorus restriction and vitamin D-substitution on secondary hyperparathyroidism is a proteinuric mouse model. Kidney Blood Press Res 2015;40:153–65.

51. Lumlertgul D, Burke TJ, Gillum DM, et al. Phosphate depletion arrests progression of chronic renal failure independent of protein intake. Kidney Int 1986;29: 658–66.

52. Koizumi T, Murakami K, Nakayama H, et al. Role of dietary phosphorus in the progression of renal failure. Biochem Biophys Res Commun 2002;295:917–21.

53. Barber PJ, Rawlings JM, Markwell PJ, et al. Effect of dietary phosphate restriction on renal secondary hyperparathyroidism in the cat. J Small Anim Pract 1999;40:62–70.

54. Geddes RF, Elliott J, Syme HM. The effect of feeding a renal diet on plasma fibroblast growth factor 23 concentrations in cats with stable azotemic chronic kidney disease. J Vet Intern Med 2013;27:1354–61.

55. Finco DR, Barsanti JA, Brown SA. Influence of dietary source of phosphorus on fecal and urinary excretion of phosphorus and other minerals by male cats. Am J Vet Res 1989;50:263–6.

56. Moe SM, Zidehsaraj MP, Chambers MA, et al. Vegetarian compared with meat dietary protein source and phosphorus homeostasis in chronic kidney disease. Clin J Am Soc Nephrol 2011;6:257–64.

57. Bijsmans ES, Jepson RE, Chang YM, et al. Changes in systolic blood pressure over time in healthy cats and cats with chronic kidney disease. J Vet Intern Med 2015;29:855–61.

58. Finco DR. Association of systemic hypertension with renal injury in dogs with induced renal failure. J Vet Intern Med 2004;18:289–94.

59. Elliott J, Syme HM. Proteinuria in chronic kidney disease in cats: prognostic marker or therapeutic target? J Vet Intern Med 2006;20:1052–3.

60. Turner JL, Brogdon JD, Lees GE, et al. Idiopathic hypertension in a cat with secondary hypertensive retinopathy associated with a high-salt diet. J Am Anim Hosp Assoc 1990;26:647–51.

61. Luckschander N, Iben C, Hosgood G, et al. Dietary NaCl does not affect blood pressure in healthy cats. J Vet Intern Med 2004;18:463–7.

62. Kirk CA, Jewell DE, Lowry SR. Effects of sodium chloride on selected parameters in cats. Vet Ther 2006;7:333–46.

63. Xu H, Laflamme DP, Long GL. Effects of dietary sodium chloride on health parameters in mature cats. J Feline Med Surg 2009;11:435–41.

64. Reynolds BS, Chetboul V, Nguyen P, et al. Effects of dietary salt intake on renal function: a 2-year study in healthy aged cats. J Vet Intern Med 2013;27:507–15.

65. Buranakarl C, Mathur S, Brown SA. Effects of dietary sodium chloride intake on renal function and blood pressure in cats with normal and reduced renal function. Am J Vet Res 2004;65:620–7.

66. Kobori H, Nangaku M, Navar LG, et al. The intrarenal renin-angiotensin system: from physiology to the pathobiology of hypertension and kidney disease. Pharmacol Rev 2007;59:251–87.

67. Jensen J, Henik RA, Brownfield M, et al. Plasma renin activity and angiotensin I and aldosterone concentrations in cats with hypertension associated with chronic renal disease. Am J Vet Res 1997;58:535–40.

68. Mitani S, Yabuki A, Taniguchi K, et al. Association between the intrarenal renin-angiotensin system and renal injury in chronic kidney disease of dogs and cats. J Vet Med Sci 2013;75:127–33.

69. Dutta UK, Lane J, Roberts LJ, et al. Superoxide formation and interaction with nitric oxide modulate systemic arterial pressure and renal function in salt-depleted dogs. Exp Biol Med 2006;231:269–76.

70. Munoz-Durango N, Vecchiola A, Gonzalez-Gomez LM, et al. Modulation of immunity and inflammation by the mineralocorticoid receptor and aldosterone. Biomed Res Int 2015;2015:652738.

71. Mathur S, Brown CA, Dietrich UM, et al. Evaluation of a technique of inducing hypertensive renal insufficiency in cats. Am J Vet Res 2004;65:1006–13.

72. Hughes KL, Slater MR, Geller S, et al. Diet and lifestyle variables as risk factors for chronic renal failure in pet cats. Prev Vet Med 2002;55:1–15.

73. Yu S, Morris JG. Sodium requirement of adult cats for maintenance based on plasma aldosterone concentration. J Nutr 1999;129:419–23.

74. Rodriguez F, Llinajs MT, Gonzalez JD, et al. Renal changes induced by cyclooxygenase-2 inhibitor during normal and low sodium intake. Hypertension 2000;36:276–81.

75. Harris RC, Breyer MD. Physiological regulation of cyclooxygenase-2 in the kidney. Am J Physiol Renal Physiol 2001;281:F1–11.

76. Brown SA, Brown CA, Crowell WA, et al. Beneficial effects of chronic administration of dietary omega-3 polyunsaturated fatty acids in dogs with renal insufficiency. J Lab Clin Med 1998;131:447–55.

77. Brown SA, Brown CA, Crowell WA, et al. Effects of dietary polyunsaturated fatty acid supplementation in early renal insufficiency in dogs. J Lab Clin Med 2000; 135:275–86.

78. Brown SA, Brown CA, Crowell WA, et al. Dietary fatty acid composition affects renal function [abstract]. In: Proceedings of the 1996 Purina Forum on Small Animal Nutrition. Santa Barbara (CA): Veterinary Practice; 1997. p. 35.

79. Simopoulos AP. The importance of the ratio of omega-6/omega-3 essential fatty acids. Biomed Pharmacother 2002;56:365–79.

80. Tonkin L, Parnell N. Evaluation of serum fatty acids in cats with chronic kidney disease [abstract]. Lakewood (CO): American College of Veterinary Internal Medicine (ACVIM); 2015.

81. Dow SW, Fettman MJ, LeCouteur RA, et al. Potassium depletion in cats: renal and dietary influences. J Am Vet Med Assoc 1987;191:1569–75.

82. Theisen SK, DiBartola SP, Radin MJ, et al. Muscle potassium content and potassium gluconate supplementation in normokalemic cats with naturally occurring chronic renal failure. J Vet Intern Med 1997;11:212–7.

83. DeSousa RC, Harrington JT, Ricanti ES, et al. Renal regulation of acid-base equilibrium during chronic administration of mineral acid. J Clin Invest 1974; 53:465–76.

84. Dow SW, Fettman MJ, Smith KR, et al. Effects of dietary acidification and potassium depletion on acid base balance, mineral metabolism and renal function in adult cats. J Nutr 1990;120:569–78.

85. Buffington CAT, DiBartola SP, Chew DJ. Effect of low potassium commercial non-purified diet on renal function of adult cats. J Nutr 1991;121:S91–2.

86. Cook NE, Rogers QR, Morris JG. Acid-base balanced affects dietary choice in cats. Appetite 1996;26:175–92.

87. Elliott J, Syme HM, Reubens E, et al. Assessment of acid-base status of cats with naturally occurring chronic renal failure. J Small Anim Pract 2003;44:65–70.

88. Kraut JA, Madias NE. Metabolic acidosis of CKD: an update. Am J Kidney Dis 2015;67(2):307–17.

89. Kopple JD, Kalantar-Zadeh K, Mehrotra R. Risks of chronic metabolic acidosis in patients with chronic kidney disease. Kidney Int Suppl 2005;95:S21–7.
90. Franch HA, Mitch WE. Catabolism in uremia: the impact of metabolic acidosis. J Am Soc Nephrol 1998;9:S78–81.
91. Franch HA, Raissi S, Wang X, et al. Acidosis impairs insulin receptor substrate-1-associated phosphoinositide 3-kinase signaling in muscle cells: consequences of proteolysis. Am J Physiol Renal Physiol 2004;287:F700–6.
92. May RC, Masud T, Logue B, et al. Metabolic acidosis accelerates whole body protein degradation and leucine oxidation by a glucocorticoid-dependent mechanism. Miner Electrolyte Metab 1992;18:245–9.
93. de Brito-Ashurst I, Varagunam M, Raftery MJ, et al. Bicarbonate supplementation slows progression of CKD and improves nutritional status. J Am Soc Nephrol 2009;20:2075–84.
94. Mehrotra R, Bross R, Wang H, et al. Effect of high-normal compared with low-normal arterial pH on protein balances in automated peritoneal dialysis patients. Am J Clin Nutr 2009;90:1532–40.
95. Taylor EJ, Adams C, Neville R. Some nutritional aspects of ageing in dogs and cats. Proc Nutr Soc 1995;54(3):645–56.
96. Bermingham EN, Weidgraaf K, Hekman M, et al. Seasonal and age effects on energy requirements in domestic short-hair cats (Felis catus) in a temperate environment. J Anim Physiol Anim Nutr 2012;97:522–30.
97. Harper EJ. Changing perspectives on aging and energy requirements: aging, body weight and body composition in humans, dogs and cats [expanded abstract]. J Nutr 1998;128:2627S–31S.
98. Laflamme DP, Gunn-Moore D. Nutrition for aging cats. Vet Clin North Am Small Anim Pract 2014;44:761–74.
99. Villaverde C, Fascetti AJ. Macronutrients in feline health. Vet Clin North Am Small Anim Pract 2014;44:699–717.
100. Laflamme DP. Sarcopenia and weight loss in the geriatric cat. In: Little S, editor. August's consultations in feline internal medicine, vol. 7. St Louis (MO): Elsevier; 2016. p. 951–6.
101. Brown SA, Finco DR, Bartges JW, et al. Interventional nutrition for renal disease. Clin Tech Small Anim Pract 1998;13:217–23.
102. Greene JP, Lefebvre SL, Wang M, et al. Risk factors associated with the development of chronic kidney disease in cats evaluated at primary care veterinary hospitals. J Am Vet Med Assoc 2014;244:320–7.
103. Markovich JE, Freeman LM, Labato MA, et al. Survey of dietary and medication practices of owners of cats with chronic kidney disease. J Feline Med Surg 2015;17:979–83.
104. Jepson RE, Brodbelt D, Vallance C, et al. Evaluation of predictors of the development of azotemia in cats. J Vet Intern Med 2009;23:806–13.
105. Graham KA, Reaich D, Channon SM, et al. Correction of acidosis in hemodialysis decreases whole-body protein degradation. J Am Soc Nephrol 1997;8:632–7.
106. Remer T. Influence of nutrition on acid-base balance – metabolic aspects. Eur J Nutr 2001;40:214–20.
107. Herron M, Buffington CAT. Environmental enrichment for indoor cats. Compend Contin Educ Vet 2010;32:E4.
108. Ellis SL, Rodan I, Carney HC, et al. AAFP and ISFM feline environmental needs guidelines. J Feline Med Surg 2013;15:219–30.

109. Quimby JM, Lunn KF. Mirtazapine as an appetite stimulant and anti-emetic in cats with chronic kidney disease: a masked placebo-controlled crossover clinical trial. Vet J 2013;197:651–5.

110. Prentiss PG, Wolf AV, Eddy HA. Hydropenia in cat and dog: ability of the cat to meet its water requirements solely from a diet of fish or meat. Am J Physiol 1959;196:25.

111. Hawthorne AJ, Markwell PJ. Dietary sodium promotes increased water intake and urine volume in cats. J Nutr 2004;134:2128S–9S.

112. Carciofi AC, Bazzoli RS, Zanni A. Influence of water content and the digestibility of pet foods on the water balance of cats. Braz J Vet Res Anim Sci 2005;42:429–34.

113. Buckley CM, Hawthorne A, Colyer A, et al. Effect of dietary water intake on urinary output, specific gravity and relative supersaturation for calcium oxalate and struvite in the cat. Br J Nutr 2011;106:S128–30.

114. Kirschvink N. Effects of feeding frequency on water intake in cats [Abstract]. Lakewood (CO): American College of Veterinary Internal Medicine (ACVIM); 2005.

115. Finco DR, Adams DD, Crowell WA, et al. Food and water intake and urine composition in cats: influence of continuous versus periodic feeding. Am J Vet Res 1986;47:1638–42.

116. Greco D, Xu H, Zanghi B, et al. The effect of feeding inversely proportional amounts of dry versus canned food on water consumption, hydration and urinary parameters in cats. [Abstract]. Proceedings 39th WSAVA Congress. Cape Town (South Africa), September 16-19, 2014.

117. Yu S, Paetau-Robinson I. Dietary supplements of vitamins E and C and b-carotene reduce oxidative stress in cats with renal insufficiency. Vet Res Commun 2006;30:403–13.

118. Jepson RE, Syme HM, Vallance C, et al. Plasma asymmetric dimethylarginine, symmetric dimethylarginine, l-arginine, and nitrite/nitrate concentrations in cats with chronic kidney disease and hypertension. J Vet Intern Med 2008;22:317–24.

119. Krofič Žel M, Tozon N, Nemec Svete A. Plasma and erythrocyte glutathione peroxidase activity, serum selenium concentration, and plasma total antioxidant capacity in cats with IRIS stages I-IV chronic kidney disease. J Vet Intern Med 2014;28:130–6.

120. Richter K, Konzack A, Pihlajaniemi T, et al. Redox-fibrosis: impact of TGFβ1 on ROS generators, mediators and functional consequences. Redox Biol 2015;6:344–52.

121. Lisowaska-Myjak B. Uremic toxins and their effects on multiple organ systems. Nephron Clin Pract 2014;128:303–11.

122. Stenvinkel P, Heimbürger O, Lindholm B, et al. Are there two types of malnutrition in chronic renal failure? Evidence for relationships between malnutrition, inflammation and atherosclerosis (MIA syndrome). Nephrol Dial Transplant 2000;15:953–60.

123. Vanholder R, Glorieux G, Lameire N. The other side of the coin: Impact of toxin generation and nutrition on the uremic syndrome. Semin Dial 2002;15:311–4.

124. Vanholder R, Glorieux G, De Smet R, et al. New insights in uremeic toxins. Kidney Int 2003;63:S6–10.

125. Levey AS, Greene T, Beck GJ, et al. Dietary protein restriction and the progression of chronic renal disease: what have all of the results of the MDRD study

shown? Modification of Diet in Renal Disease Study group. J Am Soc Nephrol 1999;10:2426–39.

126. Levey A, Greene T, Sarnak M, et al. Effect of dietary protein restriction on the progression of kidney disease: long-term follow-up of the Modification of Diet in Renal Disease (MDRD) Study. Am J Kidney Dis 2006;48:879–88.

127. Kopple J, Levey A, Greene T, et al. Effect of dietary protein restriction on nutritional status in the Modification of Diet in Renal Disease Study. Kidney Int 1997; 52:778–91.

128. Shinaberger CS, Greenland S, Kopple JD, et al. Is controlling phosphorus by decreasing dietary protein intake beneficial or harmful in persons with chronic kidney disease? Am J Clin Nutr 2008;88:1511–8.

129. Kasiske BL, Lakatua JD, Ma JZ, et al. A meta-analysis of the effects of dietary protein restriction on the rate of decline in renal function. Am J Kidney Dis 1998;31:954–61.

130. Williams AJ, Walls J. Metabolic consequences of differing protein diets in experimental renal disease. Eur J Clin Invest 1987;17:117–22.

131. Kontessis P, Jones S, Dodds R, et al. Renal, metabolic and hormonal responses to ingestion of animal and vegetable proteins. Kidney Int 1990;38:136–44.

132. Pecis M, DeAzevedo MJ, Gross JL. Chicken and fish diet reduces glomerular hyperfiltration in IDDM patients. Diabetes Care 1994;17:665–72.

133. Finco DR, Cooper TL. Soy protein increases glomerular filtration rate in dogs with normal or reduced renal function. J Nutr 2000;130:745–8.

134. Finch NC, Geddes RF, Syme HM, et al. Fibroblast growth factor 23 (FGF-23) concentrations in cats with early nonazotemic chronic kidney disease (CKD) and in healthy geriatric cats. J Vet Intern Med 2013;27:227–33.

Controversies in Veterinary Nephrology: Differing Viewpoints

Role of Dietary Protein in the Management of Feline Chronic Kidney Disease

Jennifer A. Larsen, DVM, PhD

KEYWORDS

- Feline chronic kidney disease • Dietary protein • Catabolism • Digestibility

KEY POINTS

- Many cats with chronic kidney disease (CKD) are aged, and there is concern that aged cats may have reduced protein digestive efficiency, potentially leading to risk for protein malnutrition when using diets formulated for feline CKD.
- When energy needs are not met, catabolism of body tissues occurs, leading to losses of lean body mass and likely increasing risk of morbidity and mortality in cats with CKD.
- There is no evidence that dietary protein concentrations above and beyond what is contained in feline CKD diets is beneficial in any cat, or can prevent or reverse negative energy and nitrogen balances in a cat with poor food intake.

There is no question that the role of diet in management of chronic kidney disease (CKD) is important. The 2 articles in this issue (see David J. Polzin and Julie A. Churchill, "Controversies in Veterinary Nephrology: Renal Diets Are Indicated for Cats with International Renal Interest Society Chronic Kidney Disease Stages 2 to 4: The Pro View," and Margie A. Scherk and Dottie P. Laflamme, "Controversies in Veterinary Nephrology: Renal Diets Are Indicated for Cats with International Renal Interest Society Chronic Kidney Disease Stages 2 to 4: The Con View"), are thoughtful but provide different interpretations of the current knowledge on this topic. The basics of the role of protein in nutrition are well discussed, including the contribution to urea as well as supply of essential amino acids and maintenance of normal function. However, it is clear that more research is needed to fully answer the questions raised here. As pointed out, neither clinical trials involving product testing, nor prospective research investigating dietary influences on cats with induced kidney disease provide guidance on the utility of specific nutritional strategies. Likewise, extrapolating guidance for

The author has nothing to disclose.
Molecular Biosciences, School of Veterinary Medicine, University of California, Davis, One Shields Avenue, Davis, CA 95616, USA
E-mail address: jalarsen@vmth.ucdavis.edu

management of cats with CKD from data derived from dialysis-dependent people consuming less than their protein requirements, as well as studies in other species such as dogs and rodents, also is not ideal. Further, it is prudent to exercise caution and avoid overinterpretation of partial data only available in abstracts and proceedings due to the significant limitations of evaluating such incomplete information.

The challenges and limitations of establishing protein requirements in both healthy cats and those with CKD are also well recognized. Extrapolation from serial body composition measurements (such as those obtained with dual energy X-ray absorptiometry [DEXA] and D_2O dilution techniques) is often used as a marker of adequacy of dietary protein intake in normal animals and people. However, these methods carry limitations specific to the technique used as well as the inferred acceptance that body composition is the single best way to estimate requirements. Of course, carcass analysis, the gold standard of body composition analysis, is not possible for serial measurements nor feasible or ethical for use in companion animals. In addition, carcass analysis has its own limitations and required assumptions.

Similarly, other measurements used to estimate protein requirements, such as nitrogen balance, have inherent limitations and confounding factors. The role of changes in energy intake, in addition to the separate effects of gain or loss of body weight, is important due to the impacts on nitrogen balance as an estimate of protein requirements. As such, protein requirements may not be accurately estimated due to energy intake variation as well as body weight and composition changes during the balance trial. In addition, the role of other nutrients, especially carbohydrate, which spares nitrogen, especially at lower protein intakes,[1] is an important aspect of interpreting such data. Regardless of methodology used, more accurate estimates of protein requirements may be obtained when using animals well adapted to the protein concentration in the diet and eating adequate amounts to maintain weight stability over time.

A related issue is the difficulty assessing the protein status in clinical patients. Muscle condition scoring remains subjective, and most measures of body composition or muscle catabolism are only feasible in a research setting. Imaging techniques such as computed tomography or ultrasonography to evaluate muscle mass in individuals may be developed and validated in the future in order to facilitate such clinical assessments. The lack of clear clinical data to provide guidance on both inadequate and excessive intake of dietary protein perhaps encourages a more conservative approach to the design of diets for cats with CKD. The goal is to avoid providing too little protein so that known requirements are not met, yet not allowing excessive intakes that might risk uremia and increase morbidity in this population. Provision of moderate amounts of high-quality dietary protein (meeting requirements plus a margin of safety to account for various known and unknown factors) seems warranted.

Certainly the quality of dietary protein (as reflected by the digestibility as well as the amino acid profile and amino acid bioavailability) is an important determinate in the efficiency of protein utilization. Given the potential and perhaps common essential amino acid inadequacies in some feline diets,[2] comparing protein requirement data across studies is a challenge, and unequivocal conclusions may not be possible. Amino acid bioavailability data are largely missing for common pet food ingredients, complete diets, and for companion animal species. It also should be noted that protein digestibility methodology carry limitations that were not addressed here. Use of apparent (fecal) digestibility requires many assumptions. Further, it is well established that dietary factors such as fiber type, fiber concentration, and protein concentration, as well as several other animal and study design factors influence the measurement of protein digestibility.

Many cats with CKD are aged, and there is concern that aged cats may have reduced protein digestive efficiency, potentially leading to risk for protein malnutrition when using diets formulated for feline CKD. Partial and limited data presented in conference proceedings used a defined value of 77% for low digestibility; increased incidence of low protein digestibility was associated with increasing age when comparing groups of unknown numbers of cats that were 8 to 10, 10 to 12, 12 to 14, or over 14 years of age.[3] On the other hand, published data reported in the scientific literature showed a statistical difference in protein digestibility of 3 different diets between young (approximately 3 years old) and old (approximately 11.6 years old) cats, but group mean values were never lower than 83% regardless of diet or age.[4] Another study assessing cats of 6 age groups ranging from 1 to 14 years identified only a slight trend but not a significant effect of age on protein digestibility.[5] Although it is difficult to draw firm conclusions given differences in study design, populations, diets, and other factors, the apparently minor effects of age on protein digestibility in aged cats may not have a clinically significant impact given the nutritional profiles of diets formulated for feline CKD.

The National Research Council (NRC) minimum requirements for protein and amino acids were established based on data from growing animals, nitrogen balance studies, and other parameters. The NRC recommended allowance for dietary protein concentration for adult cats represents a 25% increase over the minimum requirements to account for digestibility and bioavailability. The currently available veterinary therapeutic diets for feline CKD supply protein in concentrations at least 40% above the NRC minimum requirement for adult cats; this margin helps ensure adequate intake of protein and amino acids for the majority of cats if calorie requirements are met. In addition, these diets are formulated with known amino acid profiles and digestibility coefficients to ensure protein quality and therefore nutritional adequacy. Indeed, as noted by the pro view, studies in cats with naturally occurring CKD and fed therapeutic diets with lowered protein found no negative effect on body weight and body condition scores over more than 2 years.

Adequate food intake was noted to be a critical factor in the management of cats with CKD in both articles. Energy intake cannot be overemphasized for its important role in the feeding of cats with CKD. It is well established that dietary protein is used for energy if inadequate quantities of food are consumed, which lowers the efficiency of protein utilization for other critical needs including maintenance of lean body mass. When energy needs are not met, catabolism of body tissues occurs, leading to losses of lean body mass and likely increasing risk of morbidity and mortality in cats with CKD.

Interestingly, healthy cats sometimes are reported to adjust food intake to maintain normal protein and/or energy intakes when dietary protein concentration or energy digestibility is low.[5,6] In addition, despite being carnivores, healthy cats are remarkably metabolically flexible and can adapt to a range of fat, carbohydrate, and even protein intakes as long as requirements are met.[7-11] It is possible and would not be surprising if this adaptability for adjustments in both food intake and metabolic plasticity is compromised during illness. Therefore, identifying and addressing underlying causes for poor appetite is critical (eg, acidosis, anemia, concurrent urinary tract infection, or hypertension), in order to correct negative balances in both energy and protein. Thus far, there is no evidence that dietary protein concentrations above and beyond what is contained in feline CKD diets (which is already in excess of established requirements) is beneficial in any cat, or can prevent or reverse negative energy and nitrogen balances in a cat with poor food intake.

There are additional noteworthy and practical points raised in both articles, including an emphasis on avoiding diet change in ill cats to reduce the risk of food aversions leading to refusal of specific diets. Stabilization and improvement in general well-being should be achieved prior to introducing a new diet in order to maximize acceptance and minimize risk of food aversions.

Both viewpoints also advocated the use of feeding tubes, which are a critical component of the nutritional and medical management of advanced CKD in cats. Enteral feeding devices provide a means to ensure adequate amounts of an appropriate diet for the CKD stage, as well as a means to maintain hydration and give medications. Of course, body weight should be monitored regularly in cats with CKD. Successful dietary therapy together with avoiding oral administration of necessary medications and eliminating the need for subcutaneous fluids can increase compliance and promote the cat–owner bond, and likely prolongs lifespan with improved quality of life.

REFERENCES

1. Munro HN. General aspects of the regulation of protein metabolism by diet and by hormones. In: Munro HN, Allison JB, editors. Mammalian protein metabolism. New York: Academic Press; 1964. p. 381–481.
2. Rutherfurd SM, Rutherfurd-Markwick KJ, Moughan PJ. Available (ileal digestible reactive) lysine in selected pet foods. J Agric Food Chem 2007;55:3517–22.
3. Perez-Camargo G. Cat nutrition: what's new in the old? Comp Cont Educ Small Anim Pract 2004;26(Suppl 2A):5–10.
4. Peachey SE, Dawson JM, Harper EJ. The effect of ageing on nutrient digestibility by cats fed beef tallow-, sunflower oil- or olive oil-enriched diets. Growth Dev Aging 1999;63:61–70.
5. Taylor EJ, Adams C, Neville R. Some nutritional aspects of ageing in dogs and cats. Proc Nutr Soc 1995;54:645–56.
6. Laflamme DP, Hannah SS. Discrepancy between use of lean body mass or nitrogen balance to determine protein requirements for adult cats. J Feline Med Surg 2013;15:691–7.
7. Hoenig M, Thomaseth K, Waldron M, et al. Fatty acid turnover, substrate oxidation, and heat production in lean and obese cats during the euglycemic hyperinsulinemic clamp. Domest Anim Endocrinol 2007;32:329–38.
8. Lester T, Czarnecki-Maulden G, Lewis D. Cats increase fatty acid oxidation when isocalorically fed meat-based diets with increasing fat content. Am J Physiol 1999;277:R878–86.
9. Green AS, Ramsey JJ, Villaverde C, et al. Cats are able to adapt protein oxidation to protein intake provided their requirement for dietary protein is met. J Nutr 2008; 138:1053–60.
10. Gooding MA, Flickinger EA, Atkinson JL, et al. Effects of high-fat and high-carbohydrate diets on fat and carbohydrate oxidation and plasma metabolites in healthy cats. J Anim Physiol Anim Nutr (Berl) 2014;98:596–607.
11. Russell K, Murgatroyd PR, Batt RM. Net protein oxidation is adapted to dietary protein intake in domestic cats (Felis silvestris catus). J Nutr 2002;132:456–60.

Utilization of Feeding Tubes in the Management of Feline Chronic Kidney Disease

Sheri Ross, DVM, PhD

KEYWORDS

- Esophagostomy feeding tubes • Feline chronic kidney disease • Nutrition

KEY POINTS

- Esophagostomy feeding tubes are useful, and in many cases essential, for the comprehensive management of cats with moderate to advanced chronic kidney disease.
- Often disregarded as a long-term management option, feeding tubes should more appropriately be considered a lifelong therapeutic appliance to facilitate the global management of cats with CKD thus providing improved therapeutic efficacy and quality-of-life.
- Esophagostomy tubes facilitate the maintenance of adequate hydration, avoiding episodes of hospitalization for diuresis and hypertension associated with parenteral salt-containing hydration strategies.

The long-term use of esophagostomy feeding tubes provides the means to maintain hydration, maintain adequate nutrition, and facilitate medication administration in patients with chronic kidney disease (CKD). Many clinicians are reluctant to regard enteral feeding tubes as a long-term solution for the nutritional, hydration, and medical management of chronically ill patients, especially those with CKD. Feline patients with CKD often have a protracted disease course with a progressive decline in body condition that may lead to comorbid conditions and eventually euthanasia because of a perceived decline in quality-of-life by the owner. Proactive use of esophagostomy feeding tubes, can prevent this decline in body condition and facilitate the administration of medications and maintenance of hydration, thus increasing owner and patient compliance and minimizing episodes of hospitalization. These tubes are easily placed in a primary care clinic and consistently extend the quantity and, most importantly, the quality-of-life for patients with CKD.

The author has nothing to disclose.
Department of Hemodialysis/Nephrology/Urology, University of California Veterinary Medical Center – San Diego, 10435 Sorrento Valley Road, Suite 101, San Diego, CA 92121, USA
E-mail address: sro@ucdavis.edu

Vet Clin Small Anim 46 (2016) 1099–1114
http://dx.doi.org/10.1016/j.cvsm.2016.06.014
0195-5616/16/© 2016 Elsevier Inc. All rights reserved.

APPROPRIATE NUTRITION IS CRITICAL IN THE MANAGEMENT OF CHRONIC KIDNEY DISEASE

Dietary therapy is an extremely important component in the management of patients with CKD. Proper nutrition may forestall many of the complications associated with advancing renal disease and has been shown to improve the patient's quality and quantity-of-life.[1,2] Compared with adult maintenance diets, the diets formulated specifically for patients with CKD typically have the following nutritional features: (1) reduced protein, phosphorus, and sodium content; (2) increased potassium and B-vitamin content; (3) increased caloric density; (4) a neutral effect on acid-base balance; and (5) an increased omega-3/omega-6 polyunsaturated fatty acid ratio. Currently there is grade I evidence supporting the recommendation that cats with serum creatinine concentrations in excess of 2.0 mg/dL (International Renal Interest Society [IRIS] CKD stages mid-2 through 4) be fed a diet formulated specifically for kidney disease.[1] Similar results were observed in an earlier, nonrandomized clinical trial in cats with naturally occurring CKD, where the median survival time for cats consuming the renal diet was 633 days compared with 264 days for cats that did not transition to a renal diet.[3]

MALNUTRITION IN PATIENTS WITH CHRONIC KIDNEY DISEASE

Hyporexia secondary to CKD is encountered most commonly in the later stages of the disease, but may occur at any point in the course of progressive CKD. There are many metabolic and husbandry factors that contribute to decreased food intake (**Box 1**). Dehydration, anemia, hypokalemia, and acidemia are examples of common metabolic derangements that may contribute to a decrease in appetite in the later stages of CKD. Many of these metabolic derangements may be corrected or improved with

---

Box 1
Factors contributing to anorexia in feline chronic kidney disease

Metabolic

Uremic stimulation of vomiting center

Hypokalemia

Dehydration

Mineral and bone disorder

Metabolic acidosis

Anemia

Uremic gastritis

Hyperphosphatemia

Food and Feeding

Altered taste/smell

Forced feeding

Sudden diet changes

Medication intolerance

Food aversion

Oral lesions/dental disease

aggressive medical management. In addition, feeding practices should be reviewed with pet owners to ensure patients are offered small, frequent meals in a calm environment. Any diet changes should be made gradually (typically over 2–4 weeks for most cats) to minimize food aversion. Additionally, therapeutic diets should never be offered to a patient when hospitalized because of the high risk of developing food aversion. With advanced kidney disease, many patients, especially those with pre-existing dental disease, may develop oral ulcerations that can significantly reduce food intake (**Fig. 1**). Aggressive medical management, including topical treatment with chlorhexidine-containing oral rinses (C.E.T. 0.12% chlorhexidine rinse, Virbac Corporation Veterinary Division, Fort Worth, TX), has been useful in managing these ulcerations. Note that many dental rinses in veterinary medicine contain zinc gluconate as an additive to minimize plaque formation. Although appropriate for routine dental care, these oral solutions should be used with care in patients with advanced CKD because of the risk of inadvertent zinc toxicity.

Some patients may remain hyporexic despite correction of contributing metabolic and environmental factors. In these patients, the addition of pharmacologic appetite stimulants may be helpful to increase calorie intake. Mirtazapine (Remeron, Organon Inc, West Orange, NJ), a tetracyclic antidepressant, is used in veterinary patients for its antinausea, antiemetic, and appetite-stimulating properties. These effects are mainly mediated through antagonism of the 5-HT3 receptor. Recent pharmacodynamic and pharmacokinetic studies have demonstrated appetite-stimulating properties and determined appropriate dose rates and intervals for cats with CKD.[4] A recent study demonstrated that 1.88 mg per cat of mirtazapine administered every 48 hours to 11 cats with CKD resulted in clinically significant increases in appetite and activity. Additionally, there was a statistically significant increase in weight gain, although the clinical difference in weight change between the two groups was subtle.[5] Mirtazapine seems to be a promising adjunctive therapy for increasing caloric intake in patients with CKD, especially when nutritional support is only needed short-term and/or in cases where feeding tube placement is not an option.

In addition to appetite stimulants, antinausea medications are useful in the management of cats with CKD. Maropitant (Cerenia, Zoetis Inc, Kalamazoo, MI) is a neurokinin

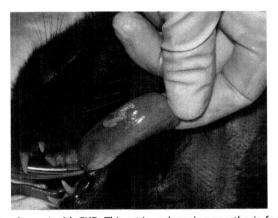

Fig. 1. Lingual ulcer in a cat with CKD. This cat is undergoing anesthesia for placement of an esophagostomy tube (E-tube). Once sedated, the extent of the sublingual ulceration secondary to the renal disease was apparent. The E-tube was placed for nutritional and hydration support, and the oral ulcerations were managed with a 0.12% chlorhexidine gluconate oral rinse.

(NK_1) receptor antagonist and inhibits vomiting via peripheral and centrally mediated effects. Preliminary use of this medication in patients with CKD has been promising, and the effects seem to extend beyond management of nausea. A recent clinical trial demonstrated that use of maropitant resulted in a clinically significant reduction in vomiting when used in cats with CKD. This was a relatively short-term study, and thus clinically significant differences in weight were not observed.[6] Anecdotally, the chronic use of low-dose (1 mg/kg/d) maropitant seems to result in increased food intake in patients that are not obviously nauseated, and an improvement in overall demeanor in some patients with CKD, whether or not they are managed with feeding tubes (**Table 1**).

CALCULATING CALORIE NEEDS

Estimation of caloric needs for patients with advanced CKD remains an issue of some controversy among nutrition experts. From a practical standpoint, any estimation of calorie requirements is only a starting point to avoid gross overfeeding or underfeeding. Monitoring a patient's clinical status and trends in their weight and lean body mass, with timely adjustment to the nutritional plan as needed, is far more important than absolute precision of the initial assessment of calorie needs. Typically, canine and feline patients should have their resting energy requirement (RER) calculated according to the following formulas:

If patient is <2.0 kg: $RER = 70 * (body\ weight\ in\ kg)^{0.75}$

If patient is >2.0 kg: $RER = (30 * [body\ weight\ in\ kg]) + 70$

Table 1
A brief formulary of some drugs commonly used in the nutritional management of feline chronic kidney disease

Medication	Indication	Dosage
Aluminum hydroxide	Hyperphosphatemia[a]	50–100 mg/kg/d divided with meals (max dose 100 mg/kg/d)
Lanthanum carbonate	Hyperphosphatemia[a]	50–100 mg/kg/d divided with meals Crush well before administration
Sodium bicarbonate	Acidosis, serum bicarbonate <18 mEq/L	60–90 mg/kg/d divided into two to three doses Administer with meals
Maropitant	Nausea/vomiting	Nausea: 2 mg/kg po, subcutaneously, or intravenously, q 24 h Chronic use: 1 mg/kg po q 24 h
Mirtazipine	Hyporexia	1.88 mg/cat q 48 h
Famotidine	Dyspepsia	0.5–1 mg/kg po, subcutaneously, or intravenously, q 24 h
Omeprazole	Dyspepsia	0.5–1 mg/kg po q 24 h (delayed-release tablets should not be split)
Sodium polystyrene sulfonate	Moderate, persistent, hyperkalemia (>6.5 mmol/L)	1000 mg/kg/d divided into two to three doses Administer with meals
0.12% Chlorhexidine gluconate oral rinse	Oral ulcerations	0.2 mL (0.1 mL into each cheek pouch) three times daily

[a] IRIS guidelines for serum phosphorous for each CKD stage: stage II, 2.7–4.5 mg/dL; stage III, <5.0 mg/dL; stage IV, <6.0 mg/dL.

Once the RER has been established, the maintenance energy requirement must be determined. In a recent review of cats with CKD being managed with esophageal feeding tubes, and thus documented and consistent caloric intake, we have demonstrated that an metabolic energy requirement (MER) equivalent to $1.4 \times$ RER is sufficient to just maintain body weight in patients with IRIS CKD stages 3 and 4 (Ross and colleagues, unpublished observations, 2015). Because most patients with CKD are typically underweight, the target MER should be increased accordingly to achieve an appropriate body composition and lean mass. In some cases, we have demonstrated patients require significantly more calories than MER calculations would predict.

ASSISTED ENTERAL FEEDING

Proactive intervention with enteral tube feeding should be considered in patients demonstrating persistent hyporexia and progressive loss of body composition and lean body mass. This is especially important in cats with CKD and hypercatabolic infectious or inflammatory comorbid diseases to prevent precipitous loss of lean body mass. Once vomiting is controlled, nasoesophageal feeding tubes provide an option for short-term (few days) nutritional and fluid support. Most cats tolerate use of nasoesophageal tubes, through which commercially available liquid renal diets may be fed. An esophagostomy tube (E-tube) or percutaneous gastrostomy tube should be considered if nutritional support is anticipated or required for more than a few days and if diets other than liquid enteral preparations are to be used.

In our experience, a large percentage of cats with IRIS CKD stages 3 and 4 fail to achieve caloric adequacy and maintain a stable body weight with *ad libitum* feeding of an appropriate therapeutic renal diet. These cats also generally fail to maintain appropriate hydration. As an adjunct to the medical management of these patients, we strongly advocate the routine use E-tubes to facilitate delivery of the nutritional therapy for CKD, and find them essential for the nutritional management of almost all patients starting hemodialysis. For the management of CKD, E-tubes facilitate the lifelong provision of stage-appropriate nutrition and hydration, and convenience for the administration of the multitude of medications these patients require, ensuring improved compliance and efficacy. E-tubes are well tolerated and easily permit feeding of a blended, therapeutic renal diet for the management of early stages of CKD. As the CKD progresses and for the management of more advanced stages of CKD, nutritional requirements generally become more restricted than can be provided by commercial therapeutic diets necessitating the use of diets formulated by a clinical nutritionist. However, these formulated diets would rarely, if ever, be sufficiently palatable to be consumed adequately by cats (or dogs) with advanced CKD (and thus would be ineffective), but they can be provided readily and efficaciously through an E-tube facilitating the management of advanced CKD.

In patients with advanced kidney disease, the metabolic causes of anorexia and vomiting lead to a decline in caloric intake and overall body condition. In desperation to see their pet eat, many owners offer any food to increase their food intake. Although the commonly touted phrase "they have to eat something" is certainly true, the quality and quantity of a patient's life is prolonged significantly if they consume an adequate amount of a stage-appropriate diet designed for CKD.[1,2] At the first signs of weight loss, owners should be encouraged to consider placement of an E-tube for lifelong nutritional support. Proactive intervention with an E-tube combats excessive catabolism, helps prevent loss of lean body mass, and facilitates the establishment of a normal body composition. E-tubes also allow for long-term provision of nutrition, hydration, and medications to facilitate all aspect of the management of CKD (**Fig. 2**).

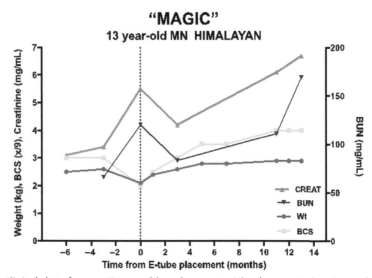

Fig. 2. Clinical data from a 13-year-old, male-castrate Himalayan cat showing a decline in body weight and body condition until placement of an E-tube at month 0. Following E-tube placement, there was a gradual increase in body weight and body condition score. Body weight remained stable after 5 months, despite progressive decline in kidney function. BCS, body condition score; BUN, blood urea nitrogen concentration; Creat, serum creatinine concentration; wt, body weight.

Although there is an initial financial commitment to placing a feeding tube, this cost often is offset by deceased number of hospitalizations required to treat episodes of acute decompensation, dehydration, and malnutrition that occur typically in patients without enteral nutritional support. Patients with enteral feeding tubes are more likely to maintain adequate hydration and nutrition to forestall acute decompensation, and the E-tube provides a means to manage minor episodes at home without intravenous fluid support, which is preferable to the cat and the owner. In addition, the presence of the tube greatly increases compliance with recommended medical management, permitting more control over metabolic complications.

Assisted enteral feeding, using either a gastrostomy tube or E-tube, has been shown to decrease morbidity and mortality in dogs and cats. Placement techniques along with associated complications and limitations also have been described for both tube types.[7–9] Traditionally, gastrostomy tubes have been preferred for chronic nutritional management, whereas E-tubes have been recommended for shorter periods (weeks), and usually only for the management of hepatic or gastrointestinal disorders. The chronic use of gastrostomy tubes for assisted feeding in the management of CKD has been described in dogs.[7] In this group of dogs, gastrostomy tubes were in place for 69 ± 91 days (range, 1–438 days) and were successful in maintaining an adequate nutritional plane in approximately half of the patients. There is a paucity of information in the literature evaluating the long-term management of CKD using E-tubes.

We have been aggressive with the use of E-tubes in the management of CKD in cats and dogs for more than 10 years. E-tubes placed for the management of CKD are typically recommended for patients with IRIS CKD stage 3 or greater because of the associated metabolic complications seen with this level of disease. Most patients that received an E-tube either maintained or improved their body condition score and body weight despite progressive renal disease (**Fig. 3**). Patients with an E-tube rarely

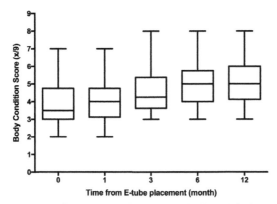

Fig. 3. Box plot of body condition score of 19 cats with chronic kidney disease over time. Time 0 indicates placement of E-tube. No significant change in body condition score was noted at the 1-month recheck. However, by 3 months the body condition score had increased and continued to increase until 6 months, when it stabilized.

required hospitalization for intravenous fluid diuresis, and supplemental hydration with subcutaneous fluid administration at home rarely is required. Dietary and medication compliance for patients with E-tubes also is greatly improved. In a recent review of our cases for the period from 2006 to 2015, cats had E-tubes in place for a longer duration than dogs. This is likely caused by the usual prolonged course of feline CKD compared with canine CKD and the respective longer survival times for cats. Of 120 feline patients that had E-tubes placed during this period, 85 cats presented with either acute kidney injury, acute on CKD, acute ureteral obstruction (managed with hemodialysis, surgery, or both), had an incomplete medical record, or died within 30 days of E-tube placement. The remaining 35 cats had E-tubes placed for management of CKD alone and had a median E-tube duration of 178 days (**Fig. 4**). The longest recorded continuous use of an E-tube in the management of feline CKD was 1893 days. This cat had regular (every 3 months) exchanges of a 14F catheter red rubber tube, using the original stoma for the entire period (**Fig. 5**).

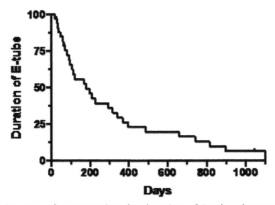

Fig. 4. Kaplan-Meier curve demonstrating the duration of E-tube placement of 34 cats. The median duration of E-tube placement was 178 days. In all but five cases, the duration of E-tube placement corresponded to survival. One cat was excluded from the graph to simplify the illustration in which the E-tube was in place for 1893 days.

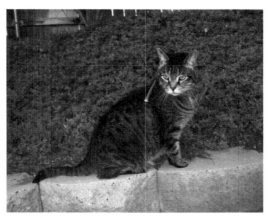

Fig. 5. Photograph of a 19-year-old cat with an E-tube. This cat had an E-tube placed at 15 years of age for the management of his CKD. At the time of his death, at the age of 21, his E-tube had been in place 1893 days, using the original stoma.

COMPLICATIONS ASSOCIATED WITH FEEDING TUBES

One of the primary concerns with E-tubes is the initial placement and requirement for general anesthesia (Appendix 1). Often patients are debilitated with a decreased ability to heal. These cats often are viewed as a significant anesthetic risk because of their debilitation and attending uremia, and therefore tube placement is abandoned or postponed. Although these are certainly considerations, their clinical condition is unlikely to improve without aggressive nutritional support. The anesthesia required for E-tube placement is brief, and most patients do surprisingly well. It is imperative that every effort be made to ensure the patient is normally hydrated and as metabolically stable as possible before undergoing anesthesia. It is also important to note these patients require longer times to recover from anesthesia. Although they may be awake and walking within an hour of the procedure, many owners note it may take up to 3 days for the cats to resume normal levels of activity. We place most E-tubes on an outpatient basis. However, we do try to place the tubes in the morning, so the patients can be monitored throughout the day. Problems during the actual placement of the tube were rare in our study population, but the spectrum of potential complications has been reported previously.[8–11] Bleeding from the insertion site was seen in three cases, but resolved within 2 hours without significant intervention.

Other complications that may be associated with feeding tubes include difficulty in placement or exchange. When placing or exchanging an E-tube it is possible the tube could course subcutaneously or into the mediastinum rather than into the esophagus. For this reason, it is necessary to obtain two-view chest radiographs to confirm proper placement before use. Likewise, after tube exchange, if there is any question as to the correct placement of the tube, radiographs should be obtained.

The most commonly encountered complication in our patient group was cellulitis or abscess formation at the insertion site. Although placement of an E-tube is not a sterile procedure, every effort should be made to keep the procedure as "clean" as possible. We have observed a decrease in the incidence of abscess formation with attention to placement technique, including the use of sterile draping and changing sterile gloves that have been contaminated in the mouth. We prescribe antibiotics (typically amoxicillin/clavulanic acid or cephalexin) for approximately 1 week postplacement of an E-tube, to help minimize the risk of infection at the site of the new stoma. Should an infection or abscess occur at the insertion site of the feeding tube, we initiate therapy with antibiotics and typically recommend hot packing the area for at least 10 minutes, two to four times daily. Most infections or abscesses resolve within a week, and rarely is it necessary or recommended to remove the tube. Even if there is severe abcessation or inflammation, it is rarely necessary to place drains or consider surgical intervention. If the inflammation is not responding as expected, a culture should be obtained to help guide antimicrobial therapy.

The second most commonly encountered complication in our study cohort was inadvertent tube removal at home. This is often the primary concern of owners considering feeding tube placement in their cats. It is important to explain to owners that inadvertent tube removal does not place their pet's life in danger. It is important also to have the cat presented for tube replacement as soon as possible following tube removal. Even with loss of recently placed tubes, a replacement tube usually is placed in the same stoma and fistulous track. However, after several hours, the stoma contracts, and it is progressively more difficult to replace a comparable sized tube. If necessary, a smaller tube may be used temporarily to maintain the stoma. After a few days the stoma enlarges around the smaller tube, and it may be exchanged for a more appropriately sized tube. This method to sequentially dilate the stoma can be used successfully to reestablish the original tube size. When the tube has been removed for several hours, the stoma may be too contracted to permit tube replacement. In these cases, we typically recommend anesthesia for placement of a new tube. In our cohort of 35 cats with CKD, there were eight episodes of tube removal, with two cats presenting for repeat tube losses. In all but one instance, the tube was replaced in the existing stoma without the need for anesthesia.

Another complication encountered was intermittent obstruction of the tube. This was a repeatable problem for certain patients, and was almost always corrected with changes in food and medication preparation or feeding practices. The most commonly encountered issues were not thoroughly crushing and dissolving medications before administration through the tube, not flushing the tube with water after the administration of medications or food, and not thoroughly blending the food to a consistency appropriate for delivery through the tube. Demonstration of proper blending and medication preparation resolved these issues in most cases. Typically we do not have owners strain the food before feeding, unless there are repetitive issues with tube obstruction. This is a cumbersome step to food preparation and was only recommended in 1 of our 35 CKD cases. Typically, straining of the food may be avoided by using a good-quality blender.

A consequence frequently observed in patients being fed with feeding tubes, particularly dogs, is the development of hyperkalemia. Many patients with advanced kidneys disease have a decreased ability to excrete a potassium load because of declining aldosterone levels and/or a decrease in distal tubular flow. Hyperkalemia may develop in patients receiving diets that are formulated with a high potassium content, particularly if they are also receiving an angiotensin-converting enzyme inhibitor or an angiotensin receptor blocker. Often, hyperkalemia develops after placement of an E-tube because the patient is now being fed to caloric requirement and thus receiving an increased potassium load compared with their intake while hyporexic. All commercially available feline therapeutic renal diets, and all but one of the canine therapeutic diets, are relatively high in potassium. Should hyperkalemia develop, the patient's diet and medication regime must be carefully evaluated. Persistent, moderate hyperkalemia (>6.5 mmol/L) usually responds readily to a reduction in dietary potassium and/or the judicious use of either a loop or thiazide diuretic precluding the coexistence of hyponatremia, which often develops with feeding a therapeutic renal diet.[12] Dietary potassium restriction typically requires an individually formulated diet by a veterinary nutritionist. If this is not feasible, a potassium binder may be used to limit the intestinal absorption of potassium from the food. Sodium polystyrene sulfonate (Kionex, KVK-Tech, Inc, Newtown, PA) is a cation exchange resin that lowers serum potassium concentration over several days. This is not an appropriate (immediate) therapy for severe hyperkalemia, and should not be used in patients with suspected ileus, bowel obstruction, or other gastrointestinal disease. The sodium polystyrene sulfonate powder is blended readily into the renal diet for administration via the E-tube.

Other medications that we commonly blend into the daily food prescription, when indicated, include aluminum hydroxide gel (Fagron US, St. Paul, MN), lanthanum carbonate tablets (Fosrenol, Shire US Inc, Wayne, PA), and sodium bicarbonate tablets (Rugby Laboratories, Livonia, MI). We have found the efficacy of the phosphorus and potassium binders is increased if they are actually blended into the daily food allotment. All other medications (angiotensin-converting enzyme inhibitors, blood pressure medications, antibiotics, and so forth) should not be blended into the food, but should be given through the tube separately to ensure accurate dosage administration and timing. Unless a medication is required to be given on an empty stomach, most may be given at the time of the feeding to simplify the overall treatment protocol.

ESOPHAGOSTOMY TUBE MAINTENANCE

When discharging patients who have received feeding tubes, it is important to explain the feeding process in detail with the owner. Our typical feeding tube instruction takes a minimum of 45 minutes. We administer a small feeding with the owner in the room. Before the discharge appointment, the owners are provided with a handout detailing the feeding process, tube maintenance, and problems that may be encountered. Owners are told to call the attending or an emergency service immediately should the tube become dislodged and not to try to replace it themselves.

Home care typically involves daily, thorough cleaning of the insertion site. We typically dispense packets of 4 × 4 gauze squares soaked in a dilute 0.5% chlorhexidine solution (not scrub) and instruct them to thoroughly clean the tube site at least once daily and allow it to air dry. This also provides an opportunity for the owners to inspect the tube site to ensure that there is no swelling or discharge.

Although many people prefer to leave feeding tubes bandaged, we find this predisposes to infection because of the moisture trapped on the skin. We typically discharge patients with a light bandage the owners are instructed to remove within the first 24 hours. Thereafter, the owners are told to clean the tube site daily. They may leave the tube site covered with a light piece of stockinette, because this provides some support to the tube and also prevents the patient from scratching at the site. Often, after several weeks, we find that owners prefer to leave the tube uncovered. This provides good airflow, and most patients by this time do not bother with the tube site.

LONG-TERM TUBE MAINTENANCE

Recently, several options for E-tubes have been made available, incorporating new features to facilitate their placement and use while minimizing tissue reactions. Traditionally, we have used and had excellent success with red rubber tubes in cats and all sizes of dogs; however, these tubes have a tendency to become stiff after 6 to 12 weeks of use and therefore require intermittent exchange. Many tubes composed

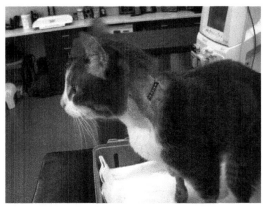

Fig. 6. Photograph demonstrating proper placement of an E-tube in the left cervical region. This red rubber feeding tube is secured with two rows of a finger-trap suture pattern.

of silicone are softer and do not require frequent exchange, but may reflux from the esophagus during episodes of vomiting. Some newly available tubes combine the durability of a silicone tube while remaining rigid enough to minimize reflux (esophagostomy feeding tube, MILA International, Inc, Florence, KY). Regardless of the tube type, we find the sutures securing the tube need to be evaluated at least every 3 months to ensure security. Exchanging or resuturing of an E-tube is a quick procedure and does not typically require sedation or anesthesia. The left cervical region is clipped, and the area around the tube insertion site is scrubbed thoroughly. A topical 2% lidocaine/prilocaine cream is then applied around the insertion site. This is allowed to sit for a minimum of 10 minutes. This provides sufficient topical analgesia to permit placement of sutures with minimal discomfort to the patient. The tube insertion site is again surgically scrubbed, the previous sutures are clipped, and the old tube is removed. After a further scrub, sterile lubricant is applied to the tip of the new tube, which is then inserted into the existing stoma. The tube is gently advanced to the desired level, and secured using a "finger-trap" suture pattern (**Fig. 6**). We routinely exchange these tubes in the context of an office visit and have very few problems. In a particularly fractious animal, sedation may be required, although this is uncommon. The new tube should slide easily into the existing stoma and should never be advanced forcibly without a wire guide. If resistance is met, the animal's head may be repositioned to facilitate passage. If there is any question about the positioning of a replacement tube, two-view thoracic radiographs should be obtained to ensure that the tube is within the esophagus.

Alternatively, a sterile, flexible vascular wire may be passed through the existing feeding tube to exit in the esophagus via a hole preplaced at the end of the tube at the time of its original placement. The old tube is removed over the wire, and the wire then serves as a guide for the passage of the new tube into the existing stoma and subcutaneous fistula. Using this technique for tube exchanges, we have maintained a single stoma for nearly 2000 days of continuous use.

SUMMARY

E-tubes are useful, and in many cases essential, for the comprehensive management of cats with moderate to advanced CKD. Although they are often disregarded as a long-term management option, they should more appropriately be considered a lifelong therapeutic appliance to facilitate the global management of cats with CKD thus providing improved therapeutic efficacy and quality-of-life. E-tubes facilitate the maintenance of adequate hydration, avoiding episodes of hospitalization for diuresis and hypertension associated with parenteral salt-containing hydration strategies. In addition E-tubes increase owner compliance by facilitating the administration of medications, which helps to mitigate the metabolic problems seen with advanced CKD. Finally, and perhaps most importantly, feeding tubes provide a means to deliver a stage-appropriate dietary prescription for cats with CKD and maintain an adequate nutritional plane in a patient that otherwise would be subject to chronic wasting.

REFERENCES

1. Ross SJ, Osborne CA, Kirk CA, et al. Clinical evaluation of dietary modification for treatment of spontaneous chronic kidney disease in cats. J Am Vet Med Assoc 2006;229(6):949–57.
2. Jacob F, Polzin DJ, Osborne CA, et al. Clinical evaluation of dietary modification for treatment of spontaneous chronic renal failure in dogs. J Am Vet Med Assoc 2003;220:1163–70.
3. Elliott J, Rawlings JM, Markwell PJ, et al. Survival of cats with naturally occurring chronic renal failure: effect of dietary management. J Small Anim Pract 2000;41: 235–42.
4. Quimby JM, Gustafson DL, Lunn KF. The pharmacokinetics of mirtazapine in cats with chronic kidney disease and in age-matched control cats. J Vet Intern Med 2011;25(5):985–9.
5. Quimby JM, Lunn KF. Mirtazapine as an appetite stimulant and anti-emetic in cats with chronic kidney disease: a masked placebo-controlled crossover clinical trial. Vet J 2013;197(3):651–5.
6. Quimby JM, Brock WT, Moses K, et al. Chronic use of maropitant for the management of vomiting and inappetence in cats with chronic kidney disease: a blinded, placebo-controlled clinical trial. J Feline Med Surg 2015; 17(8):692–7.
7. Elliott DA, Riel DL, Rogers QR. Complications and outcomes associated with use of gastrostomy tubes for nutritional management of dogs with renal failure; 56 cases (1994-1999). J Am Vet Med Assoc 2000;217(9): 1337–42.
8. Ireland LM, Hohenhaus AE, Broussard JD, et al. A Comparison of owner management and complications in 67 cats with esophagostomy and percutaneous endoscopic gastrostomy feeding tubes. J Am Anim Hosp Assoc 2003;39(3):241–6.
9. Levine PB, Smallwood LJ, Buback JL. Esophagostomy tubes as a method of nutritional management in cats: a retrospective study. J Am Anim Hosp Assoc 1997;33(5):405–10.
10. Crowe DT, Devey JJ. Esophagostomy tubes for feeding and decompression: clinical experience in 29 small animal patients. J Am Anim Hosp Assoc 1997;33(5): 393–403.
11. Devitt CM, Seim HB 3rd. Clinical evaluation of tube esophagostomy in small animals. J Am Anim Hosp Assoc 1997;33(1):55–60.
12. Segev G, Fascetti AJ, Weeth LP, et al. Correction of hyperkalemia in dogs with chronic kidney disease consuming commercial renal therapeutic diets by a potassium-reduced home-prepared diet. J Vet Intern Med 2010;24: 546–50.

APPENDIX 1: ESOPHAGOSTOMY TUBE PLACEMENT

The following is a step-by-step guide for feeding tube placement.

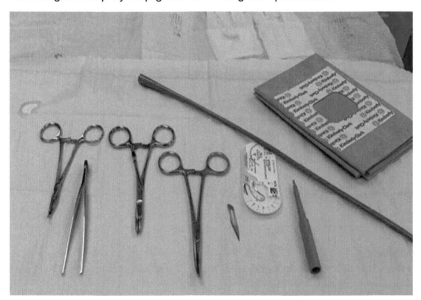

Supplies:
  Red rubber feeding tube
    14F catheter for cats and small dogs
    18F catheter for dogs
  Needle holders
  Skin biopsy punch
  Large curved Kelly (cats)
  Carmault forceps (medium-sized dogs)
  Right angle forceps (large dogs only)
  #11 scalpel blade
  Procedure drape
  Sterile lube
  Sterile gloves (two pair)

Before placement, we typically use a skin biopsy punch to make a hole in the end of the red rubber catheter. Using the skin biopsy punch ensures that the edges are tapered at the end minimizing irritation to the esophagus. A 2-mm punch works well with a 14F catheter red rubber tube and a 3-mm punch is used for an 18F catheter red rubber tube.

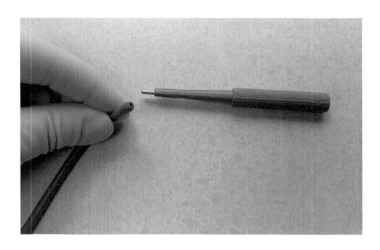

Procedure:
1. Place the patient under general anesthesia. Ensure that the endotracheal tube is in place with the cuff inflated.
2. Clip and surgically prepare the left side of the neck.
3. Visualize the jugular groove and the wing of the atlas. The insertion site for the esophagostomy-tube is dorsal to the jugular vein and approximately 2 to 3 cm caudal to the wing of the atlas.
4. A fenestrated procedure drape should be placed at this time.
5. Gently place a mouth gag to open the mouth and facilitate placement.
6. Advance curved Carmault forceps into the proximal esophagus and rotate so that the tips are pointing up.
7. Place the tips under the desired insertion site.
8. Using blunt force, push the tips of the forceps through the esophageal wall up to the skin.
9. Maintain tension and use the scalpel blade to make a small skin incision directly over the tips of the forceps. Advance the forceps though the skin incision.
10. Grasp the tip of a red rubber feeding tube with the tips of the forceps. Use the forceps to pull the tube out of the mouth.
11. Point the tip of the red rubber tube back into the mouth and advance it down the esophagus. Be careful not to wrap the feeding tube around the endotracheal tube.
12. Continue to advance the tube down the esophagus while maintaining tension on the end of the tube until you feel it "flip" into place.
13. You may premeasure the tube so that the tip is 3 cm cranial to the cardiac sphincter and mark it with an indelible marker. I typically advance the tube until I feel the cardiac sphincter and then back it out 3 cm.
14. Do NOT touch the tube with the hand that has been in the patient's mouth. Change gloves before suturing to prevent contamination.
15. Once in place, suture the tube to the neck at the insertion site. We no longer recommend a purse string suture and have found that two lateral sutures, placed perpendicular to, and just above the insertion site, provide the best hold with a decrease in the incidence of infection. Each of the lateral sutures should be secured loosely to the skin and then firmly to the tube using a finger-trap pattern.

16. A rubber stopper from a blood tube makes a great tube cap. Alternatively, a Christmas tree adapter and infusion plug may be used to stopper the tube, but this combination is cumbersome and seems to annoy patients. The rubber stoppers are light, cheap, and easily replaced.
17. A "tacking suture" may be placed loosely around the tube on the back to direct the tube caudodorsally and provide some stability.

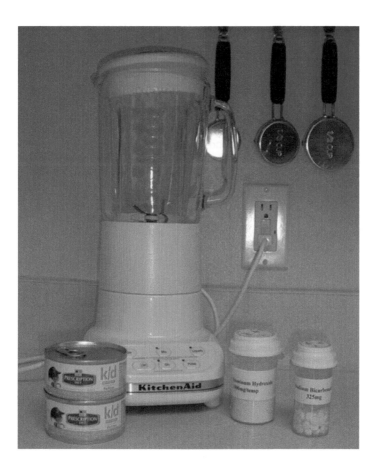

Example of a typical diet recipe for a cat with stage 4 CKD that is hyerphosphatemic and acidemic:

Weight = 5.5 kg

RER = 251 kcal/day

MER = RER × 1.4 = 352 kcal/day

Feline k/d = 183 kcal/can

Patient's Recipe
- 2 cans k/d with chicken (2 × 5.5 oz cans)
- one-quarter can water
- 500 mg aluminum hydroxide
- 650 mg sodium bicarbonate

Place all components in blender and blend well for at least 3 minutes. The final product should resemble smooth pudding. This amount is the entire food ration for this cat for 1 day if he is eating nothing on his own. Two cans of food blended with one-quarter can of water is approximately 300 mL (at 1.2 kcal/mL). The total amount varies slightly.

Generally the food should be divided into four meals daily, but over time the volume per feeding may be increased and the number of meals reduced. For example, my own cat receives 120 mL of blended food twice daily. This is a huge amount for a normal cat, but he is a very large cat, and my schedule allows for only two feedings daily. For my patients, I generally start with four feedings daily. If the patient has been eating only a small amount for some time, we may have to start with half of the calculated MER and gradually increase the volume fed over several days. It may take 1 to 2 weeks to achieve MER in some cases. Rapid or aggressive escalation of the volume fed almost always results in vomiting: unpleasant for the patient and frustrating for the owner. Go slowly.

NOTE: The doses of aluminum hydroxide and bicarbonate used previously are for illustrative purposes only. Medications and doses must be tailored to the individual patient. These are two of the very few medications that may be blended with the food. Most medications should be crushed and given through the tube separately.

Abbreviations: MER, metabolic energy requirement; RER, resting energy requirement.

Management of Proteinuria in Dogs and Cats with Chronic Kidney Disease

Shelly L. Vaden, DVM, PhD[a],*,
Jonathan Elliott, MA, VetMB, PhD, Cert SAC, MRCVS[b]

KEYWORDS

- Urine protein:creatinine ratio • Proteinuria • Hypertension • Angiotensin
- Aldosterone • Glomerular • Chronic kidney disease

KEY POINTS

- Proteinuria is a negative prognostic for chronic kidney disease and is associated with degree of functional impairment, the risk of uremic crisis, progressive worsening of azotemia, or death.
- Normal dogs and most normal cats should have a urine protein:creatinine ratio that is less than 0.4 and less than 0.2, respectively; persistent proteinuria above this magnitude warrants attention.
- Administration of angiotensin-converting enzyme inhibitors and/or angiotensin receptor blockers is considered a standard of care in dogs and cats with renal proteinuria.
- Blood pressure control and nutritional modification are important considerations and part of the standard of care for dogs and cats with renal proteinuria.
- Renal biopsy and administration of immunosuppressive agents should be considered in dogs with glomerular proteinuria that have not responded to standard therapy.

Dr S.L. Vaden has acted as a paid consultant for Heska Corporation and Idexx Ltd. She receives research grant funding from Morris Animal Foundation (D12CA-053) and the American Kennel Club Canine Health Foundation (01844). Dr J. Elliot has acted as a paid consultant for Bayer Animal Health, Boehringer Ingelheim, Elanco Animal Health, Idexx Ltd, CEVA Animal Health, Orion Inc, Nextvet Ltd, Waltham Centre for Pet Nutrition. He receives research grant funding from CEVA Animal Health, Elanco Animal Health, Zoetis Animal Health, Royal Canin and Waltham Centre for Pet Nutrition. Dr J. Elliot is also a member of the International Renal Interest Society, which receives financial support from Elanco Animal Health.
[a] Department of Clinical Sciences, College of Veterinary Medicine, North Carolina State University, 1052 William Moore Drive, Raleigh, NC 27607, USA; [b] Department of Comparative Biomedical Sciences, Royal Veterinary College, University of London, Royal College Street, London NW1 0TU, UK
* Corresponding author.
E-mail address: slvaden@ncsu.edu

PROTEINURIA AS A PROGNOSTIC INDICATOR IN CHRONIC KIDNEY DISEASE

Proteinuria is a negative prognostic indicator for both dogs and cats with chronic kidney disease. In dogs with chronic kidney disease, an initial urine protein:creatinine ratio (UPC) of greater than 1.0 was associated with a threefold greater risk of developing a uremic crisis and death.[1] The relative risk of adverse outcomes increased 1.5 times for every increase in the UPC by 1. In another canine study, proteinuria correlated with the degree of functional impairment, as measured by glomerular filtration rate; dogs with a UPC of less than 1.0 lived 2.7 times longer on average than dogs with a UPC of greater than 1.0.[2]

When nonazotemic cats were evaluated prospectively and longitudinally, proteinuria was found to be associated significantly with the development of azotemia by 12 months.[3] Both proteinuria and serum creatinine were related to shortened survival in cats with chronic kidney disease.[4,5] This was true even when cats had UPC as low as 0.2 to 0.4.

Chronic proteinuria has been shown to be associated with interstitial fibrosis as well as tubular degeneration and atrophy, although the exact mechanisms of injury are a subject of debate.[6,7] There is some evidence that reabsorbed proteins and lipids are directly toxic to the tubular epithelial cells, triggering inflammation and apoptosis. In addition, excessive lysosomal processing of proteins leads to lysosomal rupture and the intracellular release of cytotoxic enzymes. Proteinuria may increase the workload of the tubular epithelial cell beyond its capabilities. Proteinacious casts cause tubular obstruction, which further injures the cells. Glomerular injury results in decreased perfusion of the tubulointerstitium, resulting in cellular hypoxia. Increased glomerular permselectivity increases the filtration of other substances, such as transferrin, that cause additional tubular injury.

Because proteinuria is associated with negative outcomes, it is imperative that the practicing veterinarian has a thorough understanding of appropriate assessment and management of proteinuria in dogs and cats with chronic kidney disease.

NORMAL RENAL HANDLING OF PROTEIN

The glomerulus is a complex structure that functions as a filter, across which an ultrafiltrate of the plasma is formed. This filtration system, made up of the fenestrated endothelium, glomerular basement membrane, and visceral epithelial cells (podocytes), is freely permeable to water and small dissolved solutes but retains cells and most macromolecules, such as proteins. The podocyte is the most differentiated cell in the glomerulus and is essential to the filtration unit.[6] In addition to these factors, glycocalyx has been found to play an important role in maintaining glomerular permselectivity by restricting the passage of proteins.[8] The major determinant restricting passage of proteins into the filtrate is molecular size. Low-molecular-weight proteins, such as insulin and immunoglobulin fragments, pass freely through the filter, but as molecules increase in size they are retained with increasing efficiency. Only small amounts of substances larger than 60,000 to 70,000 Da pass in to the filtrate. The podocyte foot processes, epithelial slits, basement membrane, and endothelium are all rich in negatively charged glycoproteins that create an ionic charge barrier and impede the passage of negatively charged molecules more than would be expected based on their size alone. Albumin, a negatively charged protein with a molecular weight of 69,000 Da, is normally largely excluded from the filtrate. Despite this complex filtration system, the glomerulus normally leaks small quantities of albumin. Rapid endocytosis and hydrolysis of these proteins by proximal tubular cells occurs. Filtered albumin and other proteins are ultimately released to the blood as amino acids. A normal animal should excrete virtually no protein in the urine, but certainly an amount that is below the limit of detection of routine urine protein assays.[9]

LABORATORY TESTS FOR URINE PROTEIN

The urine dipstick, the sulfosalicylic turbidimetric test (SSA, Bumin test), or the UPC can be used to measure total urine protein. The urine dipstick is the most readily available test of urine protein, but is also the least reliable. Both false positives and false negatives occur. The sensitivity and specificity of the urine protein dipstick are as low as 54% and 69%, respectively, in the dog and 60% and 31%, respectively, in the cat.[10] Although the urine dipstick primarily detects albumin, it also measures globulins. The SSA is more reliable than the urine dipstick for the detection of proteinuria (both albumin and globulin); however, use of this test requires either having the appropriate reagents and standards on hand or sending the urine sample to a reference laboratory. The amount of protein present in the urine of normal dogs and cats is less than the lower limit of detection for both of these tests. When both urine dipstick and SSA test results are available, the results of the SSA test should be given greater consideration than those of the urine dipstick. Positive results with either of these tests must be interpreted in light of the urine specific gravity.

Dogs and cats with repeatable positive dipstick or SSA results in urine samples that are free of pyuria or a color change from hematuria should have urine protein losses quantified by the UPC. The UPC is determined using a quantitative test for total urine protein, the results of which are expressed as a ratio to urine creatinine, thereby eliminating the need to consider the urine specific gravity when interpreting the results. The ratio correlates well with 24-hour urine protein losses and can be measured either in-house or as a send out test. Normal dogs, female cats, and neutered male cats should have a UPC that is less than 0.2 (**Table 1**). Normal intact male cats can have a UPC of up to 0.6, most likely owing to the excretion of large amounts of cauxin.

Persistent microalbuminuria is the mildest, and often earliest, detectable form of proteinuria. Urine albumin can be measured quantitatively through a commercial reference laboratory using a species-specific assay. The urine is diluted to a standard concentration (1.010) before assay, eliminating the need to consider urine specific gravity when interpreting the test results. Alternatively, some reference laboratories report urine albumin as a ratio to creatinine (ie, milligrams of albumin to grams of creatinine). Microalbuminuria is defined as concentrations of albumin in the urine that are greater than normal, but less than the limit of detection using the urine dipstick. By this definition, the upper end of urine albumin concentrations that are still considered to be microalbuminuria is 30 mg/dL (or 300 mg albumin per gram of creatinine). Urine albumin concentrations greater than this are called overt albuminuria. Proteinuria of this magnitude can often be detected using the UPC.

Table 1		
International Renal Interest Society classification of proteinuria in dogs and cats with chronic kidney disease		
Substage	**Cat[a]**	**Dog**
Nonproteinuric	<0.2	<0.2
Borderline proteinuric	0.2–0.4	0.2–0.5
Proteinuric	>0.4	>0.5

[a] Applies to normal female and neutered male cats; normal intact male cats may have a urine protein:creatinine ratio as high as 0.6.

CLINICAL ASSESSMENT OF PROTEINURIA

Accurate assessment of proteinuria involves 3 key elements: persistence, localization, and magnitude.[11] Persistent proteinuria is defined as proteinuria that has been detected on 3 or more occasions, 2 or more weeks apart. Persistent proteinuria should be localized as being prerenal, postrenal, or renal (**Table 2**). Identifying the cause of proteinuria in an affected dog or cat is important so that appropriate therapeutic measures can be implemented. Renal proteinuria that is glomerular or tubulointerstitial in origin is the most relevant form of proteinuria when managing dogs with chronic kidney disease. However, it is important to ensure that proteinuria is not owing to prerenal or postrenal causes, because the management of these disorders varies substantially from the management of chronic kidney disease. Functional proteinuria is not very common in dogs and cats, or at least it is poorly documented.

Table 2
Categorization of potential causes of proteinuria in dogs and cats

Category	Mechanism	Potential Causes
Prerenal	Greater than normal delivery of low molecular weight plasma proteins to the normal glomerulus	• Hemoglobinuria from intravascular hemolysis • Myoglobinuria from rhabdomyolysis • Immunoglobulin light chains from multiple myeloma or lymphoma
Renal	Abnormal renal handling of normal plasma proteins caused by one of the following subcategories:	
Functional (physiologic)	Altered renal physiology in response to transient stressor	• Strenuous exercise • Fever • Seizure • Exposure to extreme heat or cold
Glomerular	Altered permselectivity of the glomerular basement membrane	Any cause of glomerular injury or dysfunction (eg, membranoproliferative glomerulonephritis, membranous nephropathy, glomerulosclerosis, amyloidosis)
Tubular[a]	Impaired tubular recovery of plasma proteins that are normally found in the glomerular filtrate	Any cause of renal tubular dysfunction (eg, acute tubular necrosis, Fanconi syndrome)
Interstitial[a]	Exudation of proteins from the interstitial space into the urinary space	Interstitial nephritis
Postrenal	Entry of protein into the urine in association with exudation of blood or serum into the lower urinary or genital tracts	• Urinary tract infection • Urolithiasis • Transitional cell carcinoma • Vaginitis

[a] Tubular and interstitial can be difficult to separate in a clinical setting and are often referred to as tubulointerstitial.

Once prerenal and postrenal causes of persistent proteinuria are eliminated, the magnitude of the proteinuria is used to help determine if renal proteinuria is glomerular or tubulointerstitial in origin. Magnitude is assessed using a quantitative test for urine protein (generally UPC but could also be urine albumin). Once prerenal and postrenal causes of proteinuria have been excluded, it is recommended that a UPC be evaluated in all dog and cats with persistent proteinuria as determined by dipstick or SSA.

The International Renal Interest Society has recommended substaging dogs and cats with chronic kidney disease on the basis of their UPC (see **Table 1**). Dogs that have renal proteinuria and a UPC of 2.0 or greater usually have glomerular disease, whereas dogs with a UPC of less than 2.0 might have either glomerular disease or tubulointerstitial disease. Glomerular diseases occur much less commonly in cats but should be suspected when the UPC is 2 or greater. Concurrent hypoalbuminuria is added evidence that glomerular disease is present.

Urine sodium-dodecyl sulfate polyacrylamide gel electrophoresis can be used to help determine if renal proteinuria is glomerular or tubulointerstitial in origin.[12] Finding predominantly low molecular weight proteins is consistent with tubulointerstitial disease whereas glomerular damage is more likely associated with a pattern of intermediate and high-molecular-weight proteins. When there is concurrent glomerular and tubulointerstitial disease, a mixture of sizes is expected. In addition to sodium-dodecyl sulfate polyacrylamide gel electrophoresis, there are certain novel biomarkers that may prove in the future to identify tubulointerstitial damage is present (eg, retinol binding protein, kidney injury molecule-1).

INHIBITION OF THE RENIN–ANGIOTENSIN–ALDOSTERONE SYSTEM TO MANAGE PROTEINURIA

Hemodynamic forces influence the transglomerular movement of proteins, and it follows that altering renal hemodynamics would be effective in reducing proteinuria.[13] The renin–angiotensin–aldosterone system (RAAS) has been the major target system for this approach to reducing proteinuria (**Fig. 1**). Agents that target RAAS include the angiotensin-converting enzyme inhibitors (ACEi), angiotensin receptor blockers (ARB),

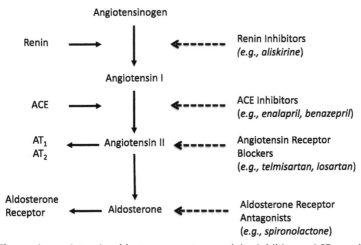

Fig. 1. The renin–angiotensin–aldosterone system and its inhibitors. ACE, angiotensin-converting enzyme.

and aldosterone receptor antagonists **(Table 3)**. Although renin inhibitors are being used in people, they have not been used to any great extent in dogs and cats. All RAAS inhibitors have antihypertensive effects although most of them only minimally reduce blood pressure (ie, 10%–15%). These drugs likely reduce proteinuria by several mechanisms in addition to the expected decrease in glomerular capillary hypertension. Likewise, the reduction in proteinuria is greater than would be expected on the basis of their antihypertensive effects alone. RAAS inhibition is considered a standard of care in dogs and cats with renal proteinuria where the UPC is less than 0.5 to 1 and greater than 0.2 to 0.4, respectively. The inhibitors of RAAS reduce proteinuria in populations of animals, but the effect in individual animals might vary. It may take trial and error with different drugs or combinations of drugs before the target antiproteinuric effect is achieved (see Monitoring Drug Therapy); some animals may never achieve target reductions.

Angiotensin-Converting Enzyme Inhibitors

Administration of ACEi has been associated positive outcomes in dogs, cats, and people with chronic kidney disease.[14–17] Enalapril significantly reduced proteinuria and

Table 3
Inhibitors of RAAS used in dogs and cats with chronic kidney disease

Class	Drug	Initial Dose	Escalating Dose Strategy
Angiotensin-converting enzyme inhibitors	Benazapril	0.25–0.5 mg/kg PO q24 h[a] Dog or cat	Increase by 0.25–0.5 mg/kg to a maximum daily dose of 2 mg/kg; can be given q12 h
	Enalapril	0.25–0.5 mg/kg PO q24 h[a] Dog or cat	Increase by 0.25–0.5 mg/kg to a maximum daily dose of 2 mg/kg; can be given q12 h
	Lisinopril	0.25–0.5 mg/kg PO q24 h[a] Dog or cat	Increase by 0.25–0.5 mg/kg to a maximum daily dose of 2 mg/kg; can be given q12 h
	Ramipril	0.125 mg/kg PO q24 h Dog	Increase by 0.125 mg/kg q24 h to a maximum of 0.5 mg/kg q24 h; usually given q24 h
	Imidapril	0.25 mg/kg PO q24 h Dog	Increase by 0.25 mg/kg q24 h to a maximum of 2 mg/kg q24 h; usually given q24 h
Angiotensin receptor blockers	Telmisartan[b]	0.5–1.0 mg/kg PO q24 h Dog Dog or cat	Increase by 0.25–0.5 mg/kg to a maximum daily dose of 5 mg/kg; usually given q24 h
	Losartan[c]	0.25–0.5 mg/kg PO q24 h Dog	Increase by 0.25–0.5 mg/kg to a maximum daily dose of 2 mg/kg; can be given q12 h
Aldosterone receptor blocker	Spironolactone[d]	0.5–2 mg/kg PO q12–24 h Dog	

Abbreviations: PO, orally; RAAS, renin–angiotensin–aldosterone system.
[a] Smaller starting doses should be used in animals with in stage 3 or 4 chronic kidney disease or if there are concurrent medical problems that have the potential to lead to dehydration or reduced appetite.
[b] Can be used a single agent or combined with an angiotensin-converting enzyme inhibitor (ACEi).
[c] Concurrent administration of an ACEi is generally recommended.
[d] Only recommended in dogs with glomerular disease that have increased serum or urine aldosterone concentrations and have failed or not tolerated an ACEi or angiotensin receptor blocker.

delayed the onset or the progression of azotemia in dogs with glomerulonephritis.[17] In dogs with partial nephrectomies, enalapril treated dogs had a reduction in glomerular and tubulointerstitial lesions following 6 months of treatment.[18] Likewise, dogs with chronic kidney disease that were given benazepril had higher glomerular filtration rates and lower UPCs when compared with a placebo-treated group.[14]

Benazepril administration was associated with reduced glomerular capillary pressure in cats with induced chronic kidney disease.[19] In cats with naturally occurring chronic kidney disease, benazepril was associated with a reduction in proteinuria, even in the subgroup of cats with an initial UPC of less than 0.2; cats with an initial UPC greater than 1 demonstrated better appetites when given benazepril versus placebo. Although these drugs reduce proteinuria in cats, studies have not yet demonstrated a positive effect on survival or progression of chronic kidney disease.

Proposed mechanisms for these effects include decreased efferent glomerular arteriolar resistance leading to decreased or normalized glomerular transcapillary hydraulic pressure, reduced loss of glomerular heparin sulfate, decreased size of the glomerular capillary endothelial pores, improved lipoprotein metabolism, slowed glomerular mesangial growth and proliferation, and inhibition of bradykinin degradation.

Initially, an ACEi is given once daily, but more than one-half of the dogs will need twice daily administration eventually and perhaps additional dosage escalations (**Fig. 2**).[17] Many veterinarians are concerned about administering an ACEi to a dog or cat that is already azotemic. In people, the renoprotective effects of ACEi are independent of the baseline renal function, and ACEi slowed progressive disease even in patients with severe renal failure.[20] In reality, it seems to be uncommon for dogs and cats to have severe worsening of azotemia (ie, >30% increase from baseline) owing to ACEi administration alone, provided that the animals are clinically stable before the introduction of these agents. Dogs that are dehydrated may be at highest risk for worsening of azotemia after initiating ACEi therapy; euvolemia should be achieved before initiating an ACEi to these patients. Furthermore, some caution is warranted when administering an ACEi to a dog or cat in late stage 3 or stage 4 chronic kidney disease, including consideration of a low initial starting dose and small incremental increases.

Many veterinarians wonder if one ACEi is better than another in animals with reduced renal function. The pharmacokinetics of ACEi are complicated, and the effects of disease on the pharmacodynamics of these drugs in not necessarily predictable. There is no scientific basis to support that one ACEi has superior pharmacodynamic action. Benazepril and its active metabolite, benazeprilat, are largely eliminated by the biliary route with a smaller fraction being excreted in the urine; impaired renal function does not affect the clearance of this drug in dogs.[21] In contrast, enalapril and its active metabolite, enalaprilat, are primarily eliminated by the kidney. Animals in late International Renal Interest Society chronic kidney disease stage 3 or 4 may require a lower dosage of enalapril to achieve target antiproteinuric effects.

Angiotensin Receptor Blockers

ARB block the angiotensin II type 1 receptor. Several ARBs have been studied extensively in people with glomerular disease and lead to a reduction in proteinuria similar to that seen with ACEi. People treated with losartan had an average reduction in proteinuria of 35% from baseline during a 3.4-year follow-up period; much of this decrease was achieved in the first 6 months of therapy.[22] In irbesartan-treated patients, every

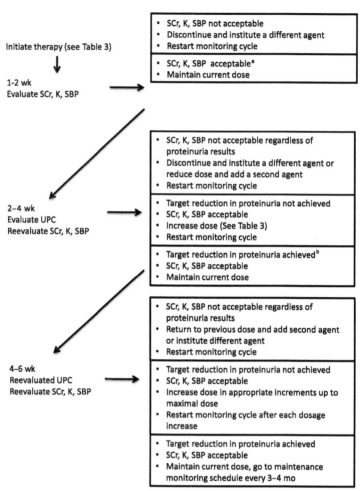

Fig. 2. Making adjustments to renin–angiotensin–aldosterone system inhibition therapy in dogs with renal proteinuria. [a] Results are acceptable when K <6.0 mEq/L, SBP >120 mm Hg, and SCr is stable or minimally increased (ie, <30% increase above baseline when stage 1 or 2 CKD, <10% when stage 3 CKD, no increase when stage 4 CKD). [b] Target reduction in proteinuria is UPC <1 (primary) or >50% reduction from baseline (secondary). CKD, chronic kidney disease; K, serum potassium; SBP, systolic blood pressure; SCr, serum creatinine; UPC, urine protein:creatinine ratio.

50% reduction in proteinuria achieved during the first 12 months of therapy reduced the risk of a negative renal outcome by more than one-half.[22]

The use of ARBs in dogs and cats with proteinuric chronic kidney disease is still being developed. The one that seems to be the most effective is telmisartan; however, losartan has been used more extensively.[23,24] Even though dogs do not seem to produce one of the major active metabolites of losartan, there is good evidence that losartan exerts pharmacodynamic effects in dogs.[25] Contrary to this, pharmacodynamic studies suggest that losartan may not be effective in cats, at least as predicted by attenuation of pressor responses.[26]

Telmisartan is more lipophilic, and has a longer half-life than losartan; its blocking effects persist for longer than would be predicted from its plasma half-life.

Furthermore, it has a higher affinity for, and dissociates more slowly from, the angiotensin-1 receptor. Therefore, it is not surprising that telmisartan was shown to be more effective in reducing proteinuria in people with diabetic nephropathy.[22] Telmisartan was as effective as amlodipine in controlling blood pressure in people with chronic kidney disease.[27] Similarly, telmisartan attenuated angiotensin 1–induced blood pressure response to a greater degree than did benazepril in normal cats.[26] If these observations are confirmed in dogs and cats, telmisartan might be the initial RAAS inhibitor of choice when proteinuria and systemic hypertension are both present. A randomized controlled clinical trial comparing the effects of telmisartan and benazepril on proteinuria in cats with naturally occurring chronic kidney disease demonstrated overall that telmisartan was as effective as benazepril in preventing an increase in UPC during a 6-month treatment period. Indeed, telmisartan reduced UPC relative to the pretreatment value at all time points evaluated in the 6-month trial whereas benazepril only reduced UPC at very early time points.[23]

Combined Therapy with Angiotensin-Converting Enzyme Inhibitors and Angiotensin Receptor Blockers

There may be an added benefit to combined administration of an ACEi and an ARB because of the inability of either class of drug to provide complete RAAS blockade when given alone.[22] Although not evaluated in dogs and cats, studies in people have suggested that these drugs may be additive or perhaps even synergistic in reducing proteinuria.[28] The dosage of each individual drug might be reduced during combined therapy, thereby reducing the likelihood of adverse effects of the individual drugs. However, the approach of combining these 2 agents must be used cautiously in light of a human study where elderly patients prescribed this combination had a higher risk of kidney failure and death.[29] Controlled studies are needed in dogs to determine if the antiprotienuric effects of ACEi and ARBs are optimized by combination therapy or monotherapy with individualized dosage escalation.

Aldosterone Breakthrough

Complete blockade of the RAAS system is generally not achieved with RAAS inhibitors. In the absence of angiotensin-converting enzyme, angiotensin II is produced by other kinases and is, therefore, not suppressed completely by an ACEi alone. Blockade of the angiotensin II type 1 receptor with an ARB may give rise to a compensatory increase in renin activity, and therefore an incomplete block of the RAAS.[30] Combination therapy increases the degree of blockade, but it still may not provide more than 75% to 80% blockade.

Serum aldosterone increases over time in some people treated even with maximal dosages of RAAS inhibitors, a phenomenon referred to as aldosterone breakthrough. The incidence of aldosterone breakthrough in people treated with RAAS inhibitors for chronic kidney disease, systemic hypertension or heart failure is between 10% and 53%.[31] Prolonged hyperaldosteronism can have adverse effects on the heart, systemic blood vessels, and glomeruli. Therefore, it is not surprising that some people that experience aldosterone breakthrough during treatment for various glomerular diseases have more negative outcomes (eg, higher magnitude proteinuria, greater reduction in glomerular filtration rate).[32,33] Preliminary studies have demonstrated that aldosterone breakthrough may occur in up to one-third of dogs with proteinuric renal diseases that are receiving RAAS inhibitors (Ames, unpublished data, 2015). More study is needed to determine if aldosterone breakthrough is associated with poorer treatment outcomes in dogs.

Aldosterone Receptor Antagonists

Aldosterone receptor antagonists have been shown to reduce proteinuria and stabilize kidney function in an additive fashion to ACEi and/or ARB in people, particularly if they have evidence of aldosterone breakthrough before adding the aldosterone receptor antagonist.[34] Eplerenone may be the drug of choice in people because the relative lack of binding to androgen and progesterone receptors produces fewer endocrine side effects. However, endocrine side effects of spironolactone in dogs are less problematic and the preference is unclear in veterinary medicine. Although spironolactone has been used most commonly in veterinary medicine, there is little evidence supporting the efficacy of this drug in dogs in the management of glomerular disease. Sprionoloactone should only be effective if serum or urine aldosterone concentrations are increased, indicative of aldosterone breakthrough. This drug could be tried in dogs that have high serum or urine aldosterone concentrations and persistent proteinuria despite treatment with an ACEi and/or ARB. The drug should not be used in cats until more is known about its efficacy and safety in this species.

Monitoring Drug Therapy

The UPC, urinalysis, systemic blood pressure, and serum albumin, creatinine. and potassium concentrations (in fasting samples) should be monitored at least quarterly in all animals being treated for proteinuric renal disease. However, patients having new drugs introduced or dosage modifications being made for drugs already being administered should be monitored more frequently (see **Fig. 2**). One to 2 weeks after an ACEi or ARB is added or changed, the UPC, serum creatinine, serum potassium, and systemic blood pressure should be evaluated to verify the recent change in therapy has not resulted in a severe worsening of renal function (ie, >30% increase in serum creatinine), a concerning increase in serum potassium concentrations, or hypotension (an unlikely occurrence with these drugs).

Day-to-day variations in the UPC occur in most dogs with glomerular proteinuria, with greater variation occurring in dogs with a UPC of greater than 4[35]; variations also occur in cats, but these have not been as well-characterized. Changes in urine protein content are most accurately measured by assessing trends in the UPC over time. Because there is greater day-to-day variation in dogs with a UPC of greater than 4, consideration should be given to either averaging 2 to 3 serial UPC or measuring a UPC in urine that has been pooled from 2 to 3 collections.[36] In 1 study, demonstration of a significant difference between serial values in proteinuric dogs required a change by at least 35% at high UPC values (near 12) and 80% at low UPC values (near 0.5).[35] Thus, a reduction in UPC near these reported magnitudes without an increase in the serum creatinine concentration is required to indicate improvement or response to therapy.

Making Therapeutic Adjustments for Renin–Angiotensin–Aldosterone System Inhibitors

An ACEi is the initial therapy prescribed for most dogs and cats with proteinuria, with the typical starting dosage of 0.5 mg/kg every 24 hours (see **Fig. 2**). However, the ARB telmisartan may soon be recommended as a reasonable alternative for an initial agent. In dogs and cats, the ideal therapeutic target is a reduction in the UPC to less than 1 without inappropriate worsening of renal function. Because this ideal target is not achieved in most animals, a reduction in UPC of 50% or greater is often the target. The degree to which worsening of renal function is tolerated will in part depend on the stage of chronic kidney disease the dog is in. Dogs with International Renal Interest

Society chronic kidney disease stages 1 and 2 can have an increase in serum creatinine of up to 30% without modifying therapy. The goal in dogs with stage 3 chronic kidney disease would be to maintain stable renal function, allowing only for a 10% increase in serum creatinine. If renal function deteriorates beyond these allowances, therapeutic adjustments may be indicated. Dogs with stage 4 chronic kidney disease are generally intolerant of worsening of renal function and any deterioration may have clinical consequences. Whereas RAAS inhibitors can be used in this subset of patients, the initial starting doses and incremental dose increases should be very low and renal function should be monitored closely; therapeutic adjustments may be needed to maintain baseline renal function.

If the target reduction in UPC is not achieved, the plasma potassium concentration is less than 6 mmol/L, and any changes in renal function decrease within the tolerable limit, dosages may be increased every 4 to 6 weeks to establish the UPC nadir. If the target reduction in UPC is not achieved with a maximal dosage an ACEi, the next step should be to add an ARB. Alternatively an ARB can be used as monotherapy in dogs who seem to be intolerant of an ACEi.

Managing Hyperkalemia

Hyperkalemia seems to be a common side effect of RAAS inhibition in dogs with kidney disease, but is probably uncommon in cats. Pseudohyperkalemia, often associated with thrombocytosis, can also occur in dogs and needs to be ruled out by measuring the potassium concentration in lithium heparin plasma before taking further action. Because of the cardiotoxic effects of potassium, dogs or cats with true hyperkalemia of greater than 5.5 mEq/L should be monitored closely; therapy should be modified if serum potassium concentrations are greater than 6 to 6.5 mEq/L. When plasma potassium concentrations are less than 6 mEq/L, an electrocardiograph should be evaluated for cardiac conduction disturbances. True hyperkalemia can be managed by reducing the ACEi or ARB drug dosage, discontinuing spironolactone administration, or by feeding diets that are reduced in potassium (note that renal diets may be supplemented with potassium). The use of an intestinal potassium binder (eg, kayexelate) has been limited in dogs. (See Sheri Ross' article, "Utilization of Feeding Tubes in the Management of Feline Chronic Kidney Disease," in this issue.) Rarely, hyperkalemia would be severe enough to warrant hemodialysis. Potassium-reduced home-prepared diets that were formulated by a veterinary nutritionist have been shown to effectively correct hyperkalemia in the long term in dogs with chronic kidney disease.[37]

MANAGEMENT OF HYPERTENSION

The kidney is one of the target organs for hypertensive damage and sustained hypertension may lead to an increased magnitude of proteinuria, rate of decline of renal function, frequency of uremic crises, and mortality.[3,38,39] The goal of antihypertensive therapy is to reduce the blood pressure so the risk of continued target organ damage is minimized (**Table 4**). Inhibitors of RAAS are generally only weak antihypertensive agents, leading to a reduction in blood pressure by only about 10% to 15%. Dogs and cats that have sustained systolic blood pressures of 160 mm Hg or greater while being administered a RAAS inhibitor have a moderate to high risk of future target organ damage and may need additional therapeutic consideration. In these animals, the first step is to increase the dose of the RAAS inhibitor. If the upper limit of the dosage range is being administered and the risk of target organ damage remains moderate to high, the next step is to add a calcium channel blocker. Amlodipine is usually recommended

Table 4
Staging of blood pressure in dogs and cats according to the risk for future target organ damage

Blood Pressure Stage	Systolic (mm Hg)	Diastolic (mm Hg)
Normotensive – risk none to minimal	<150	<95
Borderline hypertensive – low risk	150–159	95–99
Hypertensive – moderate risk	160–179	110–119
Severely hypertensive - high risk	≥180	≥120

with a starting dose of 0.2 to 0.4 mg/kg every 24 hours but can be incrementally increased to a total daily dose of 0.75 mg/kg, which can be divided to every 12 hours. There is evidence that amlodipine will activate the RAAS system; therefore, it should not be used as monotherapy for the management of hypertension in dogs.[40] However, in cats monotherapy may be more appropriate because giving multiple drugs makes it more difficult to achieve compliance. Amlodipine alone may bring the UPC down to less than 0.2 in hypertensive cats, and amlodipine-induced increases in plasma renin activity are not associated with an increase in aldosterone in cats.[41]

Systolic blood pressure should be monitored during therapy and maintained greater than 120 mm Hg in treated dogs and cats. High salt intake should be avoided, although salt restriction alone will not reduce blood pressure adequately.

DIET

In animal models of chronic kidney disease, the magnitude of proteinuria can be reduced by dietary modification, specifically by modifying the polyunsaturated fatty acid ratio and protein content.[13] Dietary supplementation with n-3 polyunsaturated fatty acids or feeding a diet that has a reduced n-6/n-3 ratio that is, close to 5:1, as found in most commercially available renal diets is expected to alter the long-term course of renal injury and decrease the magnitude of proteinuria. It is generally accepted that feeding a renal diet that is modified in protein content reduces intraglomerular capillary pressure as well as the magnitude of proteinuria and the generation of uremic toxins. However, the magnitude of this reduction in proteinuria is small. Renal diet alone should not be expected to reduce proteinuria adequately in most animals.

RENAL BIOPSY

Nearly 60% of dogs with glomerular proteinuria will have either immune complex–mediated glomerulonephritis or amyloidosis,[42] both of which may represent an aberrant or excessive immune or inflammatory response to an infectious, neoplastic or inflammatory condition. Cats rarely get glomerulonephritis; however, it should be anticipated that individual cats could develop glomerulonephritis secondary to a concurrent systemic disease. Therefore, in dogs or cats with glomerular proteinuria it is indicated to pursue extended diagnostic testing, the extent of which might vary depending on patient characteristics and potential exposure to regional infectious agents.[43] It is possible that complete or partial resolution of proteinuria will follow successful treatment of any causative systemic diseases.

Renal biopsy should be considered in animals with persistent glomerular range proteinuria that do not have any contraindications to renal biopsy and have not responded to standard therapy.[43] Some of the more common contraindications to biopsy include chronic kidney disease with a serum creatinine of greater than 5 mg/dL, uncontrolled hypertension, pyelonephritis, renal cystic disease, coagulopathy, hydronephrosis, and severe anemia. When biopsy samples are processed correctly and evaluated by an experienced nephropathologist, clinical decisions regarding the diagnosis, treatment, and prognosis can be made from the information obtained through renal biopsy in dogs. Experienced personnel should be involved with procuring, preparing, and interpreting the renal biopsy that has been processed for light, electron, and immunofluorescence microscopy.[43]

From a therapeutic standpoint, the primary purpose of the renal biopsy is to determine if there is an active immunopathogenesis ongoing in the glomeruli and if immunosuppressive therapy is indicated or not. Finding electron dense deposits in subendothelial, subepithelial, intramembranous, or mesangial locations of the glomerulus by electron microscopy or demonstrating positive and unequivocal immunofluorescent staining for immunoglobulins and/or complement in an immune complex or antiglomerular basement membrane pattern of deposition in peripheral capillary loops or the mesangial compartment with immunofluorescence microscopy provides compelling evidence to initiate a trial of immunosuppressive therapy.[44] Probable evidence of an immunopathogenesis can be documented by light microscopy with one of the following: red granular staining of capillary walls with Masson trichrome, spikes along the glomerular basement membrane or holes within the glomerular basement membrane with Jones Methenamine sliver stain. These findings would be expected in just less than 50% of dogs with glomerular disease.[42] When renal biopsy results are not available, it becomes more difficult to make a decision about using immunosuppressive treatment because approximately 50% of dogs with glomerular disease would be expected not to have an immunopathogenesis of their disease. Consensus recommendations are to consider immunosuppressive drugs in the treatment of dogs with glomerular disease when (1) the source of proteinuria is clearly glomerular in origin, (2) the drugs are not otherwise contraindicated, (3) the dog's breed and age of disease onset are not suggestive of a familial nephropathy, (4) amyloidosis has been deemed unlikely, (5) the serum creatinine is greater than 3.0 mg/dL or progressively increasing, or (6) the serum albumin is less than 2.0 g/dL.[45]

IMMUNOSUPPRESSIVE AGENTS

Empirical administration of immunosuppressive or antiinflammatory therapy has been recommended for dogs that have no known contraindications for the specific drugs being considered and have severe, persistent, or progressive glomerular disease in which there is renal biopsy-supported evidence of immune-mediated pathogenesis.[44] Dogs with more severe disease or rate of progression should be treated more aggressively than those with relatively stable disease. Single agent or combination therapy for rapid onset of immunosuppression should be considered in dogs with high magnitude proteinuria with hypoalbuminemia, nephrotic syndrome, or rapidly progressive azotemia.[44] Mycophenolate mofetil or cyclophosphamide, with or without short-term administration of glucocorticoids, has been suggested as the first choice. Glucocorticoids should be limited to short-term therapy because of the association with corticosteroid excess and proteinuria. Dogs with stable or more slowly progressive disease that have only partial or no response to standard therapy might be given drugs that have a either a rapid or a more delayed onset of action, such as mycophenolate mofetil, chlorambucil, or cyclophosphamide. Cyclosporine has also been suggested as a first choice for stable or slowly progressive dogs. It is important to note that cyclosporine is the only drug that has been studied prospectively in dogs with glomerular disease and was found to be of no benefit, although there were flaws in the design of that study.[46]

All dogs treated with immunosuppressive therapy for their glomerular disease should be monitored closely. Treatment should be discontinued or adjusted if adverse drug effects develop. In the absence of adverse effects, 8 to 12 weeks of initial therapy should be provided before changing the course of treatment. If the therapeutic response is suboptimal at the end of 8 to 12 weeks, an alternate drug protocol should be considered. However, if after 3 to 4 months a therapeutic response has not been achieved, consideration should be given to discontinuing immunosuppressive drug administration. If after this time, a response has been noted, the drug dose or schedule should be tapered to one that maintains the response without worsening of proteinuria, azotemia or clinical signs.[44]

REFERENCES

1. Jacob F, Polson DJ, Osborne CA, et al. Evaluation of the association between initial proteinuria and morbidity rate or death in dogs with naturally occurring chronic renal failure. J Am Vet Med Assoc 2005;226:393–400.
2. Wehner A, Hartmann K, Hirschberger J. Associations between proteinuria, systemic hypertension and glomerular filtration rate in dogs with renal and non-renal diseases. Vet Rec 2008;162:141–7.
3. Jepson RE, Brodbelt D, Vallance C, et al. Evaluation of predictors of the development of azotemia in cats. J Vet Intern Med 2009;23:806–13.
4. Syme HM, Markwell PJ, Pfeiffer DU, et al. Survival of cats with naturally occurring chronic renal failure is related to severity of proteinuria. J Vet Intern Med 2006;20:528–35.
5. King JN, Tasker S, Gunn-Moore DA, et al. Prognostic factors in cats with chronic kidney disease. J Vet Intern Med 2007;21:906–16.
6. Toblli JE, Bevione P, DiGennaro F, et al. Understanding the mechanisms of proteinuria: therapeutic implications. Int J Nephrol 2012;2012:1–13.
7. Pollock CA, Poronnik P. Albumin transport and processing by the proximal tubule: physiology and pathophysiology. Curr Opin Nephrol Hypertens 2007;16:359–64.
8. Singh A, Satchell SC, Neal CR, et al. Glomerular endothelial glycocalyx constitutes a barrier to protein permeability. J Am Soc Nephrol 2007;18:2885–93.
9. Maack T. Renal handling of proteins and polypeptides. Compr Physiol 2011;2039–82. http://dx.doi.org/10.1002/cphy.cp080244.
10. Grauer GF, Moore LE, Smith AR, et al. Comparison of conventional urine protein test strips and a quantitative ELISA for the detection of canine and feline albuminuria [abstract]. J Vet Intern Med 2004;18:418–9.
11. Lees GE, Brown SA, Elliot J, et al. Assessment and management of proteinuria in dogs and cats: 2004 ACVIM forum consensus statement (small animal). J Vet Intern Med 2005;19:377–85.
12. Nabity MB. Urinary biomarkers of chronic kidney disease in veterinary medicine: where do we stand? Paper presented at the American College of Veterinary Pathologists/American Society of Veterinary Clinical Pathology Concurrent Annual Meetings. Baltimore, October 30–November 3, 2010.
13. Brown S, Elliot J, Francey T, et al. Consensus recommendations for standard therapy of glomerular disease in dogs. J Vet Intern Med 2013;27:S27–43.
14. Tenhundfeld J, Wefstaedt P, Nolte JA. A randomized controlled clinical trial of the use of benazepril and heparin for the treatment of chronic kidney disease in dogs. J Am Vet Med Assoc 2009;234:1031–7.

15. King JN, Gunn-Moore DA, Tasker S, et al. Tolerability and efficacy of benazepril in cats with chronic kidney disease. J Vet Intern Med 2006;20:1054–64.
16. Mizutani H, Koyama H, Watanabe T, et al. Evaluation of the clinical efficacy of benazepril in the treatment of chronic insufficiency in cats. J Vet Intern Med 2006;20: 1074–9.
17. Grauer GF, Greco DS, Getzy DM, et al. Effects of enalapril vs placebo as a treatment for canine idiopathic glomerulonephritis. J Vet Intern Med 2000;14:526–33.
18. Brown SA, Finco DR, Brown CA, et al. Evaluation of the effects of inhibition of angiotensin converting enzyme with enalapril in dogs with induced chronic renal insufficiency. Am J Vet Res 2003;64:321–7.
19. Brown SA, Brown CA, Jacobs G, et al. Effects of the angiotensin converting enzyme inhibitor benazepril in cats with induced renal insufficiency. Am J Vet Res 2001;62:375–83.
20. Ryan MJ, Tuttle KR. Elevations in serum creatinine with RAAS blockade: why isn't it a sign of kidney injury? Curr Opin Nephrol Hyperten 2008;17:443–9.
21. Lefebvre HP, Laroute V, Concordet D, et al. Effects of renal impairment on the disposition of orally administered enalapril, benazepril, and their active metabolites. J Vet Intern Med 1999;13:21–7.
22. Bakris G, Burgess E, Weir M, et al. Telmisartan is more effective than losartan in reducing proteinuria in patients with diabetic nephropathy. Kidney Int 2008;74: 364–9.
23. Sent U, Gossl R, Elliot J, et al. Comparison of efficacy of long-term oral treatment with telmisartan and benazepril in cats with chronic kidney disease. J Vet Intern Med 2015;29:1479–87.
24. Bugbee AC, Coleman AE, Wang A, et al. Telmisartan treatment of refractory proteinuria in a dog. J Vet Intern Med 2014;28:1871–4.
25. Christ DD, Wong PC, Wong YN, et al. The pharmacokinetics and pharmacodynamics of the angiotensin II receptor antagonist losartan potassium (DuP 753/ MK 954) in the dog. J Pharm Exp Ther 1992;268:1199–205.
26. Jenkins TL, Coleman AE, Schmiedt CW, et al. Attenuation of the pressor response to exogenous angiotensin by angiotensin receptor blockers and benazepril hydrochloride in clinically normal cats. Am J Vet Res 2015;76:807–13.
27. Nakamura T, Inoue T, Suzuki T, et al. Comparison of renal and vascular protective effects between telmisartan and amlodipine in hypertensive patients with chronic kidney disease and mild renal insufficiency. Hypertens Res 2007;31:841–50.
28. Linas SL. Are two better than one? Angiotensin-converting enzyme inhibitors plus angiotensin receptor blockers for reducing blood pressure and proteinuria in kidney disease. Clin J Am Soc Nephrol 2008;3:S17–23.
29. McAlister FA, Zhang J, Tonelli M, et al. The safety of combining angiotensin-converting enzyme inhibitors with angiotensin-receptor blockers in elderly patients: a population-based longitudinal analysis. Can Med Assoc J 2011;183: E309–11.
30. Laverman GD, Navis GJ, Henning RH, et al. Dual blockade of renin-angiotensin system blockade at optimal doses for proteinuria. Kidney Int 2002;62:1020–5.
31. Bomback AS, Klemmer PJ. The incidence and implications of aldosterone breakthrough. Nat Clin Pract Nephrol 2007;3:486–92.
32. Horita Y, Taura K, Taguchi T, et al. Aldosterone breakthrough during therapy with angiotensin-converting enzyme inhibitors and angiotensin II receptor blockers in proteinuria patients with immunoglobulin A nephropathy. Nephrology 2006;11: 462–6.

33. Schjoedt KJ, Andersen S, Rossing P, et al. Aldosterone escape during blockade of the renin-angiotensin-aldosterone system in diabetic nephropathy is associated with enhanced decline in glomerular filtration rate. Diabetologia 2004;47: 1936–9.

34. Bianchi S, Bigazzi R, Campese VM. Long-term effects of spironolactone on proteinuria and kidney function in patients with chronic kidney disease. Kidney Int 2006;70:2116–23.

35. Nabity MB, Boggess MM, Kashtan CE, et al. Day-to-day variation in the urine protein:creatinine ratio in female dogs with stable glomerular proteinuria caused by X-linked hereditary nephropathy. J Vet Intern Med 2007;21:425–30.

36. LeVine DN, Zhang D, Harris T, et al. The use of pooled versus serial urine samples to measure urine protein:creatinine ratios. Vet Clin Path 2010;39:53–6.

37. Segev G, Fascetti AJ, Weeth LP, et al. Correction of hyperkalemia in dogs with chronic kidney disease consuming commercial renal therapeutic diets by a potassium-reduced home-prepared diet. J Vet Intern Med 2010;24:546–50.

38. Finco D. Association of systemic hypertension with renal injury in dogs with induced renal failure. J Vet Inter Med 2004;18:289–94.

39. Brown S, Atkins C, Bagley R, et al. Guidelines for the identification, evaluation, and management of systemic hypertension in dogs and cats. J Vet Intern Med 2007;21:542–58.

40. Atkins CE, Rausch WP, Gardner SY, et al. The effect of amlodipine and the combination of amlodipine and enalapril on the renin-angiotensin-aldosterone system in the dog. J Vet Pharmacol Therap 2007;30:394–400.

41. Jepson RE, Syme JM, Elliot J. Plasma renin activity and aldosterone concentrations in hypertensive cats with and without azotemia and in response to treatment with amlodipine besylate. J Vet Intern Med 2014;28:144–55.

42. Schneider SM, Cianciolo RE, Nabity MB, et al. Prevalence of immune-complex glomerulonephridities in dogs biopsied for suspected glomerular disease: 501 cases (2007-2012). J Vet Intern Med 2013;27:S67–75.

43. Littman MP, Daminet S, Grauer GF, et al. Consensus recommendations for the diagnostic investigation of dogs with suspected glomerular disease. J Vet Intern Med 2013;27:S19–26.

44. Segev G, Cowgill LD, Heiene R, et al. Consensus recommendations for immunosuppressive treatment of dogs with glomerular disease based on established pathology. J Vet Intern Med 2013;27:S44–54.

45. Pressler B, Vaden S, Gerber B, et al. Consensus recommendations for immunosuppressive treatment of dogs with glomerular disease absent a pathologic diagnosis. J Vet Intern Med 2013;27:S55–9.

46. Vaden SL, Breitschwerdt E, Armstrong PJ, et al. The effects of cyclosporine versus standard care in dogs with naturally occurring glomerulonephritis. J Vet Intern Med 1995;9:259–66.

Update on Mineral and Bone Disorders in Chronic Kidney Disease

Jonathan D. Foster, VMD

KEYWORDS

- Renal secondary hyperparathyroidism • Fibroblast growth factor 23
- Renal osteodystrophy • Hyperphosphatemia

KEY POINTS

- Phosphorus retention occurs early in chronic kidney disease, resulting in elevated serum concentrations of fibroblast growth factor 23 and parathyroid hormone.
- Increased serum concentrations of fibroblast growth factor 23 and parathyroid hormone lead to a constellation of syndromes called bone and mineral disorders in chronic kidney disease and also contribute to progression of kidney disease.
- Minimizing phosphorus retention through dietary therapy and medical intervention can improve these hormone elevations and may prevent or mitigate subsequent consequences.

MINERAL AND BONE DISORDERS IN CHRONIC KIDNEY DISEASE

Disturbances of mineral metabolism, including calcium, phosphorus, and magnesium, are common in patients with chronic kidney disease (CKD). Because of deranged renal handling of these minerals, and particularly phosphorus, aberrations in concentrations of parathyroid hormone (PTH), fibroblast growth factor 23 (FGF-23), and calcitriol develop. These alterations and the multiple clinical syndromes they lead to are collectively called CKD–mineral and bone disorder (CKD-MBD).[1–4] A summary of known, suspected, and unreported manifestations of CKD-MBD in dogs and cats is listed in **Box 1**.

Renal Secondary Hyperparathyroidism

The central force driving this process is continued intake of phosphorus exceeding the diminished capacity of the kidneys to excrete phosphorus due to reduced glomerular filtration rate (GFR) consequent to CKD.[5] Phosphorus retention initially stimulates FGF-23 production from osteoclasts and then in later stages of CKD phosphorus

Disclosures: The author has nothing to disclose.
Department of Clinical Studies, University of Pennsylvania School of Veterinary Medicine, 3900 Delancey Street, Philadelphia, PA 19104, USA
E-mail address: fosterjo@vet.upenn.edu

Box 1
Consequences of chronic kidney disease–mineral and bone disorder in dogs and cats

Known to occur

Renal secondary hyperparathyroidism

Accelerated progression of kidney disease

Increased mortality rate

Renal osteodystrophy

Cardiac arrhythmia

Extraskeletal calcification

Hypocalcemia

Hypercalcemia

Hypomagnesemia

Hypermagnesemia

Likely to occur

Decreased bone density

Vessel calcification

Not recognized

Pulmonary hypertension

Atherosclerosis

Valvular calcification

Tertiary hyperparathyroidism

Impaired skeletal response to PTH

Adynamic bone disease

---

retention, and ultimately hyperphosphatemia, promotes increased synthesis of PTH. FGF-23 needs α-klotho as a coreceptor for most of its actions, although some klotho-independent actions are emerging.[6] α-Klotho is expressed primarily in the kidney and parathyroid glands. FGF-23 binds to the FGF-1 receptor and α-klotho to downregulate the two main sodium-linked phosphate transporters responsible for phosphorus reabsorption in the proximal tubule of the kidney (NPT2a and NPT2c). Reduced reabsorption of phosphorus thereby increases phosphate excretion. FGF-23 also inhibits phosphate absorption from the intestine indirectly by inhibiting the conversion of 25-hydroxycholecalciferol (calcidiol) to 1,25 dihydroxycholecalciferol (calcitriol). In addition, FGF-23 decreases the synthesis of PTH from the parathyroid gland. Similar to FGF-23, PTH also inhibits renal phosphorus reabsorption through downregulation of NPT2a and NPT2c.[7] However, in contrast to the action of FGF-23, PTH increases the synthesis of calcitriol from calcidiol. Calcitriol will result in increased calcium and phosphorus absorption from the gastrointestinal tract (GI) tract. The primary role of PTH is to maintain serum ionized calcium (iCa) concentration; the increased renal excretion of phosphorus is a secondary activity. FGF-23 seems to be mainly involved with serum phosphorus regulation.

Patients with mild reduction in GFR retain sufficient functional nephrons to effectively respond to these increased hormone concentrations. Because FGF-23 and

PTH increase renal phosphorus excretion, their activity keeps the serum phosphorus concentration within the reference range. This relationship is called the *trade-off hypothesis*; serum phosphorus is maintained in the normal range at the expense of elevated FGF-23 and PTH activity. The trade-off is that an increased concentration of these hormones has deleterious effects. Decreased serum calcitriol and increased serum phosphorus concentrations lead to hypocalcemia, the major stimulus for PTH secretion. This process begins early in CKD; as kidney disease progresses, the aberrations in serum phosphorus, calcium, FGF-23, PTH, and calcitriol concentrations typically increase in magnitude. Studies have confirmed some dogs with International Renal Interest Society (IRIS) CKD stage 1 have evidence of renal secondary hyperparathyroidism.[8]

A summary of the pathophysiology of renal secondary hyperparathyroidism is displayed in **Fig. 1** and can be summarized as followed:

Decreased GFR → phosphorus retention → increased serum FGF-23 → decreased calcitriol synthesis → hypocalcemia → increased serum PTH

Cats have been shown to have elevated serum FGF-23 concentration before the development of azotemia, confirming that phosphorus retention occurs early in CKD (before azotemia) and FGF-23 may be a good marker of subclinical CKD.[9] Most cats had normal serum phosphorus concentration in this study. Both cats and dogs with CKD have been demonstrated to have elevations in PTH preceding hyperphosphatemia. One study showed 36% of IRIS CKD stage 1 dogs had renal secondary hyperparathyroidism, whereas only 18% had hyperphosphatemia.[8] Elevations in serum FGF-23 or PTH concentration likely suggest the presence of phosphorus retention, even in normophosphatemic patients. The prevalence of hyperparathyroidism

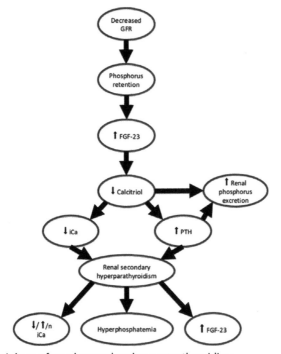

Fig. 1. Pathophysiology of renal secondary hyperparathyroidism.

increased with the IRIS CKD stage of CKD, such that 100% of IRIS CKD stage 4 dogs were found to have renal secondary hyperparathyroidism. Similar results were demonstrated in cats, whereby serum PTH and FGF-23 concentrations increased with advancing severity of CKD.[10,11] Notably, increases in FGF-23 occurred before increases in PTH. Serum FGF-23 concentration was found to be an independent predictor of CKD progression in cats, whereas serum PTH, creatinine, and phosphorus concentrations were not.[12] Hyperphosphatemia has been associated with accelerated progression of CKD in cats in another study.[13] High serum PTH concentrations contribute to morbidity and mortality in people with CKD; however, this has not been evaluated in veterinary patients.[14] Parathyroidectomy in an experimental model of canine kidney failure did result in lower serum PTH concentration compared with dogs who had induced kidney failure without parathyroidectomy.[15] The parathyroidectomized dogs trended toward a higher survival rate, although it did not reach statistical significance.

Renal Osteodystrophy

PTH stimulates osteoclast activity in order to release calcium into blood, helping to correct hypocalcemia. An unintended consequence is the release of phosphorus from bone as well. The chronic elevation in serum PTH concentration seen in patients with CKD-MBD can lead to numerous bone disorders, collectively referred to as renal osteodystrophy. Renal osteodystrophy includes a spectrum of skeletal abnormalities in humans, including osteomalacia, osteopenia, osteoporosis, osteitis fibrosa, and adynamic bone disease. PTH-mediated bone resorption has been reported in dogs and can range from focal to generalized bone loss and can progress to fibrous osteodystrophy, whereby demineralized bone is replaced by fibrous tissue.[16] For unknown reasons, the mandibles and maxilla are preferentially affected in canine renal osteodystrophy.[17] As fibrous tissues replace bone, there may be osseous swelling, facial deformity, and bone malleability, commonly referred to as rubber jaw (**Fig. 2**). Cats can also be affected by renal osteodystrophy; however, only 3 case reports exist in the literature and none of these cats has maxillofacial deformity.[18–20] Patients of any age may develop renal osteodystrophy; however, younger dogs are more often reported to have bony swellings of their maxilla and mandible, presumably due to incomplete skeletal maturation and concurrent juvenile renal disease.[16] There is emerging evidence that dogs and cats with CKD have decreased cortical bone density compared with nonazotemic, age-matched controls (Segev and Shipov, unpublished data, 2016).

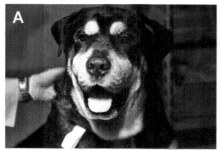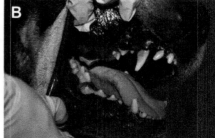

Fig. 2. An 8-year-old castrated male Rottweiler with IRIS CKD stage 3 (*A*) who has bilateral renal osteodystrophy of the maxilla (*B*). Pertinent laboratory values: serum phosphorus 6.8 (reference interval [RI] 2.8–6.1 mg/dL), ionized calcium 1.27 (RI 1.25–1.45 mmol/L), calcidiol 23 (RI 60–215 nmol/L), PTH 26.9 (RI 0.5–5.8 pmol/L).

Vessel and Tissue Mineralization

Increased serum concentrations of calcium and phosphorus may lead to soft tissue mineralization.[21–23] The serum calcium-phosphorus product has long been used as a surrogate to assess the risk of mineralization; however, some have criticized that this approach inappropriately simplifies the process of dystrophic mineralization.[24] A recent study demonstrated dogs with CKD and a total calcium-phosphorus product greater than 70 mg^2/dL^2 had a higher mortality rate than those with a lower calcium-phosphorus product.[23] Similar results were found in an experimental model of canine CKD whereby survival was associated with an ionized calcium-phosphorus product.[15]

Vascular calcification is common in people with CKD and is associated with increased morbidity and mortality.[25,26] The pathogenesis is incompletely understood, but disturbed calcium and phosphorus metabolism remains a central hypothesis. Cardiovascular calcification may affect the arterial media, atherosclerotic plaques, myocardium, and heart valves. End results include systemic hypertension, pulmonary hypertension, and increased risk of cardiovascular complications. Although systemic hypertension is considered a key component of veterinary cardiovascular-renal disorder, the prevalence and significance of vascular calcification in dogs and cats remains unknown.[27] Thoracic radiographs can often demonstrate calcification of the descending aorta and other large vessels in affected patients (**Fig. 3**).

TREATMENT OF CHRONIC KIDNEY DISEASE MINERAL AND BONE DISORDER

The syndrome of CKD-MBD can only be cured by renal transplantation. Therefore, for most veterinary patients the triggers and effects of CKD-MBD need to be medically managed. Phosphorus is considered the key player in CKD-MBD, as its retention stimulates synthesis of FGF-23 and PTH, which have been associated with increased mortality rates in people.[28,29] Recently, FGF-23 was shown to be an independent predictor of mortality in cats with CKD.[12] This study did not find PTH to be a predictor, suggesting that FGF-23 may play a large role driving the consequences of renal secondary hyperparathyroidism and progressive kidney dysfunction. Growing evidence indicates that increasing serum FGF-23 concentration in early stages of CKD are at least partially responsible for maintaining serum phosphorus within the normal range. Early

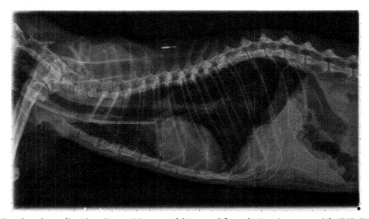

Fig. 3. Aortic mineralization in an 11-year-old spayed female Persian cat with IRIS CKD stage 5. A hemodialysis catheter is located in the right jugular vein and cranial vena cava as part of stabilization before renal transplantation.

management of serum FGF-23 concentration may prevent the premature decrease in serum 1,25-vitamin D3 and the subsequent increase in serum PTH.[30] This management may result in better survival outcomes and slower progression of CKD; however, this has not been evaluated in veterinary patients.

The goals of therapy are to prevent a positive phosphorus balance, optimize calcium metabolism, offset the consequences of abnormal vitamin D metabolism, prevent extraskeletal calcification, maintain skeletal health, and lessen risk factors that contribute to the increased mortality and accelerated disease progression in patients with CKD. The treatment required to achieve these are different in each patient. Patients' severity of CKD, serum concentrations of phosphorus, ionized calcium, PTH, calcitriol, and FGF-23 need to be evaluated to help create the best treatment plan. Therapy should be aimed at minimizing phosphorus retention, normalizing hyperphosphatemia, correcting calcium derangements, and normalizing serum FGF-23 and PTH concentrations.

The initial steps in managing CKD-MBD are to facilitate a balance between phosphorus intake and renal phosphorus excretion. In 2006, IRIS CKD generated targets for serum phosphorus concentration that are most appropriate for the stage of CKD (Table 1). These recommendations are based on clinical experience and supported by data from cats with experimentally induced renal disease, whereby maintaining a serum phosphorus concentration between 4 and 5 mg/dL was renoprotective.[31] Additionally, one study in dogs with CKD demonstrated an association between serum phosphorus and PTH concentrations and suggested serum phosphorus concentrations greater than 4.5 to 5.5 mg/dL fairly accurately predict the existence of renal secondary hyperparathyroidism.[8]

People with advanced CKD are medically managed to obtain a serum PTH concentration 2- to 9-fold higher than the reference range.[32] This high target PTH concentration is to help prevent adynamic bone disease, a condition of low bone turnover due to skeletal resistance to PTH. This disease has not been recognized in animals. The target PTH concentration for people with earlier stages of CKD is unknown; however, it has been suggested that therapy be instituted in early stages of CKD when PTH is minimally elevated and serum phosphorus concentration is normal.[30] If a phosphorus-restricted diet alone is insufficient to correct the elevated PTH concentration, phosphate binders should be administered, even if the phosphorus concentration is within the target range.[32] The target serum PTH concentration for animals with CKD is unknown. Parathyroidectomy in dogs with experimentally induced CKD resulted in lower serum PTH concentrations and a trend towards longer survival compared with dogs with normal parathyroid function; however, survival did not reach statistical significance.[15] Studies are needed to determine the optimal PTH target in animals with CKD.

Although currently there is no commercially available assay for FGF-23, serum PTH concentration can be measured in both dogs and cats. Serum PTH concentration

Table 1	
Serum phosphorus targets	
IRIS CKD Stage	Target Serum Phosphorus Concentration (mg/dL)
1	No recommendation
2	2.5–4.5
3	2.5–5.0
4	2.5–6.0

should be measured in patients with unexplained soft tissue or vascular calcification, evidence of renal secondary osteodystrophy, or decreased radiographic bone density regardless of absence of azotemia or hyperphosphatemia. Some dogs with IRIS CKD stage 1 have renal secondary hyperparathyroidism despite a normal serum phosphorus concentration.[8] Similar findings have been shown in cats with stage 2 CKD.[11] The serum PTH concentration can be measured in animals with any stage of CKD to determine if hyperparathyroidism is present.

The ideal timing for reassessment of the serum iCa and phosphorus concentrations has not been evaluated in veterinary medicine. Rechecking these values 4 to 6 weeks after initiation of dietary or medical therapy seems appropriate.

Dietary Therapy

Feeding a phosphorus-restricted diet is the first step in the management of recombinant human PTH. Several studies have demonstrated that feeding renal diets are associated with prolonged survival times in dogs and cats with CKD.[33–36] These diets have been shown to reduce serum concentrations of phosphorus,[34,36] PTH,[10] and FGF-23.[37] Because PTH and FGF-23 can be elevated before the development of hyperphosphatemia, phosphorus-restricted diets are indicated for patients with evidence of CKD-MBD (see **Box 1**) and increased serum PTH concentration, even if their serum phosphorus concentration is within the IRIS CKD target range. Hypophosphatemia is rarely encountered when a renal diet is fed to a patient without hyperphosphatemia.

Phosphate Binders

Many patients with CKD will have persistent hyperphosphatemia despite being fed a phosphorus-restricted renal diet. These patients still have a positive phosphorus balance due to diminished renal excretion, which can be offset by preventing GI absorption of phosphorus, through the use of a phosphate binder. Phosphate is absorbed in the small intestines via passive diffusion and by active transport mediated by the sodium-dependent phosphate transporter NaPi-IIb (NPT2b). The expression of this transporter is upregulated by calcitriol.[38]

In people, the use of phosphate binders in patients with CKD with normal serum phosphate levels has been associated with improved control of secondary hyperparathyroidism without corresponding changes in serum phosphate levels.[30] Although such studies have not been performed in veterinary medicine, phosphate binder therapy is likely warranted in patients with elevated serum FGF-23 or PTH despite normophosphatemia.

When determining the most appropriate phosphate binder, consideration should also be given to the serum calcium concentration. Free or iCa is the biologically active form of calcium and is the only form monitored and regulated by the interplay of PTH, calcitriol, and calcitonin. The serum total calcium concentration is poor at predicting the iCa, a phenomenon that is even more discordant in animals with CKD.[39] Corrected calcium, a formula that accounts for decrease in total calcium due to hypoalbuminemia, should also not be used to predict the calcium status of dogs and cats. In dogs with hypoalbuminemia, serum total calcium concentration overestimates hypocalcemia and underestimates normocalcemia, where corrected calcium over represents normocalcemia and underestimates hypocalcemia.[40] Dogs with CKD may have ionized hypocalcemia, hypercalcemia, or normocalcemia.[41] Much of the variability in serum total calcium concentration in dogs with CKD is due to alterations in the complexed fraction of calcium.[42] Therefore, serum iCa must be measured to accurately assess the calcium status of patients with CKD. By evaluating the serum phosphorus and iCa concentrations, appropriate therapeutics can be chosen (**Fig. 4**).

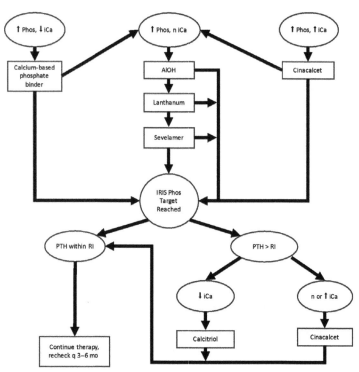

Fig. 4. Suggested algorithm for managing CKD-MBD. AIOH, aluminum hydroxide; n, normal; Phos, serum phosphorus concentration; RI, reference interval.

It is prudent to remember that all phosphate binders, with the exception of niacinamide, work via inhibiting dietary phosphate absorption in the GI tract. Therefore, they are only effective when administered concurrently with meals. Giving a phosphate binder to an anorexic patient or in the absence of food within the GI tract will have negligible effects. Animals that graze on food throughout the day, rather than receiving discrete meals, may pose more of a challenge to administer phosphate binders. These drugs need to administered whenever food is being consumed to have the maximal effect. For animals that graze continuously on dry food, some phosphate binders (such as powdered aluminum hydroxide) can be mixed with the food. Although many of these drugs are tasteless, some dogs and cats will become averse to their diet when the drug is added. In such cases, the phosphate binder can be administered mixed with canned food as a treat or can be directly administered orally to patients after they eat. Transitioning animals that graze on food to eating 2 or 3 discrete meals per day may increase the likelihood of successful phosphate-binder administration.

Treating Hyperphosphatemic, Hypocalcemic Patients

The goal of therapy for these patients would be to decrease the serum phosphorus concentration into the target range specific for their IRIS CKD stage as well as normalization of the serum iCa concentration. Calcium-based binders (acetate and carbonate) are the main therapeutic indicated for these patients, as they are effective and relatively inexpensive. Calcium acetate is more effective at binding phosphate than calcium carbonate; however this may not be appreciated clinically. Calcium citrate has also been used as a phosphate-binder, but citrate can enhance intestinal calcium, as well as aluminum absorption. This may result in aluminum toxicity when administered concurrently with aluminum hydroxide. Because large doses of calcium-based phosphate binders are often required to reduce the serum phosphorus concentration, the necessary dosage may lead to hypercalcemia. Use of calcium-based phosphate binders is contraindicated in patients with hypercalcemia or extraskeletal/vascular calcification.

If calcium-based phosphate binders are effective in correcting serum ionized hypocalcemia, but hyperphosphatemia persists, additional therapy is needed as suggested below.

Treating Hyperphosphatemic, Normocalcemic Patients

The goal of therapy for these patients is to maintain the normal serum iCa concentration, while decreasing the serum phosphorus concentration. Calcium-based phosphate binders could be considered in these patients; however, they will often cause hypercalcemia when given in sufficient doses required to control the serum phosphorus. Typically, other therapeutics are needed.

Aluminum hydroxide (AlOH) is considered a potent phosphate binder, although clinically many patients with IRIS CKD stage III to IV need additional phosphate binders to control the serum phosphorus concentration. This binder is considered to be the first-line phosphate binder by many veterinary nephrologists. The daily dosage of AlOH should not exceed 90 to 100 mg/kg/d in both dogs and cats. Clinical experience has shown that many animals will have persistent hyperphosphatemia despite this therapy; therefore, many practitioners use the maximal dosage of AlOH (90–100 mg/kg/d) as the starting dosage. Concurrent administration of citrate (potassium citrate, calcium citrate, and so forth) should be performed cautiously, as citrate increases the intestinal absorption of aluminum. If concurrent administration is needed, a lower dose of AlOH should be used or preferably a nonaluminum phosphate binder. Aluminum toxicity has been reported in 2 dogs who were receiving high dosages of AlOH (126 and 200 mg/kg/d).[43] Manifestations of toxicity include neurologic signs (ataxia, altered peripheral reflexes, decreased menace response, and so forth) and a microcytic anemia. Treatment of aluminum toxicity involves chelation therapy with deferoxamine and extracorporeal removal with hemodialysis. Administering a daily dose of AlOH less than 100 mg/kg/d has not been associated with toxicity. If hyperphosphatemia persists after 4 to 6 weeks of AlOH therapy, the dosage should be increased; or if the maximal dose is already being administered, an additional phosphate binder should be used.

Lanthanum is often used as a second- or third-line phosphate binder. Like aluminum, lanthanum is a rare metal, which forms insoluble complexes with phosphorus within the intestinal lumen. The capacity of this compound to bind phosphorus in vitro is similar to that of AlOH and is greater than that of calcium acetate, calcium carbonate, and sevelamer.[44] The combination of a phosphorus-restricted diet and lanthanum therapy was effective in lowering FGF-23 concentrations in people with CKD.[45] A very small fraction of ingested lanthanum is absorbed from the GI tract; trace amounts are detectable in various tissues, including liver and bone. Although the consequences of lanthanum absorption and tissue deposition are unknown, there have been no adverse effects observed in people. Lanthanum is hepatically excreted. Doses of 2000 mg/kg of lanthanum have been administered to dogs for 3 months without adverse effects.[44] A tolerability study of lanthanum carbonate octahydrate demonstrated adverse effects (vomiting and anorexia) in healthy cats when the dose reached 2000 mg/kg.[46] This study demonstrated increased fecal phosphorus excretion due to lanthanum administration; however, no change in serum phosphorus concentration was observed. A retrospective study of lanthanum administration to dogs and cats with renal failure identified no significant adverse effects at dosages up to 312 mg/kg/d in cats and 174 mg/kg/d in dogs (Hendricks and Foster, unpublished data, 2016). One dog developed diarrhea, potentially due to lanthanum; another developed pancreatitis unlikely related to lanthanum. No adverse effects were observed in cats. Lanthanum administration was associated with reduction in serum phosphorus concentration in these patients.

Sevelamer (linked with either hydrochloride or carbonate) is a synthetic hydrogel of cross-linked poly-allylamine, which binds phosphorus within the lumen of the GI tract and reduces its absorption. It can be used in place of or in addition to lanthanum for patients with refractory hyperphosphatemia. Sevelamer hydrochloride (HCl) can cause metabolic acidosis from gastric carbon dioxide production and has also been shown to reduce serum cholesterol by 20% to 30%. Sevelamer carbonate causes lower GI side effects and is more commonly used.

The dose of sevelamer can be escalated to achieve serum phosphorus targets.[47] When large dosages of sevelamer are needed to control hyperphosphatemia, it is cheaper to use lanthanum.[48] Sevelamer has been shown to reduce FGF-23 concentrations in people with CKD.[30]

Sevelamer carbonate and sevelamer HCl have been reported to interfere with levothyroxine absorption leading to a condition of hypothyroidism in human patients previously well compensated with a given replacement dose.[49] Sevelamer can also bind furosemide and cyclosporine, thus, reducing their GI absorption.

Recently, 2 new iron-containing phosphate binders, ferric citrate and sucroferric oxyhydroxide, have entered the market for people with CKD. Three additional drugs (iron magnesium hydroxyl carbonate, PT20, SBR759) are currently in development.[50] Similar to other phosphate binders, these drugs reduce GI absorption of phosphorus. Ferric citrate has been demonstrated to have an efficacy similar to sevelamer in reducing serum phosphorus. Ferric citrate has been demonstrated to reduce FGF-23 concentration and has inconsistent effects on PTH (studies show no change, reduction, or increase).[51] These drugs are also effective oral iron supplements. One study showed ferric citrate increased serum ferritin, total iron saturation, and hemoglobin concentration while reducing serum phosphorus in people with CKD.[52] Iron-based phosphate binders reduce the need for erythropoietin-stimulating agents and parenteral iron supplementation.[53] These medications are expensive and have not been evaluated in dogs and cats with CKD. Currently, they are quite expensive and, therefore, cost prohibitive to most owners.

Niacinamide (also known as nicotinamide) and niacin are the principal forms of vitamin B3. Despite structural similarities and equivalent nutritional properties, niacinamide and niacin have differing actions and adverse effect profiles. Although niacinamide can cause GI discomfort and reportedly lowers platelet counts, it does not cause flushing, which is commonly seen with niacin. Niacinamide decreases phosphate uptake by inhibiting sodium/phosphorus cotransporters in the renal proximal tubule (Na/Pi2a) and intestine (Na/Pi2b). This drug has been effective in lowering serum phosphorus concentration and low-density lipoprotein concentrations in people; however, its use in hyperphosphatemic animals has not been evaluated.[54–56] Niacinamide has been used for decades as therapy for autoimmune skin diseases in dogs and is generally well tolerated.[57] Rarely, GI intolerance is observed. No studies have been published evaluating its phosphorus-lowering effect in dogs. The use of niacinamide may be considered for patients with a serum phosphorus concentration greater than the IRIS CKD target range despite a conventional approach (diet, AlOH, lanthanum, and sevelamer) or for those pets whose owners cannot afford lanthanum or sevelamer.

Sucralfate was recently evaluated for its efficacy as a phosphate binder in cats, both healthy and with CKD.[58] A total of 500 mg of sucralfate by mouth every 8 hours did not result in decreased serum phosphorus concentration in healthy cats and normophosphatemic cats with CKD. Side effects were common, including vomiting, dehydration, constipation, and worsening of azotemia. The use of sucralfate as a phosphate binder cannot be recommended at this time.

Treating Hyperphosphatemic, Hypercalcemic Patients

The combination of hyperphosphatemia and hypercalcemia is uncommon in veterinary patients with CKD but will be encountered. Calcium-based phosphate binders are contraindicated in these patients. The phosphate binders that are indicated for treating patients who are normocalcemic could be considered here; however, most of these drugs have minimal effect on the serum calcium concentration (**Table 2**). Calcimimetics are a potent class of drugs that can effectively lower both the serum phosphorus and ionized calcium concentrations.

Calcimimetic drugs act directly on the calcium sensing receptor (CaSR) in the parathyroid gland to reduce PTH secretion. Cinacalcet is the representative drug of and most potent suppressor of PTH production among the class. The drug is absorbed quickly, such that peak concentrations occur within approximately 2 to 6 hours in people. Serum PTH concentrations fall inversely with the increase in serum cinacalcet concentration. However, as the drug concentration declines and the level of CaSR activation diminishes, the serum PTH concentration subsequently increases toward predose values during the remainder of the day. Despite the change in PTH throughout the day, the serum calcium concentration does not show similar fluctuations in people receiving cinacalcet. In humans it is generally recommended that PTH be measured 12 hours after cinacalcet administration. Calcimimetics also lower serum calcium concentration; therefore, they should not be used in patients with ionized hypocalcemia. If hypocalcemia should occur with cinacalcet therapy, the dosage could be reduced if the target PTH has been achieved or patients may receive concurrent treatment with vitamin D analogues or calcium supplements.

After 1 to 2 weeks of cinacalcet therapy, the serum concentrations of phosphorus and ionized calcium can be reassessed. Serum PTH concentration is recommended to be rechecked 1 to 4 weeks after drug initiation or a change in dosage. To minimize the possibility of hypocalcemia, the initial dosage of cinacalcet is low (approximately 0.5 mg/kg once daily), and subsequent doses are increased every 2 to 3 weeks until the serum phosphorus and calcium concentrations are controlled or a maximum dosage of 3 mg/kg/d is achieved. These dosages are extrapolated from human therapy. This drug has not been evaluated in veterinary medicine, although clinical experiences suggest it is well tolerated and effective. Nausea and vomiting are the most common adverse effects.

CONTROLLING SERUM PARATHYROID HORMONE CONCENTRATION

After the serum phosphorus concentration has been restored to the IRIS CKD target range, it is recommended to assess the serum PTH concentration. It is safe to assume that patients with CKD with a serum phosphorus concentration greater than 5.5 mg/dL will have renal secondary hyperparathyroidism.[8] Measuring PTH before the correction of hyperphosphatemia may not be economically justified in many patients, as it is

Table 2
Effects of drugs used to manage chronic kidney disease–mineral and bone disorder

Drug	Target	Efficacy	Phosphorus	Calcium	PTH	FGF-23	Dosage	Advantages	Adverse Effects
Calcium-based binders	GI phosphorus absorption	+ to ++++	↓	↑	↓	↓	60–150 mg/kg/d	Inexpensive	Hypercalcemia
Aluminum hydroxide	GI phosphorus absorption	++++	↓	↔	↔	↓	90 mg/kg/d	Inexpensive	Aluminum toxicity
Lanthanum	GI phosphorus absorption	+++	↓	↔	↔	↓	60–200 mg/kg/d		Systemic absorption
Sevelamer	GI phosphorus absorption	+++	↓	↔	↔	↓	30–135 mg/kg/d[a]		GI upset Reduces levothyroxine, furosemide, cyclosporine absorption
Ferric citrate	GI phosphorus absorption	+++	↓	↔	↔	↓	85–125 mg/kg/d[a]	Bioavailable oral iron supplement	No clinical experience
Calcitriol	Vitamin D receptor	++	↑	↑	↓	↑	2.0–5.0 ng/kg q24h		Hypercalcemia
Cinacalcet	Calcium sensing receptor	+++	↓	↓	↓	↓	Initial: 0.5 mg/kg q24h Max: 1.5 mg/kg q8h[a]		GI upset Hypocalcemia

The symbol (+) indicates the potent grade. The arrows indicate the expected result to (↓, decrease; ↑, increase; ↔, both) the blood value.
[a] Dose extrapolated from human recommendations.

reasonable to presume PTH will be elevated and correction of hyperphosphatemia may result in improvement in serum PTH concentration.

The ideal range for the serum PTH concentration is unknown in veterinary patients with CKD. The established reference range for dogs and cats has been determined from assessing nonazotemic animals.[59] Median serum PTH concentration in dogs with CKD has been demonstrated to be 10-fold higher than the upper limit of the reference range.[60] Currently, many clinicians strive to return the serum PTH concentration to within the reference range for healthy animals, which may be quite challenging to accomplish in patients with advanced CKD. Additionally, it is unknown if this target is too low and could be associated with adverse effects. Complications, such as adynamic bone disease, can occur in people with excessive PTH suppression; however, this condition has not been investigated for animals. It is unknown if animals with CKD develop such a disorder, as they may not live long enough for symptoms to develop.

Correcting hyperphosphatemia may improve the serum PTH concentration. It is reasonable to wait to measure PTH until the serum phosphorus concentration is within the IRIS CKD target range. If the serum PTH concentration is elevated despite adequate control of phosphorus, additional therapies can be introduced to normalize PTH. Such therapies are certainly indicated for patients with symptoms of CKD-MBD (see **Box 1**). Patients with ionized hypocalcemia would most benefit from calcitriol therapy. Those with hypercalcemia would be more appropriately treated with cinacalcet. For patients with a normal serum ionized calcium concentration, either drug could be used. Despite the paucity of research evaluating their effects in dogs and cats with CKD, the research in people suggests a more predictable reduction in PTH with cinacalcet therapy than calcitriol. Therefore, the author recommends the usage of cinacalcet for normocalcemic patients.

Vitamin D Analogues

Both phosphate and FGF-23 reduce calcitriol production via inhibition of 1-α-hydroxylase in the kidneys. Because phosphorus retention and/or hyperphosphatemia stimulate FGF-23 production, correction of hyperphosphatemia may promote calcitriol synthesis by suppressing both 1-α-hydroxylase inhibitors. The reduction in functional renal mass characteristic of advanced CKD may also limit renal calcitriol synthesis. Dogs with CKD have been shown to have lower serum calcitriol concentrations compared with healthy controls; however, few dogs with CKD had levels less than the reference range.[60] Another study found that, compared with normal control dogs, calcitriol concentrations were significantly lower in dogs with IRIS CKD stages 3 and 4, whereas calcitriol concentrations in dogs with IRIS CKD stages 1 and 2 did not differ from normal dogs.[8] One study found 35% of cats with CKD had calcitriol concentrations less than the reference range.[10] Decreased calcitriol concentrations contribute to development of secondary hyperparathyroidism (see **Fig. 1**).

Because calcitriol increases the GI absorption of calcium and phosphorus, investigators have suggested the serum phosphorus concentration to be less than 6 mg/dL before initiating calcitriol therapy.[61] However, this suggestion has been replaced with the recommendation that phosphorus be controlled to the concentration identified for each IRIS CKD stage. If calcitriol therapy results in increased GI phosphorus absorption, the serum phosphorus concentration may increase greater than the recommended target range and necessitate the use of higher dosages of phosphate binders. For this reason, calcitriol should not be considered first-line therapy for hyperphosphatemic hypocalcemic patients.

Similar to naturally occurring disease in people, dogs with experimentally induced CKD have demonstrated a diminished osteoclast response to PTH.[62] Thus, uremic dogs will have a reduction in PTH-mediated osteoclastic bone reabsorption and, thereby, less calcium and phosphate is released into blood compared with nonuremic dogs. Administration of calcitriol to these patients increased the PTH-mediated release of calcium from bone, thereby, increasing the serum calcium concentration. However, it is unknown if this is due to a direct effect of calcitriol on osteoclasts or through increased activity of PTH.

A meta-analysis examining the effects of vitamin D compounds in human patients with CKD found that they did not reduce the risk of death or vascular calcification; compared with placebo, calcitriol *increased* the risks of hypercalcemia and hyperphosphatemia while inconsistently reducing PTH levels.[63] However, other studies have shown improved mortality rates in people.[64] In a study in humans with renal secondary hyperparathyroidism, intravenous calcitriol administration resulted in increased FGF-23 concentrations.[65] Less is known regarding the risks and benefits of calcitriol in veterinary patients. Daily calcitriol (2.5 ng/kg by mouth every 24 hours) and intermittent calcitriol administration (8.75 ng/kg by mouth every 84 hours) did not reduce serum PTH concentrations in healthy cats and those with CKD.[66] The 22-oxacalcitriol reduced serum PTH concentration in dogs with experimentally induced CKD but not in healthy controls.[67] A 2005 abstract reported survival benefits of calcitriol supplementation to dogs with CKD.[68] Median survival time was 365 days for the calcitriol treatment group and 250 days for the placebo-treated group. A survey of veterinarians regularly using oral calcitriol therapy in their canine and feline patients with CKD found that most thought calcitriol therapy improved clinical signs and prolonged survival.[69] Further evaluation of calcitriol therapy is clearly needed in veterinary medicine.

It is recommended that calcitriol be administered at an oral dosage of 2.0 to 2.5 ng/kg every 24 hours.[70] Hypercalcemia is possible with high dosages and regular monitoring of ionized calcium is essential. The dosage may be increased to a maximum of 5 ng/kg ever 24 hours. It should not be given with meals, as it increases intestinal calcium and phosphorus absorption.

Calcimimetics

The administration of cinacalcet is described earlier. Despite its efficacy in reducing serum PTH concentration, cinacalcet did not significantly reduce the risk of death or major cardiovascular events compared with placebo in people with end-stage renal disease requiring maintenance hemodialysis.[71]

Hemodialysis

Phosphorus is removed during hemodialysis; in people, approximately 800 to 1200 mg can be removed during a single intermittent hemodialysis treatment.[72] Despite a normal diet and conventional 3-times-per-week dialysis schedules, the use of phosphorus binders is almost universally required in people to control hyperphosphatemia. Therefore, chronic hemodialysis does not remove enough phosphorus to negate the need for additional phosphorus-lowering therapies, which is an outcome observed with veterinary patients as well. Phosphorus behaves as a middle-weight solute, despite its molecular weight of 95 Da. Serum phosphorus concentration decreases rather markedly during the first hour of dialysis, and then the serum phosphorus concentration is relatively well maintained, even during long dialysis sessions. Prolonged weekly dialysis time (often >30 hours) is needed to negate the need for oral phosphate binders, which is an accomplishment only achieved with at-home nocturnal dialysis. Currently, this is not an option for veterinary patients.

SUMMARY

Recent advancements in our understanding of the interplay between phosphorus, calcium, PTH, and FGF-23 has shifted the focus away from renal secondary hyperparathyroidism being the only worrisome complication to the spectrum of CKD-MBD. The central concept to much of the pathophysiology is phosphorus retention. Therefore, a large part of the therapy for CKD-MBD is focused on restoring a normal phosphorus balance through reduced intake. However, it would be shortsighted to exclude the management of serum calcium and calcitriol concentrations. Commercial assays are currently available for canine and feline PTH measurement; it is hoped that FGF-23 assays will become readily available in the near future. Despite the improved understanding of CDK-MBD pathophysiology, veterinary medicine lacks rigorous evaluation of the efficacy of most interventions for this disorder. Future research into cardiovascular complications, bone heath, and overall mortality are needed to refine our treatment goals and to improve clinical outcomes.

REFERENCES

1. Rosol TJ, Capen CC. Pathophysiology of calcium, phosphorus, and magnesium metabolism in animals. Vet Clin North Am Small Anim Pract 1996;26(5):1155–84.
2. Humphrey S, Kirby R, Rudloff E. Magnesium physiology and clinical therapy in veterinary critical care. J Vet Emerg Crit Care 2014;25(2):210–25.
3. Toll J, Erb H, Birnbaum N, et al. Prevalence and incidence of serum magnesium abnormalities in hospitalized cats. J Vet Intern Med 2002;16(3):217–21.
4. Dhupa N, Proulx J. Hypocalcemia and hypomagnesemia. Vet Clin North Am Small Anim Pract 1998;28(3):587–608.
5. Geddes RF, Finch NC, Syme HM, et al. The role of phosphorus in the pathophysiology of chronic kidney disease. J Vet Emerg Crit Care 2013;23(2):122–33.
6. Fukumoto S, Shimizu Y. Fibroblast growth factor 23 as a phosphotropic hormone and beyond. J Bone Miner Metab 2011;29(5):507–14.
7. Biber J, Hernando N, Forster I. Phosphate transporters and their function. Annu Rev Physiol 2013;75:535–50.
8. Cortadellas O, Fernández del Palacio MJ, Talavera J, et al. Calcium and phosphorus homeostasis in dogs with spontaneous chronic kidney disease at different stages of severity. J Vet Intern Med 2010;24(1):73–9.
9. Finch NC, Geddes RF, Syme HM, et al. Fibroblast growth factor 23 (FGF-23) concentrations in cats with early nonazotemic chronic kidney disease (CKD) and in healthy geriatric cats. J Vet Intern Med 2013;27(2):227–33.
10. Barber PJ, Elliott J. Feline chronic renal failure: calcium homeostasis in 80 cases diagnosed between 1992 and 1995. J Small Anim Pract 1998;39(3):108–16.
11. Geddes RF, Finch NC, Elliott J, et al. Fibroblast growth factor 23 in feline chronic kidney disease. J Vet Intern Med 2013;27(2):234–41.
12. Geddes RF, Elliott J, Syme HM. Relationship between plasma fibroblast growth factor-23 concentration and survival time in cats with chronic kidney disease. J Vet Intern Med 2015;29(6):1494–501.
13. Chakrabarti S, Syme HM, Elliott J. Clinicopathological variables predicting progression of azotemia in cats with chronic kidney disease. J Vet Intern Med 2012;26(2):275–81.
14. Natoli JL, Boer R, Nathanson BH, et al. Is there an association between elevated or low serum levels of phosphorus, parathyroid hormone, and calcium and mortality in patients with end stage renal disease? A meta-analysis. BMC Nephrol 2013;14(1):88.

15. Finco DR, Brown SA, Crowell WA, et al. Effects of parathyroidectomy on induced renal failure in dogs. Am J Vet Res 1997;58(2):188–95.

16. Davis EM. Oral manifestations of chronic kidney disease and renal secondary hyperparathyroidism: a comparative review. J Vet Dent 2015;32(2):87–98.

17. Sarkiala EM, Dambach D, Harvey CE. Jaw lesions resulting from renal hyperparathyroidism in a young dog–a case report. J Vet Dent 1994;11(4):121–4.

18. Mattson A, Fettman MJ, Grauer GF. Renal secondary hyperparathyroidism in a cat. J Am Anim Hosp Assoc 1993;29(4):345–50.

19. Jackson HA, Barber PJ. Resolution of metastatic calcification in the paws of a cat with successful dietary management of renal hyperparathyroidism. J Small Anim Pract 1998;39(10):495–7.

20. Gnudi G, Bertoni G, Luppi A, et al. Unusual hyperparathyroidism in a cat. Vet Radiol Ultrasound 2001;42(3):250–3.

21. Nagode LA, Chew DJ. Nephrocalcinosis caused by hyperparathyroidism in progression of renal failure: treatment with calcitriol. Semin Vet Med Surg (Small Anim) 1992;7(3):202–20.

22. Block GA, Hulbert-Shearon TE, Levin NW, et al. Association of serum phosphorus and calcium x phosphate product with mortality risk in chronic hemodialysis patients: a national study. Am J Kidney Dis 1998;31(4):607–17.

23. Lippi I, Guidi G, Marchetti V, et al. Prognostic role of the product of serum calcium and phosphorus concentrations in dogs with chronic kidney disease: 31 cases (2008-2010). J Am Vet Med Assoc 2014;245(10):1135–40.

24. O'Neill WC. The fallacy of the calcium-phosphorus product. Kidney Int 2007; 72(7):792–6.

25. Blacher J, Guerin AP, Pannier B, et al. Arterial calcifications, arterial stiffness, and cardiovascular risk in end-stage renal disease. Hypertension 2001;38(4):938–42.

26. Moe SM, Chen NX. Mechanisms of vascular calcification in chronic kidney disease. J Am Soc Nephrol 2008;19(2):213–6.

27. Pouchelon J-L, Atkins CE, Bussadori C, et al. Cardiovascular-renal axis disorders in the domestic dog and cat: a veterinary consensus statement. J Small Anim Pract 2015;56(9):537–52.

28. Gutiérrez OM, Mannstadt M, Isakova T, et al. Fibroblast growth factor 23 and mortality among patients undergoing hemodialysis. N Engl J Med 2008;359(6): 584–92.

29. Tentori F, Blayney MJ, Albert JM, et al. Mortality risk for dialysis patients with different levels of serum calcium, phosphorus, and PTH: the Dialysis Outcomes and Practice Patterns Study (DOPPS). Am J Kidney Dis 2008;52(3):519–30.

30. Oliveira RB, Cancela ALE, Graciolli FG, et al. Early control of PTH and FGF23 in normophosphatemic CKD patients: a new target in CKD-MBD therapy? Clin J Am Soc Nephrol 2010;5(2):286–91.

31. Ross LA, Finco DR, Crowell WA. Effect of dietary phosphorus restriction on the kidneys of cats with reduced renal mass. Am J Vet Res 1982;43(6):1023–6.

32. Kidney disease: Improving Global Outcomes (KDIGO) CKD-MBD Work Group. KDIGO clinical practice guideline for the diagnosis, evaluation, prevention, and treatment of chronic kidney disease-mineral and bone disorder (CKD-MBD). Kidney Int Suppl 2009;76:S1–130.

33. Plantinga EA, Everts H, Kastelein AMC, et al. Retrospective study of the survival of cats with acquired chronic renal insufficiency offered different commercial diets. Vet Rec 2005;157(7):185–7.

34. Elliott J, Rawlings JM, Markwell PJ, et al. Survival of cats with naturally occurring chronic renal failure: effect of dietary management. J Small Anim Pract 2000; 41(6):235–42.

35. Jacob F, Polzin DJ, Osborne CA, et al. Clinical evaluation of dietary modification for treatment of spontaneous chronic renal failure in dogs. J Am Vet Med Assoc 2002;220(8):1163–70.

36. Ross SJ, Osborne CA, Kirk CA, et al. Clinical evaluation of dietary modification for treatment of spontaneous chronic kidney disease in cats. J Am Vet Med Assoc 2006;229(6):949–57.

37. Geddes RF, Elliott J, Syme HM. The effect of feeding a renal diet on plasma fibroblast growth factor 23 concentrations in cats with stable azotemic chronic kidney disease. J Vet Intern Med 2013;27(6):1354–61.

38. Christakos S, Lieben L, Masuyama R, et al. Vitamin D endocrine system and the intestine. Bonekey Rep 2014;3:496.

39. Schenck PA, Chew DJ. Prediction of serum ionized calcium concentration by use of serum total calcium concentration in dogs. Am J Vet Res 2005;66(8):1330–6.

40. Sharp CR, Kerl ME, Mann F. A comparison of total calcium, corrected calcium, and ionized calcium concentrations as indicators of calcium homeostasis among hypoalbuminemic dogs requiring intensive care. J Vet Emerg Crit Care 2009; 19(6):571–8.

41. Kogika MM, Lustoza MD, Notomi MK, et al. Serum ionized calcium in dogs with chronic renal failure and metabolic acidosis. Vet Clin Pathol 2006;35(4):441–5.

42. Schenck PA, Chew DJ. Determination of calcium fractionation in dogs with chronic renal failure. Am J Vet Res 2003;64(9):1181–4.

43. Segev G, Bandt C, Francey T, et al. Aluminum toxicity following administration of aluminum-based phosphate binders in 2 dogs with renal failure. J Vet Intern Med 2008;22(6):1432–5.

44. Hutchison AJ. Calcitriol, lanthanum carbonate, and other new phosphate binders in the management of renal osteodystrophy. Perit Dial Int 1999;19(Suppl 2): S408–12.

45. Isakova T, Barchi-Chung A, Enfield G, et al. Effects of dietary phosphate restriction and phosphate binders on FGF23 levels in CKD. Clin J Am Soc Nephrol 2013;8(6):1009–18.

46. Schmidt BH, Dribusch U, Delport PC, et al. Tolerability and efficacy of the intestinal phosphate binder Lantharenol® in cats. BMC Vet Res 2012;8(1):14.

47. Chen N, Wu X, Ding X, et al. Sevelamer carbonate lowers serum phosphorus effectively in haemodialysis patients: a randomized, double-blind, placebo-controlled, dose-titration study. Nephrol Dial Transplant 2014;29(1):152–60.

48. Keith MS, Wilson RJ, Preston P, et al. Cost-minimization analysis of lanthanum carbonate versus sevelamer hydrochloride in US patients with end-stage renal disease. Clin Ther 2014;36(9):1276–86.

49. Iovino M, Iovine N, Petrosino A, et al. Sevelamer carbonate markedly reduces levothyroxine absorption. Endocr Metab Immune Disord Drug Targets 2014;14(3): 206–9.

50. Schmid H, Lederer SR. Novel iron-containing phosphate binders for treatment of hyperphosphatemia. Expert Opin Pharmacother 2015;16(14):2179–91.

51. Iguchi A, Kazama JJ, Yamamoto S, et al. Administration of ferric citrate hydrate decreases circulating FGF23 levels independently of serum phosphate levels in hemodialysis patients with iron deficiency. Nephron 2015;131(3):161–6.

52. Block GA, Fishbane S, Rodriguez M, et al. A 12-week, double-blind, placebo-controlled trial of ferric citrate for the treatment of iron deficiency anemia and

reduction of serum phosphate in patients with CKD Stages 3-5. Am J Kidney Dis 2015;65(5):728–36.

53. Nakanishi T, Hasuike Y, Nanami M, et al. Novel iron-containing phosphate binders and anemia treatment in CKD: oral iron intake revisited. Nephrol Dial Transplant 2015 [pii:gfv268].

54. Cheng SC, Young DO, Huang Y, et al. A randomized, double-blind, placebo-controlled trial of niacinamide for reduction of phosphorus in hemodialysis patients. Clin J Am Soc Nephrol 2008;3(4):1131–8.

55. Rennick A, Kalakeche R, Seel L, et al. Nicotinic acid and nicotinamide: a review of their use for hyperphosphatemia in dialysis patients. Pharmacotherapy 2013; 33(6):683–90.

56. Borolossy El R, Wakeel El LM, Hakim El I, et al. Efficacy and safety of nicotin-amide in the management of hyperphosphatemia in pediatric patients on regular hemodialysis. Pediatr Nephrol 2015;31(2):1–8.

57. White SD, Rosychuk RA, Reinke SI, et al. Use of tetracycline and niacinamide for treatment of autoimmune skin disease in 31 dogs. J Am Vet Med Assoc 1992; 200(10):1497–500.

58. Quimby J, Lappin M. Evaluating sucralfate as a phosphate binder in normal cats and cats with chronic kidney disease. J Am Anim Hosp Assoc 2016;52(1):8–12.

59. Pineda C, Aguilera-Tejero E, Raya AI, et al. Feline parathyroid hormone: validation of hormonal assays and dynamics of secretion. Domest Anim Endocrinol 2012; 42(4):256–64.

60. Gerber B, Hässig M, Reusch CE. Serum concentrations of 1,25-dihydroxychole-calciferol and 25-hydroxycholecalciferol in clinically normal dogs and dogs with acute and chronic renal failure. Am J Vet Res 2003;64(9):1161–6.

61. de Brito Galvao JF, Nagode LA, Schenck PA, et al. Calcitriol, calcidiol, parathy-roid hormone, and fibroblast growth factor-23 interactions in chronic kidney dis-ease. J Vet Emerg Crit Care 2013;23(2):134–62.

62. Jacob AI, Gavellas G, Canterbury J, et al. Calcemic and phosphaturic response to parathyroid hormone in normal and chronically uremic dogs. Kidney Int 1982; 22(1):21–6.

63. Palmer SC, McGregor DO, Macaskill P, et al. Meta-analysis: vitamin D com-pounds in chronic kidney disease. Ann Intern Med 2007;147(12):840–53.

64. Duranton F, Rodriguez-Ortiz ME, Duny Y, et al. Vitamin D treatment and mortality in chronic kidney disease: a systematic review and meta-analysis. Am J Nephrol 2013;37(3):239–48.

65. Nishi H, Nii-Kono T, Nakanishi S, et al. Intravenous calcitriol therapy increases serum concentrations of fibroblast growth factor-23 in dialysis patients with sec-ondary hyperparathyroidism. Nephron Clin Pract 2005;101(2):c94–9.

66. Hostutler RA, DiBartola SP, Chew DJ, et al. Comparison of the effects of daily and intermittent-dose calcitriol on serum parathyroid hormone and ionized calcium concentrations in normal cats and cats with chronic renal failure. J Vet Intern Med 2006;20(6):1307–13.

67. Takahashi F, Furuichi T, Yorozu K, et al. Effects of i.v. and oral 1,25-dihydroxy-22-oxavitamin D(3) on secondary hyperparathyroidism in dogs with chronic renal failure. Nephrol Dial Transplant 2002;17(Suppl 10):46–52.

68. Polzin D, Ross SJ, Osborne C, et al. Clinical benefit of calcitriol in canine chronic kidney disease. J Vet Intern Med 2005;19:433.

69. Nagode LA, Chew DJ, Podell M. Benefits of calcitriol therapy and serum phos-phorus control in dogs and cats with chronic renal failure. Both are essential to

prevent of suppress toxic hyperparathyroidism. Vet Clin North Am Small Anim Pract 1996;26(6):1293–330.

70. Polzin DJ. Evidence-based step-wise approach to managing chronic kidney disease in dogs and cats. J Vet Emerg Crit Care (San Antonio) 2013;23(2):205–15.

71. EVOLVE Trial Investigators, Chertow GM, Block GA, Correa-Rotter R, et al. Effect of cinacalcet on cardiovascular disease in patients undergoing dialysis. N Engl J Med 2012;367(26):2482–94.

72. Daugirdas JT. Removal of phosphorus by hemodialysis. Semin Dial 2015;28(6): 620–3.

Does Secondary Renal Osteopathy Exist in Companion Animals?

Gilad Segev, DVM*, Hagar Meltzer, DVM, Anna Shipov, DVM

KEYWORDS

- Dog • Cat • Mineral density • Quality • Bone • Hyperparathyroidism

KEY POINTS

- Renal secondary hyperparathyroidism is common in dogs and cats with chronic kidney disease.
- Renal osteodystrophy occurs in dogs and cats with chronic kidney disease and bone quality is reduced in these animals.
- In the cortical bone, material properties, bone geometry, and mechanical properties are affected.
- Bone mass is reduced in cancellous bone of animals with chronic kidney disease.

INTRODUCTION
Renal Secondary Hyperparathyroidism

Secondary hyperplasia of the parathyroid glands, resulting in increased parathyroid hormone (PTH) blood concentration, is an inevitable consequence of chronic kidney disease (CKD) in human and veterinary patients. The pathophysiology of this multifactorial syndrome, known as renal secondary hyperparathyroidism (SHPT), is complex. Progressive loss of functional nephrons leads to a decrease in the glomerular filtration rate, resulting in phosphorus retention, which promotes PTH secretion, by a direct stimulatory effect on the parathyroid gland, and more importantly, by binding free calcium, resulting in decreased ionized calcium concentration. PTH decreases phosphorus reabsorption in the renal tubules and restores normophosphatemia, but only to a certain point. As the disease progresses and glomerular filtration rate continues to decline, phosphorus retention becomes more severe and further triggers PTH secretion, which in turn promotes bone resorption and release of calcium and phosphorus to the circulation.[1,2] Vitamin D also plays a pivotal role in the pathophysiology of renal SHPT. Calcitriol, the active

The authors have nothing to disclose.
Koret School of Veterinary Medicine, The Hebrew University of Jerusalem, Hertzel Street, Rehovot 76100, Israel
* Corresponding author.
E-mail address: gilad.segev@mail.huji.ac.il

form of vitamin D, is formed by 1α-hydroxylation of 25-hydroxy-cholecalciferol in the kidney. Decreased functional renal mass and phosphorous retention result in decreased 1α-hydroxylase activity, hereby limiting calcitriol production. Calcitriol, in addition to promoting intestinal calcium absorption, is a major suppressor of PTH secretion. Therefore, reduced calcitriol levels contribute to the progression of renal SHPT, by promoting hypocalcemia and by decreasing the inhibitory effect of calcitriol on PTH secretion.[1,2] An additional, more recently identified key player in the development of renal SHPT, is fibroblast growth factor (FGF)-23, a hormone produced mainly by osteoblasts and osteocytes, which promotes renal phosphorous excretion. FGF-23 is secreted in response to hyperphosphatemia, early in the course of CKD. It downregulates 1α-hydroxylase activity, thus further decreasing calcitriol levels and worsening renal SHPT.[3,4] Increased serum FGF-23 concentration has been demonstrated as one of the earliest metabolic derangements in patients with CKD, often elevated while patients are still normophosphatemic and have normal PTH concentrations.[5]

Prevalence of renal secondary hyperparathyroidism in patients with chronic kidney disease

In humans, renal SHPT develops early in the course of CKD, and has been reported to affect 40% and 80% of patients with stage III and IV CKD, respectively.[6] Renal SHPT is also prevalent among cats and dogs with CKD. A 20-fold increase in PTH concentration was documented in a study of dogs with experimental CKD compared with healthy dogs.[7] A more recent study demonstrated SHPT is a common metabolic complication, documented in 76% and 84% of dogs and cats with naturally occurring CKD, respectively, and is present in all animals with International Renal Interest Society (IRIS) CKD stage IV disease.[8,9] In another survey, renal SHPT was documented in 47% of asymptomatic cats, being the only biochemical evidence of CKD.[9] PTH concentrations were higher in nonazotemic cats that subsequently developed azotemia within 12 months compared with cats that remained nonazotemic, and the increase in PTH occurred before changes in plasma calcium or phosphorous concentrations were detected.[10] FGF-23 blood concentration also increases in cats with CKD and were positively correlated with the IRIS stage.[11]

Bone Abnormalities Associated with Renal Secondary Hyperparathyroidism

Renal osteodystrophy

Persistently elevated PTH concentration increases bone resorption by activating osteoclasts, thereby leading to an imbalance in the bone remodeling process and consequently to decreased bone quality. This phenomenon is generally referred to as renal osteodystrophy (ROD), a complex disorder of bone, resulting from the individual and combined actions of metabolic and hormonal abnormalities that occur in CKD. ROD was defined by the National Kidney Foundation as a constellation of bone disorders, present or exacerbated by CKD, that lead to abnormal mineral metabolism, bone fragility, and fractures.[12] The definition was refined by the "Kidney Disease: Improving Global Outcomes Committee," and a new term, CKD–mineral and bone disorder was coined to refer more broadly to the skeletal and extraskeletal manifestations of the mineral disorders in CKD. The broader CKD–mineral and bone disorder is defined as a systemic disorder of mineral and bone metabolism caused by CKD and manifested by either one or a combination of (1) abnormalities of calcium, phosphorous, PTH, or vitamin D metabolism; (2) abnormalities of bone turnover, mineralization, linear growth, volume, or strength; or (3) vascular or other soft tissue calcification.[13,14]

METHODS TO ASSESS BONE QUALITY

The overall mechanical behavior of whole bone is determined by its morphology and architecture (ie, the amount and spatial distribution of bone material), and by the intrinsic properties of the bone material itself. It may be inferred that bone fragility is reduced in at least three different ways: increase bone mass (larger bones are able to carry more load), effective distribution of bone mass (put more bone tissue where mechanical demands are higher), or improve the material properties of the bone (ie, bone is stronger at the tissue level).[15]

The ability of bone to resist fracture is the most important factor in defining bone quality, because a broken bone can fulfill but few, if any, of its functions. Fractures occur as a result of a catastrophic structural failure of the whole bone, which is initiated at the material level. Bones may fail because they are too weak, too flexible, do not absorb enough energy, and/or are not resistant enough to repetitive loading. Each one of these parameters (strength, stiffness, toughness) is evaluated by mechanical testing. The combination of these properties, rather than each independently, defines the resistance to fracture. Enhancing one property over the other might be detrimental to the overall mechanical performance of the bone. For example, increased mineralization increases stiffness of the bone but at the same time it decreases toughness.

There are numerous methods to assess bone quality including bone morphometry, assessment of bone mineral density (BMD) and porosity, and an array of mechanical testing of the bone. This article describes the most common methods to assess bone quality.

Bone Mineral Density

BMD is the amount of mineral present within the bone. It is considered the most important determinant of bone quality and is the current clinical standard to predict fracture risk.[16] BMD is measured by several methods, including dual-energy X-ray absorptiometry, which measures areal BMD (in grams per square centimeter) or quantitative computer tomography (CT)/high-resolution micro-CT analysis, which measure volumetric BMD (in grams per cubic centimeter). An exponential inverse correlation exists between BMD and probability of fracture, and even a small increase in BMD (5%–8%) can improve bone strength by more than 60%.[17] However, mounting evidence indicates that BMD alone cannot predict the risk of fracture in a given bone. Bone architecture and microarchitecture, bone turnover rate, and the amount of microdamage all affect bone quality and may play a role in the bone's ability to resist fracture.[18]

Porosity

Porosity is another major determinant of bone quality. It represents the sum of all voids within the bone, which includes osteocytic lacunae, canaliculi, blood vessels, and resorption cavities (**Fig. 1**). There is a nonlinear inverse correlation between the porosity and the stiffness of the bone.[19]

Mechanical Assessment of Bone Quality: Bending Tests

Bones can be tested mechanically in compression, tension, bending, or torsion. Bending tests are one of the most common methods to test the mechanical properties of bones.[20] In the bending test, the bone (whole bone or a prepared bone specimen) is loaded in bending until failure.

Bending tests are either three-point or four-point bending experiments. In three-point bending, a bone specimen is positioned on two supports, and a

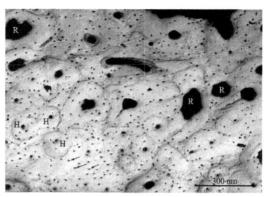

Fig. 1. Light microscopy of a feline bone depicting several secondary osteons with their central haversian canal (H). Resorptive lesions (R) are the largest cavities within the bone. Arrows indicate lacunae.

single-pronged loading device is applied to the opposite surface of the specimen, precisely in the middle of the two supports (**Fig. 2**). This central loading point is the point in which maximal load occurs, and at this location the bone ultimately fractures. Four-point bending tests use the same principles, but the load is applied by two loading prongs instead of one, located at an equal distance from either side of the midpoint. This configuration guarantees the specimen is loaded in pure bending with almost no shear stresses.[20,21]

The experimental procedure during a bending test involves induction of displacement of the loading prongs, which causes deformation of the specimen, while measuring the force required to induce this displacement yielding a load-deformation curve. This curve is subsequently converted to a stress-strain curve, from which inherent properties of the bone material are derived.[21] These properties include, for example, the Young's modulus, which is a measurement of the stiffness of a material (ie, the resistance to bending deformation), and energy to fracture, which represents the bone's toughness.

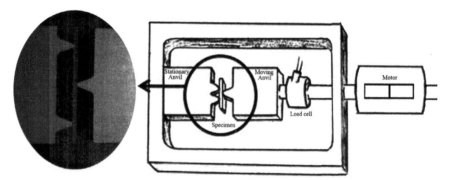

Fig. 2. Mechanical testing (three-point bending test). A bone specimen is held between two anvils. A moving anvil (with one prong) is attached to a motor that advances the anvil toward the stationary anvil (with two prongs) resulting in deformation of the tested specimen. The load required to advance the anvil is measured by a load cell.

RENAL OSTEODYSTROPHY IN HUMAN AND ANIMALS WITH CHRONIC KIDNEY DISEASE

Renal Osteodystrophy in Human Patients with Chronic Kidney Disease

Analysis of bone biopsy from the iliac crest is currently the gold standard for diagnosing and classifying ROD.[12] Because studies in humans are restricted to noninvasive or minimally invasive procedures, the precise microstructural, compositional, and mechanical bone changes that occur during ROD are not entirely known. Mild manifestations of ROD are usually observed early in the course of the disease (as early as stage II), and worsen as kidney function deteriorates. The type and nature of ROD may vary from one patient to another and encompasses a spectrum from severely suppressed to markedly elevated bone turnover. The two major types of ROD recognized in human patients are high-turnover bone disease (osteitis fibrosa) and low-turnover bone disease (adynamic bone disease), both of which are associated with increased bone fragility. Some patients suffer from one of these types predominantly, whereas others have a mixed type of bone disease. Osteomalacia also may be present.[22]

In high-turnover bone disease, increased PTH concentration enhances osteoclast activity, leading to increased bone resorption. Bone abnormalities include increased number of resorption cavities, enlarged haversian canals, and marked fibrosis involving the bone marrow.[22] Additional osteoporotic alterations include endocortical resorption, trabecular perforation, cortical thinning, and increased cortical porosity.[12]

The mechanisms underlying the development of low-turnover bone disease are not fully understood, but it generally is not associated with high PTH levels (ie, not mediated by renal SHPT). Adynamic bone disease is characterized by a defect in bone matrix formation and mineralization and a decrease in the number of osteoclasts and osteoblasts on bone surfaces. These changes are associated with an increased risk of overt fractures and microfractures. The reported prevalence of adynamic bone disease in dialysis-dependent patients with CKD varies between 15% and 60%.[22]

Bone abnormalities in all types of ROD greatly increase the risk of pathologic fractures, which are associated with excess morbidity, mortality, and health care costs. The United States Renal Data reveals that the risk for hip fracture is about four-fold higher among human hemodialysis patients compared with the general population, with the risk correlated to the duration on renal-replacement therapy.[23] Moderate-to-severe kidney disease is associated with more than a two-fold increase in hip fracture, demonstrating that patients with CKD who do not yet require renal-replacement therapy are also at an increased risk of fragility fractures.[12] Furthermore, outcomes of fractures are significantly worse in the CKD population compared with the general population, with a two- to three-fold increase in mortality following hip fractures.[14] The risk of fracture in patients with CKD has been linked directly to the severity of renal SHPT, and is reported to increase by 9% with each 200-pg/mL increase in PTH concentration and by 72% with PTH concentrations greater than 900 pg/mL.[24]

Bone Abnormalities in Veterinary Patients with Chronic Kidney Disease

Although renal SHPT is highly prevalent among cats and dogs with CKD, its effects on their bone metabolism have not been thoroughly studied. There are several case reports of cats and dogs with CKD suffering from bone abnormalities. Most reports are of young growing dogs with renal dysplasia. This is most likely because bones of young animals are more sensitive to the effects of PTH. Findings include thinning of the cortices and severe bone demineralization, with the skull and mandible most severely affected. These abnormalities often lead to pathologic jaw fractures and teeth loosening.[25,26] A case report of a cat with CKD and parathyroid hyperplasia demonstrated cortical bone lysis and cystic bone lesions, most severe in the femoral diaphysis.[27] Despite these few anecdotal reports, clinical signs associated with ROD are generally considered uncommon in dogs and cats with CKD.[25] It is possible that veterinary patients with CKD do not live long enough for skeletal changes to become clinically evident. However, with the advancement of medical management and growing availability of hemodialysis for veterinary patients, the effects of CKD on bone might become more clinically important.

Recently, two case-control studies were designed to evaluate the effect of CKD on bone quality of dogs and cats.[28,29] In the first study, 13 cats with IRIS CKD stage III and IV were compared with cats that died or were euthanized because of reasons unrelated to the urinary system (control animals). Similarly, nine dogs diagnosed with IRIS CKD stage III and IV were compared with age, sex, and body weight matched control animals. Both the cortical and the cancellous bone were evaluated.

Material Properties of the Cortical Bone

The two main determinants of bone strength (porosity and BMD)[19] were found to be altered in animals with CKD compared with control animals. The BMD of cats with CKD was lower by 4.8% compared with control animals. BMD is a major determinant of bone quality and the current clinical standard to predict fracture risk in patients with osteoporosis.[16] Even a small decrease in BMD substantially decreases the stiffness of the bone and increases fracture risk,[30] because the relationship between these two bone characterizes is exponential.[31,32] Indeed, there is an inverse correlation between low BMD and fracture risk in human dialysis patients.[16]

BMD in human patients with CKD varies, depending on the type of ROD; it may be normal or even high in adynamic bone disease, whereas it is generally low in high-turnover disease.[12] The BMD is 4.2% lower in predialysis patients with CKD compared with control subjects,[33] and 17.5% lower in patients beginning hemodialysis.[34] A recent longitudinal study that tracked changes in cortical bone in 53 human patients with CKD, found a significant decrease in BMD over time,[35] implying the length of the disease plays a role in the expected decrease in BMD. The shorter disease length might account for the more subtle changes documented in animals with CKD.

Porosity, another major determinant of bone quality, is the sum of all voids within the bone, including osteocytic lacunae, blood vessels, and resorption cavities. The overall porosity was significantly higher in dogs with CKD compared with control animals, but only tended to be higher in cats with CKD. Both dogs and cats affected with CKD had a significantly higher density of resorption cavities compared with healthy control animals (**Fig. 3**). Resorption cavities represent the largest pores in the bone, and when present in high density, bone strength is decreased because these cavities are a defect in the bone causing weakening and deterioration of bone quality.[36] Resorptive cavities are formed normally by osteoclasts as part of the remodeling process to remove damaged bone and replace it with new bone. The remodeling process is carried out by a multicentric unit, which is a group of cells comprised of osteoclasts that erode bone and form the resorption cavities, and osteoblasts that fill the bone defect with new bone matrix. Under normal conditions bone resorption and formation are approximately equal, and bone mass is maintained. SHPT leads to an imbalance of the remodeling process, causing more bone to be resorbed and less bone to be formed, leaving part of the resorption cavities not filled with new bone. Models indicate that resorption cavity size and location are important factors in determining bone quality, and the effect of cavities is larger than can be expected from simple bone loss.[37] This effect could be caused by stress concentrating effects of these cavities,

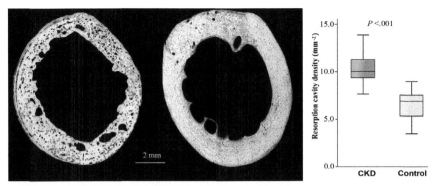

Fig. 3. Two cross-sections of bone; the left is from a cat with chronic kidney disease and the right is from a control cat. Note the increased number and size of resorption cavities in the bone of the chronic kidney disease affected cat. The box plot on the right depicts the density of resorptive cavities of cats with chronic kidney disease compared with control cats.

increasing the risk of bone failure at that point. Thus, higher resorption cavity density in the bone of patients with CKD is expected to negatively affect bone ability to resist fracture by increasing the porosity and by serving as stress risers. The higher porosity and higher density of resorptive lesions found in animals with CKD should be taken into consideration when traumatic or pathologic fractures occur in these animals.

Additional structural features that have been shown to affect cortical bone quality include osteon size and density, haversian canal size, and several other microarchitechture changes.[38] Light microscopy of bones from dogs with CKD revealed smaller lacunae.[29] It is accepted that osteocytes play a crucial role in maintaining material properties of bone by regulating the modeling and remodeling processes.[39] The morphologic changes documented may affect the osteocyte-canalicular system and impair cell-to-cell communication. This change can reduce the effectiveness of the osteocytes' role in mechanosensing and damage repair and could perhaps point to one of the mechanisms leading to cortical bone deterioration.

Bone Geometry

The geometry of the bone has been evaluated only in cats, because there is a large variability in bone size among different dog breeds. Micro-CT analysis of cortical bone of the femoral diaphysis of cats with CKD showed significantly lower cortical cross-sectional area (ie, smaller cortical area) and a 17% decrease in cortical thickness.[28] These findings suggest not only are the material properties of the bone in cats with CKD reduced, but also its mass is decreased, as reflected by smaller and narrower cortexes. Intuitively, narrower cortices and bones with lower cortical area have reduced flexural stiffness and are expected to fail (break) at lower loads.

Mechanical Properties of the Cortical Bone

The mechanical performance of whole bones depends on their geometry and the material properties of the bone matter. The most commonly assessed property of the bone material is the Young's modulus, which reflects the stiffness of the bone (the bones' ability to resist bending forces). Bones of cats with CKD had inferior mechanical properties compared with control animals; in particular they demonstrated a lower Young's modulus (by 13%), lower yield stress, and lower ultimate stress (ie, the bones were able to withstand smaller stresses before yielding and breaking). These differences were not apparent in bones from dogs with CKD. Similar to cats, human patients with CKD also have inferior mechanical bone properties compared with healthy patients, as reflected by a decreased Young's modulus (by 11.9%) in patients with high-turnover ROD.[40]

PROPERTIES OF CANCELLOUS BONE

Cancellous bone represents approximately 20% of the skeletal mass and is found in the epiphyseal regions of long bones and in flat and irregular bones. It is made of the same constituents as cortical bone but has a different spatial distribution and considerably higher porosity. In some bones, like the vertebrae, the proportion of cancellous bone is very high compared with the cortical bone.

The contribution of cancellous bone to overall mechanical properties of the whole bone is controversial[41–43]; however, it is believed it improves the bones' structural strength and assists in load distribution (energy dissipation). The lumbar vertebrae are a common place for cancellous bone analysis because of the high proportion of cancellous bone and because pathologic fractures are common in this site. Cancellous bone is assessed mainly by evaluating its bone volume (ie, the proportion of the bone volume compared with the overall volume) and trabecular thickness. Analysis of cancellous bone in cats with CKD revealed deterioration in cancellous bone quality as reflected by significantly lower trabecular thickness and bone volume (bone volume/total volume) (**Fig. 4**). Furthermore, the effect on cancellous bone was multisited and shown to occur in the vertebral bodies and in the long bones (distal femur). These findings in cats (reduced trabecular thickness and bone volume/total volume) negatively affect bone quality and were shown to be associated with increased risk for fracture.[44]

Species Differences

These studies of dogs and cats revealed similarities between the two species; however, some differences were also documented. Bone abnormalities of cats were demonstrated in all levels tested (material properties, geometry, and mechanical properties). In dogs, abnormalities were more subtle and were not documented in all aspects tested. Some of the differences between dogs and cats are likely related to the progression rate of the disease. Because SHPT is one of the early consequences of CKD, it is likely that cats, as humans, are exposed to the metabolic derangements associated with the disease for years, as opposed to dogs in which CKD often

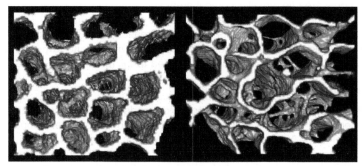

Fig. 4. Cancellous bone of a cat with chronic kidney disease (*right*) and a cat without chronic kidney disease (*left*). Note the overall reduction in bone mass in the affected cat and the lower trabecular thickness.

progresses over a shorter period of time. Therefore, in dogs, despite physiologic similarities in mineral metabolism, the effects on bone quality are less pronounced.

DOGS AND CATS AS A MODEL FOR RENAL OSTEODYSTROPHY IN HUMANS

Most studies use rodents to investigate the effects of renal SHPT on bone quality. The rat is one of the most commonly used animals in models for the human disease; however, there are marked differences between rat and human bone. Rodent bones are remarkably different from human bones in terms of type, architecture, structure, and biology, of which, most dramatically, rodent cortical bone does not remodel.[45] Moreover, findings in rats are not always consistent with regard to changes in BMD and mechanical properties,[46–48] which partly explains the shortcomings of this model. Dogs and cats can serve as an alternative and superior model for ROD in human patients. Both canine and feline adult skeletons show many structural similarities to the human bone. The cortex consists mostly of secondary osteons and remodels continuously as does the human bone.[46–49] Other advantages to study ROD in dogs and cats is that the disease occurs naturally (vs chemically, genetically, or surgically induced in laboratory animals), its prevalence is high in cats, and the disease has clinicopathologic similarities to human ROD. Canine and feline bones have technical advantages for study over rodent bones. Reliable measurement of material bone properties requires precise and accurate mechanical testing of carefully prepared geometric samples of cortical bone, such as beams or cubes. Such testing is difficult to achieve in rodents because of the small size of their bones; therefore rodent bones are often tested by three-point bending technique applied to whole bones, which is hampered by various technical limitations.[50,51] Canine and feline bones have much thicker cortices, which allow preparation of cortical bone beams for more accurate and reliable assessments using four-point bending testing.

SUMMARY

Secondary renal osteopathy exists in companion animals. Changes are more pronounced in cats compared with dogs, most likely caused by a longer disease course, but occur in both species. The documented changes further justify the need to control phosphorous concentration and to prevent SHPT in the management of CKD in dogs and cats. It is yet to be determined what is the clinical significance of these finding (if any) and whether interventions aimed to control this inevitable complication (eg, phosphorous control, administration of vitamin D derivatives) can negate, at least to some extent, the deterioration in bone quality of animals with CKD. Further studies assessing bone quality of dogs and cats with CKD are warranted because the aforementioned studies were based on a small number of animals with naturally occurring kidney disease. Variability of the severity and the chronicity of the disease existed among the animals, and therefore some of the statistical comparisons made were likely underpowered.

These studies provide evidence that dogs and cats with CKD have decreased bone quality. Until proven otherwise, the fracture risk of animals with CKD should be considered higher and fixation methods should take into account the lower bone quality of these patients.

REFERENCES

1. Khan S. Vitamin D deficiency and secondary hyperparathyroidism among patients with chronic kidney disease. Am J Med Sci 2007;333:201–7.

2. Saliba W, El-Haddad B. Secondary hyperparathyroidism: pathophysiology and treatment. J Am Board Fam Med 2009;22:574–81.
3. Nabeshima Y. The discovery of alpha-Klotho and FGF23 unveiled new insight into calcium and phosphate homeostasis. Cell Mol Life Sci 2008;65:3218–30.
4. Parker VJ, Gilor C, Chew DJ. Feline hyperparathyroidism: pathophysiology, diagnosis and treatment of primary and secondary disease. J Feline Med Surg 2015; 17:427–39.
5. Ketteler M, Biggar PH, Liangos O. FGF23 antagonism: the thin line between adaptation and maladaptation in chronic kidney disease. Nephrol Dial Transplant 2013;28:821–5.
6. Bolasco P. Treatment options of secondary hyperparathyroidism (SHPT) in patients with chronic kidney disease stages 3 and 4: an historic review. Clin Cases Miner Bone Metab 2009;6:210–9.
7. Slatopolsky E, Caglar S, Pennell JP, et al. On the pathogenesis of hyperparathyroidism in chronic experimental renal insufficiency in the dog. J Clin Invest 1971; 50:492–9.
8. Cortadellas O, Fernandez del Palacio MJ, Talavera J, et al. Calcium and phosphorus homeostasis in dogs with spontaneous chronic kidney disease at different stages of severity. J Vet Intern Med 2010;24:73–9.
9. Barber PJ, Elliott J. Feline chronic renal failure: calcium homeostasis in 80 cases diagnosed between 1992 and 1995. J Small Anim Pract 1998;39:108–16.
10. Finch NC, Syme HM, Elliott J. Parathyroid hormone concentration in geriatric cats with various degrees of renal function. J Am Vet Med Assoc 2012;241:1326–35.
11. Geddes RF, Finch NC, Elliott J, et al. Fibroblast growth factor 23 in feline chronic kidney disease. J Vet Intern Med 2013;27:234–41.
12. Nickolas TL, Leonard MB, Shane E. Chronic kidney disease and bone fracture: a growing concern. Kidney Int 2008;74:721–31.
13. Babayev R, Nickolas TL. Bone disorders in chronic kidney disease: an update in diagnosis and management. Semin Dial 2015;28:645–53.
14. Salam SN, Eastell R, Khwaja A. Fragility fractures and osteoporosis in CKD: pathophysiology and diagnostic methods. Am J Kidney Dis 2014;63:1049–59.
15. Currey JD. Bone strength: what are we trying to measure? Calcif Tissue Int 2001; 68:205–10.
16. Jamal SA, Hayden JA, Beyene J. Low bone mineral density and fractures in long-term hemodialysis patients: a meta-analysis. Am J Kidney Dis 2007;49:674–81.
17. Turner CH. Bone strength: current concepts. Ann N Y Acad Sci 2006;1068: 429–46.
18. Bouxsein ML. Bone quality: where do we go from here? Osteoporos Int 2003; 14(Suppl 5):S118–27.
19. Schaffler MB, Burr DB. Stiffness of compact bone: effects of porosity and density. J Biomech 1988;21:13–6.
20. Sharir A, Barak MM, Shahar R. Whole bone mechanics and mechanical testing. Vet J 2008;177:8–17.
21. Turner CH, Burr DB. Basic biomechanical measurements of bone: a tutorial. Bone 1993;14:595–608.
22. National Kidney Foundation. K/DOQI clinical practice guidelines for bone metabolism and disease in chronic kidney disease. Am J Kidney Dis 2003;42:S1–201.
23. Alem AM, Sherrard DJ, Gillen DL, et al. Increased risk of hip fracture among patients with end-stage renal disease. Kidney Int 2000;58:396–9.
24. Danese MD, Kim J, Doan QV, et al. PTH and the risks for hip, vertebral, and pelvic fractures among patients on dialysis. Am J Kidney Dis 2006;47:149–56.

25. Vanbrugghe B, Blond L, Carioto L, et al. Clinical and computed tomography features of secondary renal hyperparathyroidism. Can Vet J 2011;52:177–80 [quiz: 180].
26. Davis EM. Oral manifestations of chronic kidney disease and renal secondary hyperparathyroidism: a comparative review. J Vet Dent 2015;32:87–98.
27. Gnudi G, Bertoni G, Luppi A, et al. Unusual hyperparathyroidism in a cat. Vet Radiol Ultrasound 2001;42:250–3.
28. Shipov A, Segev G, Meltzer H, et al. The effect of naturally occurring chronic kidney disease on the micro-structural and mechanical properties of bone. PLoS One 2014;9:e110057.
29. Shipov S, Shahar R, Shugar N, et al. The effect of naturally occurring chronic kidney disease on the micro-structural and mechanical properties of bone in dogs [abstract]. In: The 38rd Symposium of Veterinary Medicine. Israel, December 28, 2015.
30. Yenchek RH, Ix JH, Shlipak MG, et al. Bone mineral density and fracture risk in older individuals with CKD. Clin J Am Soc Nephrol 2012;7:1130–6.
31. Wasnich RD, Ross PD, Davis JW, et al. A comparison of single and multi-site BMC measurements for assessment of spine fracture probability. J Nucl Med 1989;30: 1166–71.
32. Currey JD. The effect of porosity and mineral content on the Young's modulus of elasticity of compact bone. J Biomech 1988;21:131–9.
33. Rix M, Andreassen H, Eskildsen P, et al. Bone mineral density and biochemical markers of bone turnover in patients with predialysis chronic renal failure. Kidney Int 1999;56:1084–93.
34. Pecovnik Balon B, Hojs R, Zavratnik A, et al. Bone mineral density in patients beginning hemodialysis treatment. Am J Nephrol 2002;22:14–7.
35. Nickolas TL, Stein EM, Dworakowski E, et al. Rapid cortical bone loss in patients with chronic kidney disease. J Bone Miner Res 2013;28:1811–20.
36. Seeman E. Structural basis of growth-related gain and age-related loss of bone strength. Rheumatology 2008;47(Suppl 4):iv2–8.
37. Vanderoost J, van Lenthe GH. From histology to micro-CT: measuring and modeling resorption cavities and their relation to bone competence. World J Radiol 2014;6:643–56.
38. Yeni YN, Brown CU, Wang Z, et al. The influence of bone morphology on fracture toughness of the human femur and tibia. Bone 1997;21:453–9.
39. Lanyon LE. Osteocytes, strain detection, bone modeling and remodeling. Calcif Tissue Int 1993;53(Suppl 1):S102–6 [discussion: S106–7].
40. Malluche HH, Porter DS, Monier-Faugere MC, et al. Differences in bone quality in low- and high-turnover renal osteodystrophy. J Am Soc Nephrol 2012;23:525–32.
41. Fields AJ, Eswaran SK, Jekir MG, et al. Role of trabecular microarchitecture in whole-vertebral body biomechanical behavior. J Bone Miner Res 2009;24:1523–30.
42. Homminga J, Weinans H, Gowin W, et al. Osteoporosis changes the amount of vertebral trabecular bone at risk of fracture but not the vertebral load distribution. Spine 2001;26:1555–61.
43. Barak MM, Weiner S, Shahar R. The contribution of trabecular bone to the stiffness and strength of rat lumbar vertebrae. Spine 2010;35:E1153–9.
44. Nickolas TL, Stein E, Cohen A, et al. Bone mass and microarchitecture in CKD patients with fracture. J Am Soc Nephrol 2010;21:1371–80.
45. Shipov A, Zaslansky P, Riesemeier H, et al. Unremodeled endochondral bone is a major architectural component of the cortical bone of the rat (Rattus norvegicus). J Struct Biol 2013;183:132–40.

46. Cao H, Nazarian A, Ackerman JL, et al. Quantitative (31)P NMR spectroscopy and (1)H MRI measurements of bone mineral and matrix density differentiate metabolic bone diseases in rat models. Bone 2010;46:1582–90.

47. Iwasaki Y, Kazama JJ, Yamato H, et al. Changes in chemical composition of cortical bone associated with bone fragility in rat model with chronic kidney disease. Bone 2011;48:1260–7.

48. Jokihaara J, Jarvinen TL, Jolma P, et al. Renal insufficiency-induced bone loss is associated with an increase in bone size and preservation of strength in rat proximal femur. Bone 2006;39:353–60.

49. Miller MA, Chin J, Miller SC, et al. Disparate effects of mild, moderate, and severe secondary hyperparathyroidism on cancellous and cortical bone in rats with chronic renal insufficiency. Bone 1998;23:257–66.

50. van Lenthe GH, Voide R, Boyd SK, et al. Tissue modulus calculated from beam theory is biased by bone size and geometry: implications for the use of three-point bending tests to determine bone tissue modulus. Bone 2008;43:717–23.

51. Torcasio A, Van Oosterwyck H, van Lenthe GH. The systematic errors in tissue modulus of murine bones when estimated from three-point bending. J Biomech 2008;41:S14.

Update on Medical Management of Clinical Manifestations of Chronic Kidney Disease

CrossMark

Jessica M. Quimby, DVM, PhD

KEYWORDS

- Appetite • Anemia • Hypokalemia • Hypertension • Constipation • Renal disease

KEY POINTS

- Although chronic kidney disease is a progressive disease, multiple secondary medical derangements can be identified and treated with the hope of increasing quality of life and longevity.
- Blood pressure should be assessed in all patients with chronic kidney disease, as hypertension is common and should be medically addressed.
- Hypokalemia is common in feline chronic kidney disease patients and should be identified and medically addressed.
- Maintenance of body condition and nutritional management of chronic kidney disease is an important part of management, and antiemetics and appetite stimulants can be useful tools.
- Constipation can occur secondary to CKD and should be identified and managed.

MANAGEMENT OF HYPERTENSION
Introduction/Etiology/Epidemiology

Systemic hypertension seems to be common in dogs (31%–54%) and cats (20%–65%) with chronic kidney disease (CKD), but the exact pathophysiologic relationship is unknown.[1–3] Hypertension in veterinary patients with CKD is generally considered to be a sequela of CKD as opposed to an etiology of CKD as it is in humans, but this idea is still controversial. Although the pathophysiology of hypertension secondary to CKD is considered multifactorial and poorly understood, factors thought to be involved in the process include impaired sodium excretion and activation of the renal-angiotensin-aldosterone system, increased sympathetic tone,

Disclosure Statement: The author is a consultant for Zoetis and Aratana Therapeutics.
Department of Clinical Sciences, Colorado State University, 300 West Drake Road, Fort Collins, CO 80523, USA
E-mail address: jquimby@colostate.edu

Vet Clin Small Anim 46 (2016) 1163–1181
http://dx.doi.org/10.1016/j.cvsm.2016.06.004
vetsmall.theclinics.com
0195-5616/16/$ – see front matter © 2016 Elsevier Inc. All rights reserved.

structural changes to vasculature, endothelial dysfunction, reduced bioavailability of the vasodilator nitric oxide, and increased production of the vasoconstrictor endothelin.[1] Systemic hypertension is important to identify and address in CKD patients because of numerous deleterious effects such as progression of CKD and proteinuria, left ventricular hypertrophy and subsequent cardiac impairment, ocular disease including retinal vascular tortuosity and hemorrhage, hyphema, blindness caused by retinal detachment, and neurologic sequelae including encephalopathy, vascular events, seizures, and death.[1,2,4–7]

Patient Evaluations

All dogs with renal proteinuria or azotemia should be assessed for hypertension. Elderly cats, particularly those with CKD, should be screened routinely at initial CKD diagnosis and throughout the course of the disease, as approximately 10% will have hypertension at a later date.[8] A variety of devices are available for evaluation of blood pressure in veterinary patients. At this time, there is no clear consensus on the most accurate and reliable methodology; however, Doppler and high-definition oscillometric devices seem to be most commonly recommended. Guidelines for obtaining blood pressure in veterinary patients are outlined in **Box 1.**

Box 1
Recommended procedure for obtaining blood pressure

The calibration of the blood pressure device should be verified twice annually.

The blood pressure measurement procedure should be standardized.

The environment should be isolated, quiet, away from other animals, and ideally with the owner present.

The patient should be allowed to equilibrate to the environment for 5 to 10 minutes before assessment.

The patient should be gently restrained in ventral or lateral recumbency to limit the distance from the heart base to the cuff.

The cuff should be approximately 40% of the circumference of the cuff site in dogs and 30% to 40% in cats.

The cuff may be placed on a limb or tail but should continue to be measured in the same location each time.

An experienced, trained technician should perform all blood pressure measurements.

The patient should be calm and motionless.

The first measurement should be discarded, and at least 3, preferably 5 to 7, consecutive consistent (<20% variability) values should be obtained.

Measurements should be averaged to obtain the final reading.

The process should be repeated if there is doubt about the readings.

A standard form in the medical record should be used to record the cuff size and location, patient temperament, values obtained and final average reading, and rational for any excluded values.

Adapted from Brown S, Atkins C, Bagley R, et al. Guidelines for the identification, evaluation, and management of systemic hypertension in dogs and cats. J Vet Intern Med 2007;21:544; with permission.

Unless blood pressure is greater than 200 mm Hg or evidence of target organ damage is seen, blood pressure should be rechecked on 2 to 3 occasions to rule out white coat hypertension.[9,10] The patient should be classified according to their risk of target organ damage according to the International Renal Interest Society (IRIS) CKD blood pressure substaging system (**Table 1**).

Once hypertension has been confirmed and classified, the decision to initiate therapy is based on the degree of hypertension and the animal's IRIS CKD stage. When blood pressure is greater than 200 mm Hg or evidence of target organ damage is seen, therapy is immediately initiated. Patients with CKD stage 2 to 4 and blood pressure consistently greater than 160 mm Hg are candidates for treatment. Antihypertensive therapy should be considered for IRIS stage I patients with arterial blood pressure consistently greater than 180 mm Hg.[11]

Treatment Recommendations

It is unknown what the optimal arterial blood pressure is for patients with CKD. A general guideline is to reduce the blood pressure to less than 150 mm Hg.[4,12] Aggressive reduction of blood pressure is only necessary in patients experiencing ocular and neurologic complications, otherwise it may take weeks, particularly in dogs, to achieve adequate control.[13] Treatment strategies for cats and dogs differ slightly based on the efficacy of currently available antihypertensive medications.

Amlodipine is documented to be an effective treatment for hypertension in the cat and is the drug of choice in this species.[12,14,15] Angiotensin-converting enzyme inhibitors (ACEIs) have not been demonstrated to adequately reduce blood pressure in cats when used as a sole therapy.[16] Amlodipine is prescribed at an initial dose of 0.625 mg for cats weighing less than 5 kg and 1.25 mg in cats greater than 5 kg. Alternative formulations of the drug have been explored including transdermal amlodipine and a chewable form, which may provide some degree of efficacy.[12,17] Amlodipine has also been documented to decrease proteinuria in cats.[14]

Currently used antihypertensive medications in dogs include ACEIs (enalapril and benazepril), calcium channel blockers (amlodipine), or angiotensin receptor blockers, such as telmisartan or losartan.[18] These medications are thought to be most effective at reducing hypertension in dogs, although most dogs require multiple medications, and few studies have been done in this area. ACEIs are found to reduce intraglomerular hypertension and proteinuria and thus are commonly used in dogs, as proteinuria is a hallmark of canine CKD. Typical starting doses are 0.25 to 0.5 mg/kg every 12 to

Table 1			
International Renal Interest Society blood pressure stages for dogs and cats			
IRIS BP Stage	Systolic BP (mm Hg)	Diastolic BP (mm Hg)	Risk of Target Organ Damage
Normotension	<150	<95	Minimal
Borderline hypertension	150–159	95–99	Mild
Hypertension	160–179	100–119	Moderate
Severe hypertension	>180	>120	Severe

Abbreviation: BP, blood pressure.
Adapted from Brown S, Atkins C, Bagley R, et al. Guidelines for the identification, evaluation, and management of systemic hypertension in dogs and cats. J Vet Intern Med 2007;21:548; with permission.

24 hours with increases based on effect on blood pressure up to 2 mg/kg/d. In dogs, amlodipine doses range from 0.1 to 0.5 mg/kg/d and are combined with an ACEI. Recommended doses for angiotensin receptor blockers in dogs range from telmisartan, 1 mg/kg/d, to losartan, 0.125 mg/kg in azotemic dogs and 0.5 mg/kg in nonazotemic dogs.[18]

Sodium restriction is not recommended in veterinary patients, as blood pressure is not responsive to sodium restriction/loading; however, this finding has not been adequate assessed in patients with naturally occurring CKD.[16,18] Given the current information available, avoidance of high-sodium diets is recommended, but active sodium restriction is not.[16] It is currently unknown if subcutaneous fluids are contraindicated in hypertensive patients owing to concerns for volume and sodium loading. It is likely best to restrict subcutaneous fluids therapy in hypertensive patients to those who actively struggle with dehydration.[16]

Evaluation of Outcome/Complications

Blood pressure should be rechecked within 7 to 10 days after initiating therapy. In cats, if adequate blood pressure control has not been achieved, the amlodipine dose is typically doubled. In dogs, if blood pressure control has not been achieved with ACEIs, then amlodipine is added as a second medication.[16,18] Monitoring renal values and electrolytes is also important; ACEIs can decrease glomerular filtration rate and result in increasing azotemia, in which case therapy should be reassessed. Hyperkalemia is also a common side effect of ACEIs in dogs and may limit the dose that can be administered.[18]

MANAGEMENT OF HYPOKALEMIA
Introduction/Etiology/Epidemiology

Hypokalemia is a common finding in cats with stage 2 and 3 CKD with approximately 20% to 30% of cats affected.[19,20] Hypokalemia is less common in stage 4 CKD cats because of markedly decreased glomerular filtration[11] and is typically less common in dogs because of ACEI therapy for proteinuria. Regulation of electrolyte balance is a major function of the kidney. Potassium is freely filtered at the glomerulus, and then depending on systemic needs is titrating accordingly further along the nephron via reabsorption and excretion. Although the exact mechanism by which marked hypokalemia in feline CKD patients occurs is poorly understood, it is likely caused by a combination of increased urinary loss from polyuria resulting in less opportunity for reabsorption, inadequate dietary intake, and activation of the renin-angiotensin-aldosterone system. Chronic metabolic acidosis associated with CKD also encourages intracellular potassium depletion from intracellular influx of excess hydrogen ions and concomitant efflux of potassium.[6] In humans, hypokalemia level less than 4 meq/L is associated with increased risk for end-stage disease and mortality.[21,22] In rodent models, hypokalemia results in impaired renal angiogenesis, capillary loss, and decreased vascular endothelial growth factor.[23] In cats, experimental diets inadequate in potassium are found to result in the development renal dysfunction[24,25]; however, hypokalemia has not been found to be a risk factor for disease progression or outcome in CKD cats.[26,27]

Patient Evaluations

Cats with CKD should be routinely screened for hypokalemia. Mild hypokalemia may not be associated with clinical signs, and clinically relevant hypokalemia can often be missed because of the lack of electrolyte readings on in-house chemistry analyzers. Moderate hypokalemia (2.5–3.0 meq/L) may result in muscle weakness, lethargy, inappetence, and constipation, and severe hypokalemia (<2.5 meq/L) may result in hypokalemic myopathy including cervical ventroflexion and plantigrade stance (**Fig. 1**).[11]

Treatment Recommendations

Feline renal diets are supplemented with potassium and contain an average 0.7% to 1.2% potassium on a dry matter basis, whereas canine renal diets are not (typically, 0.4%–0.8% dry matter basis).[28] Since the introduction of potassium-supplemented renal diets, clinical presentation of profound hypokalemia in cats seems to be less common, but this has not been scientifically evaluated. Potassium supplementation is recommended in hypokalemic animals, and the oral route is the safest and preferred route in stable patients. Based on the possible renal effects of hypokalemia and how poorly representative serum potassium is in the face of metabolic acidosis,[29] some clinicians advocate prophylactic supplementation even when serum potassium is in the low normal range, with a goal of maintaining serum potassium levels greater than 4 mg/dL. However, the value of prophylactic potassium supplementation has not yet been established. Potassium supplementation may be provided orally as potassium gluconate (1–4 meq per cat twice daily) or potassium citrate (40–75 mg/kg orally divided twice daily), to effect.[13,30] Potassium citrate has the added advantage of being an alkalinizing agent; however, the degree to which it is effective for metabolic acidosis has not been evaluated. In decompensated patients in the hospital, potassium chloride is used to supplement intravenous fluids. Potassium chloride is not recommended as an oral supplement because it is acidifying and unpalatable but may be added to subcutaneous fluids at concentration up to 30 meq/L (higher concentrations can be associated with irritation).[6]

Evaluation of Outcome/Complications

When hypokalemic myopathy is present, it generally resolves within 1 to 5 days of initiation of oral or parenteral supplementation.[11] After correction of hypokalemic myopathy, potassium supplementation is adjusted based on clinical signs and serum potassium concentrations. In more stable and more mildly affected animals, serum

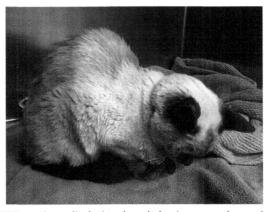

Fig. 1. Stage IV CKD patient displaying hypokalemic myopathy and moderate muscle wasting.

potassium should be rechecked 7 to 10 days after initiating potassium supplementation and dosing titrated accordingly. It has not been assessed whether all hypokalemic CKD cats require long-term potassium supplementation, but clinical impressions are that most cats will.[31] If hypokalemia seems particularly refractory to supplementation, additional medical conditions such as hyperaldosteronism and other causes for profound polyuria (ie, pyelonephritis) should be considered.

MANAGEMENT OF ANEMIA
Introduction/Etiology/Epidemiology

Anemia of CKD is typically characterized as normocytic, normochromic, or nonregenerative in nature. Approximately 30% to 65% of cats with CKD will have anemia as their disease progresses.[32] Red blood cell (RBC) production is regulated by the hormone erythropoietin, which is produced in the peritubular interstitial cells of the inner renal cortex and outer medulla. As kidney disease progresses, the number of hormone-producing cells decreases and anemia can result. Additionally, uremia has a negative effect on the lifespan of circulating RBCs. Although recent studies found that gastric ulceration is less common in dogs and cats than in humans, chronic low-grade gastrointestinal hemorrhage from mucosal friability and uremic thrombocytopathia may also contribute to anemia, and iron deficiency may be noted.[32,33] Iron deficiency can be absolute or functional and in feline CKD patients was recently found to more likely be functional.[34] The acute-phase protein hepcidin is a key regulator in iron homeostasis. Hepcidin is upregulated in inflammatory environments and leads to sequestration of iron with cells and tissues. In addition to the activities of hepcidin, proinflammatory cytokines also inhibit erythropoiesis in inflammatory states. Considering CKD in cats is histopathologically characterized by inflammatory infiltrate, a chronic inflammatory state likely plays a role in the anemia associated with the disease.

Some studies identify anemia as a negative predictor of survival in CKD.[26] Moderate-to-severe anemia has the potential to affect quality of life in CKD patients because of weakness, lethargy, and inappetence. Anemia triggers adaptations that can be detrimental, including increased release of norepinephrine, renin, angiotensin II, and aldosterone, which can lead to increased heart workload and hypertension. Anemia may also cause left heart enlargement, which could predispose patients to heart failure and fluid overload.[32] Furthermore, anemia has the potential to exacerbate progression of CKD. Hypoxia is thought to be a large player in the progression of CKD. Because of inflammatory infiltrate and expansion of interstitium, tubular cells already have compromised access to peritubular capillary blood supply. If what blood manages to reach the overworked remnant tubular cells is oxygen poor because of anemia, then the cells are starved further of nutrients and oxygen supply. Hypoxia results in fibrosis, tubular cell transdifferentiation, and activation of fibroblasts, further exacerbating the disease state.[35] Therefore, for multiple reasons, it is important that anemia be identified in CKD patients and managed appropriately.

Patient Evaluations

The decision to address anemia in the CKD patient is typically based on the degree of anemia, the likelihood of it correcting on its own, and the extent to which the patient is thought to be clinically affected. Although variable from patient to patient, typical cutoffs for strongly considering therapy are less than 20% in cats and dogs. Clinical signs such as weakness, lethargy, and inappetence would be supportive of a need to address anemia.

Treatment Recommendations

Options for treating anemia of CKD include correcting underlying factors contributing to anemia, blood transfusion, and administration of erythrocyte-stimulating agents (ESAs). Gastrointestinal hemorrhage, infection, or chronic inflammation are common underlying conditions contributing to anemia and should be addressed when possible. Identification and treatment of systemic infections may help improve anemia; urinary tract infections are particularly relevant in CKD patients, and urine should be screened accordingly. Chronic gastrointestinal hemorrhage is suspected when melena, elevated blood urea nitrogen, iron deficiency, or anemia disproportionate to level of azotemia is noted. Empirical treatment with acid suppressants and sucralfate with a subsequent increase in hematocrit support the diagnosis.

ESAs are commonly used to supplement the deficient erythropoietin hormone. Available ESAs include recombinant human erythropoietin darbepoetin alfa (Aranesp) or epoetin alfa (Epogen, Procrit). Darbepoetin is a longer-acting form of erythropoietin and is thought to have less association with antierythropoietin antibodies and pure red cell aplasia than the previously used Epogen.[36] Darbepoetin is currently the product of choice, but expense can limit its use for some owners (Walmart Specialty Pharmacy 877-453-4566, 1 mL vial [25 mg/mL] about $190). Therapy with Darbepoetin consists of an induction phase and a maintenance phase (**Fig. 2**). The recommended starting dose is 1 µg/kg subcutaneous (SQ) once weekly until the low end of the normal

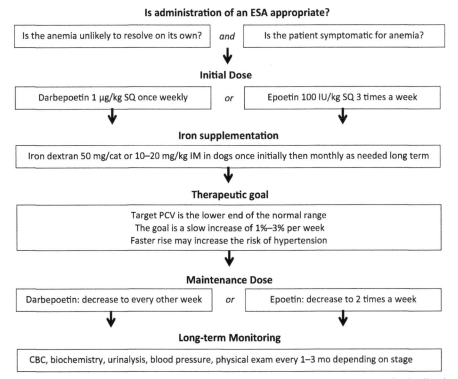

Is administration of an ESA appropriate?

| Is the anemia unlikely to resolve on its own? | *and* | Is the patient symptomatic for anemia? |

↓

Initial Dose

| Darbepoetin 1 µg/kg SQ once weekly | *or* | Epoetin 100 IU/kg SQ 3 times a week |

↓

Iron supplementation

| Iron dextran 50 mg/cat or 10–20 mg/kg IM in dogs once initially then monthly as needed long term |

↓

Therapeutic goal

Target PCV is the lower end of the normal range
The goal is a slow increase of 1%–3% per week
Faster rise may increase the risk of hypertension

↓

Maintenance Dose

| Darbepoetin: decrease to every other week | *or* | Epoetin: decrease to 2 times a week |

↓

Long-term Monitoring

| CBC, biochemistry, urinalysis, blood pressure, physical exam every 1–3 mo depending on stage |

Fig. 2. Decision flowchart for use of erythropoietin-stimulating agents. PCV, packed cell volume. (*Adapted from* Chalhoub S, Langston C, Eatroff A. Anemia of renal disease: what it is, what to do and what's new. J Feline Med Surg 2011;13:629–40.)

packed cell volume (PCV) range is reached, typically occurring within 3 to 4 weeks. Injections are then decreased to once every 2 to 3 weeks as needed to maintain PCV.[32]

Stimulating erythropoiesis is associated with a high iron demand and because of the functional iron deficiency associated with CKD, iron supplementation is recommended when therapy is initiated, as well as every few months through the course of therapy. Iron injections (iron dextran 50 mg intramuscularly in cats, 10–20 mg/kg intramuscularly in dogs, typically well tolerated) are considered more ideal that oral iron supplementation, as the latter tends to be bitter and likely to exacerbate an already poor appetite and is poorly absorbed from the gastrointestinal tract.[32] B vitamins are necessary for RBC synthesis, and the degree to which they are deficient in CKD patients and an active contributor to anemia is poorly understood. Given their benign nature, supplementation is unlikely to be harmful, but no information about efficacy currently exists. However, B vitamins are not considered effective as sole therapy for anemia.[32]

Evaluation of Outcome/Complications

Blood pressure and PCV should be checked weekly during the initiation period; hypertension associated with a rapid increase in PCV is the main side effect. Other reported side effects include pure red cell aplasia, arthralgia, fever, seizures, polycythemia, and iron deficiency.[32] Previous estimates of treatment success in cats were 60% to 65%.[32] Treatment failure may stem from inadequate dose, owner compliance, gastrointestinal GI bleeding, iron deficiency, B vitamin deficiency, concurrent infection or inflammation, aluminum toxicity, inhibition of erythropoiesis by ACE inhibitors, or bone marrow dysfunction. Typical trouble-shooting steps include increasing the dose, stopping ACEI- and aluminum-based therapies (aluminum hydroxide, sucralfate), treating for gastrointestinal bleeding or infection, and additional supplementation of iron and B vitamins. If no response is seen, then assessment of bone marrow is indicated.[32]

MANAGEMENT OF UREMIC DYSREXIA, NAUSEA, AND VOMITING
Introduction/Etiology/Epidemiology

Clinical signs of nausea, vomiting, and dysrexia are common in patients with CKD. In a recent survey of owners of cats with CKD, 43% of respondents reported abnormal appetite in their cat, necessitating 77% of those owners to coax the pet to eat more than 50% of the time.[37] Adequate caloric support is crucial for chronically ill patients, and there is evidence that CKD results in an increased metabolic state, making adequate nutrition even more of a challenge.[38] In humans, CKD protein energy wasting and poor body condition is associated with decreased survival, even in patients on dialysis.[39] Poor body condition score is also associated with a poorer prognosis dogs and cats with CKD.[40,41] In a recent study, cats were found to have lost weight before CKD diagnosis and continued to losing weight during the disease process.[41] A recent study assessing quality-of-life parameters in CKD cats found that CKD cats scored significantly lower than healthy young or geriatric cats in the categories of "appetite" and "liking food."[42] Additionally, poor appetite is perceived as a significant quality-of-life concern and can cause significant emotional distress to owners.[43]

Uremic toxins are sensed by the chemoreceptor trigger zone of the area postrema in the brain, which subsequently stimulates emesis by the vomiting center. Experimental ablation of the area postrema inhibits uremic vomiting in dogs with total nephrectomy illustrating the involvement of this structure in the pathophysiology of the disease.[44] It has long been thought that uremia has effects on the intestinal tract, such as hyperacidity, uremic gastritis, and ulceration that lead to further unwillingness to eat, but our understanding of the relevance of this pathophysiology to cats and dogs is incomplete. Cats with CKD are found to have elevated concentrations of gastrin that increase with the severity of renal failure,[45] but the relationship between gastrin, gastric acid secretion, and gastric pathology has not been fully described. Gastrin is excreted by the kidneys, and it is hypothesized that as renal function declines, hypergastrinemia develops, resulting in gastric hyperacidity.[45] However, cats that have gastrin-secreting tumors with levels of hypergastrinemia similar to those found in cats with CKD have significant gastric conditions, but this finding has not been shown in cats with CKD.[33,46] In human CKD, the development of gastric hyperacidity seems to be inconsistent and may be related to the presence of *Helicobacter* spp infection.[47] In a recent study evaluating the type and prevalence of histopathologic lesions in the stomach of cats with CKD, gastric fibrosis and mineralization were found to be prominent alterations rather than the uremic gastropathy lesions previously described in dogs and humans (uremic gastritis, ulceration, vascular injury, edema).[33] Additionally, uremic gastropathy is found to be not as severe in dogs as that described in humans. Gastrointestinal hemorrhage in cats and dogs with CKD may be more attributable to factors such as uremic thrombocytopathia rather than overt ulcerative lesions, which appear to be relatively rare.[32] Therefore, the administration of gastric protectants such as sucralfate may not be justified, unless obvious clinical evidence of gastrointestinal hemorrhage such as melena is appreciated.

In addition to buildup of uremic toxins and alterations in the gastrointestinal tract, the basic pathophysiology of appetite regulation may be significantly abnormal in animals with CKD. Appetite regulation is complex and involves a multitude of signaling compounds, but a refined summary is that regulation comprises orexigenic substances that activate the hunger center (ie, ghrelin) and anorexigenic substances that activate the satiety center of the brain (ie, leptin, cholecystokinin, obestatin, des-acyl ghrelin).[48] In humans, CKD is associated with an increased accumulation of anorexigenic substances secondary to decreased glomerular filtration rate without a concomitant increase in orexigenic substances such as ghrelin. Additionally, anorexigenic substances are found to be significantly higher in CKD patients with poor body condition than those with normal body condition.[48]

Patient Evaluations

Serial evaluations of nutritional status are a key part of CKD patient management, and a nutritional plan should be performed for every patient. Awareness of these parameters and tools for assessment have been made available owing to a global nutritional initiative by World Small Animal Veterinary Association.[49] A nutritional assessment should include body weight, body condition score, muscle mass score, adequacy of caloric intake (including open-ended questions about how the pet is eating), and a complete dietary history (including pet food, treats, supplements, and items used to give medications). In obese patients with inadequate muscle mass, body condition score often does not adequately describe muscle loss.[50] Assessment of muscle mass is particularly important in CKD patients, as it can have a profound effect on serum creatinine levels and affect the interpretation of the severity of disease and have notable implications for the nutritional status of the patient. Minimally, a score of adequate muscle mass or mild, moderate, or severe muscle loss should be determined based on epaxial, skull, scapular, and iliac musculature and documented in the medical record at each visit (see **Fig. 1**).[50,51]

Treatment Recommendations

Several antiemetic/antinausea therapies are available that may be helpful in ameliora-tion of nausea and vomiting associated with CKD (**Table 2**). These include the 5HT$_3$ receptor antagonists ondansetron and dolasetron and the NK$_1$ receptor antagonist maropitant citrate. These drugs work at the chemoreceptor trigger zone and vomiting center in the brain where uremic toxins are sensed and at receptors in the gastrointes-tinal tract. Maropitant is commonly used for acute vomiting; however, a pharmacoki-netic and toxicity study in cats indicated that longer-term use appears safe and anecdotally it is typically used for long-term therapy in chronically ill patients.[52] A recent study assessed the efficacy of maropitant for management of chronic vomiting and inappetence in cats with CKD.[53] When given daily for 2 weeks, maropitant was found to palliate vomiting associated with CKD, however, did not appear to signifi-cantly improve appetite or result in weight gain in cats with stage II and III CKD within the timeframe of the study.[53]

Ondansetron was found to be twice as effective as metoclopramide in palliating ure-mic nausea and vomiting in human CKD patients.[2] Pharmacokinetic studies in cats found that oral bioavailability of ondansetron is poor in this species (about 35%) and the half-life is very short (approximately 1 hour) making it most appropriately an every-8-hour medication.[54] Subcutaneous ondansetron had a slightly longer half-life of 3 hours. A pharmacokinetic study in dogs found that the oral bioavailability of ondansetron was very poor (<10%) indicating this may not be an appropriate route of administration.[55] Ondansetron is also not appropriate as a transdermal medication, as a study assessing transdermal absorption in cats found no detectable blood levels after administration.[56] Dolasetron is traditionally recommended as a once-daily medi-cation at doses of 0.5 to 1 mg/kg. However, a recent study exploring pharmacoki-netics and pharmacodynamics of subcutaneous dolasetron in cats found no measureable drug after just 12 hours and a failure to block xylazine-induced vomit-ing.[57] Additional studies are likely needed to determine how to best use this medica-tion in companion animals.

Although more commonly used as an appetite stimulant, mirtazapine also shows antiemetic properties, acting at the 5HT$_3$ receptor similar to ondansetron.[58] Several studies describe successful palliation of nausea and vomiting in human patients; particularly cancer patients undergoing chemotherapy.[59,60] In cats, mirtazapine was found to significantly reduce vomiting associated with CKD.[61]

Table 2			
Common medications used in medical management of appetite			
	Receptor	**Location of Action**	**Dose**
Maropitant	NK-1	Emetic center, CRTZ, GI	1 mg/kg IV/SQ q 24 h 2 mg/kg PO q 24 h
Dolasetron	5HT$_3$	CRTZ, GI afferent	0.5–1 mg/kg SQ q 24 h?
Ondansetron	5HT$_3$	CRTZ, GI afferent	1 mg/kg IV, SQ, PO q 8 h
Mirtazapine	5HT$_3$	CRTZ, GI afferent	Cats: 1.87 mg/cat q 24 h in normal cats, q 48 h in kidney or liver disease. Dogs: 0.6–1 mg/kg q 12 h.
Cyproheptadine	H1	Various	2–4 mg per cat q 12–24 h

Abbreviations: CRTZ, chemoreceptor trigger zone; GI, gastrointestinal; IV, intravenous; PO, orally; q, every.

In addition to addressing uremic nausea and vomiting, appetite stimulants can also be used to encourage food intake, particularly in late-stage patients and in patients in which a feeding tube is not desirable to the owner. Cyproheptadine has been used for some time as an appetite stimulant and has anecdotal efficacy in many patients; however, its efficacy has never been scientifically evaluated. Mirtazapine has become more commonly used, and recent exploration of its pharmacodynamics and pharmacokinetics has provided information for more effective use in animals.[62–64] Pharmacodynamic studies in cats illustrate that it can be a potent appetite stimulant, but higher doses are more commonly associated with side effects (hyperexcitability, vocalization, tremors).[65] Smaller, more frequent doses are recommended. Pharmacokinetic studies have found that the half-life is short enough that it could be administered daily in normal cats. Dose recommendations are 1.88 mg every 24 hours in cats without liver or kidney disease and 0.6 to 1 mg/kg once to twice daily in dogs without liver or kidney disease. In dogs, twice-daily dosing may be required because of short half-life compared with other species.[62] Renal disease delays clearance in CKD cats; thus, every-other-day administration is recommended.[63] The effect of liver disease on the metabolism of the drug in cats and dogs is currently unknown. In humans, liver disease delays elimination by 30%, and reduced dosing intervals are recommended.[58] A placebo-controlled, double-masked crossover clinical trial found that mirtazapine was an effective appetite stimulant in cats with CKD and resulted in significantly increased appetite and weight.[61] Mirtazapine also is amenable to transdermal administration and is found to achieve both appropriate serum levels and appetite stimulation in healthy cats.[66] Although clinical studies in cats with CKD are forthcoming, starting doses for transdermal application in CKD are anecdotally successful at 1.89 to 3.75 mg every other day. Owners should be aware that mirtazapine and cyproheptadine cannot not be administered concurrently; cyproheptadine is used as an antidote for serotonin effects of mirtazapine overdose and, thus, negates efficacy of the latter.

Future availability of the ghrelin agonist capromorelin may also provide additional opportunities to address appetite in dogs and cats with CKD by targeting the pathophysiology of appetite regulation. In both human and rodent studies, administration of ghrelin resulted in increased appetite and energy intake in patients with CKD.[48] In recent studies, administration of capromorelin resulted in increased appetite, food intake, and weight in normal and inappetent dogs and increased food intake and weight in laboratory cats.[67–69]

The exact role of hypergastrinemia in contributing to gastric hyperacidity or gastric lesions in cats and dogs with CKD is still unclear. Limiting gastric acidity with the use of H_2 blockers like famotidine or proton pump inhibitors such as omeprazole anecdotally appears to palliate inappetence in some CKD patients; however, as previously mentioned, both the degree of hyperacidity present in CKD and the efficacy of these medications for management of patients with CKD remain unproven. Recent studies of the effect of omeprazole on the gastric pH in normal cats indicates that at 1 mg/kg twice daily, it is superior to famotidine in its ability to inhibit acid production.[70] Twice-daily administration seems to be superior to once-daily administration.[71] However, proton pump inhibitors have recently been linked to an increased risk of kidney disease in humans.[72] The applicability of this finding to veterinary patients is currently unknown.

Evaluation of Outcome/Complications

As previously discussed, nutritional assessment of the patient should occur at each visit. Follow-up should also include an assessment of response to medical management of appetite. A recent study describing the most common side effects from mirtazapine (hyperexcitability, vocalization, agitation) also determined that the most common doses at which these occurred was 3.75 mg as well as accidental administration of an entire 15-mg tablet.[65] Based on this information, the recommended initial starting dose is 1.87 mg with titration up to effect, and the medication should be dispensed in the smallest available size to avoid accidental overdose. Owners should be educated to monitor for these side effects, and a call back within 24 to 48 hours should be made to allow for dose optimization. Follow-up should also include discussion regarding the pet's compliance to medication administration both orally and in the food. If food intake is affected by medications added to the ration, then an alternative plan should be made for administration.

Care should be taken to select the appropriate patients for appetite enhancement, as learned food aversion is thought by most to be prevalent, particularly in cats.[73] Learned food aversion occurs when the patient associates nausea, pain, or other physical manifestations of disease with the act of eating or the sight or scent of food. Even after the underlying illness is resolved, this aversion may remain. Therefore, it is critical that patients that are overtly nauseous (eg, drooling, gagging, turning away from food), particularly in hospital or in acute illness, are not forced to eat lest food aversion be created.[73] If the patient is too nauseous or critical to even consider oral feeding or has not responded to appetite encouragement after 3 to 5 days, placement of an enteral feeding tube should be considered. Nasoesophageal, esophageal, or gastrotomy tube can be chosen depending on the type and duration of feeding desired.[74] Esophageal feeding tubes can be a valuable tool for long-term management of CKD, as food, medications, and water can be easily given without stressing the patient. Additionally, many clinicians feel that prescription renal diets should not be fed in hospital during a crisis lest an aversion be created to the diet desired for long-term management. The best candidates for pharmacologic enhancement of appetite are patients leaving the hospital with their acute crisis resolved and patients with chronic disease in the home environment.

MANAGEMENT OF CONSTIPATION
Introduction/Etiology/Epidemiology

The prevalence of constipation associated with CKD has not been reported; however, anecdotally it seems to be a prevalent medical concern particularly in cats. The etiology of constipation associated with CKD is likely a dysfunction of water balance. As the kidney fails to provide appropriate urine concentrating ability and the patient fights with chronic subclinical dehydration, water is reabsorbed from the colon to compensate. Additionally, hypokalemia may play a role in altered colonic motility. In humans, hypokalemia is found to contribute to decreased gastrointestinal motility by weakening the basic electric rhythm of intestinal smooth muscle, an abnormality that responds favorably to supplementation.[75] Use of phosphate binders may also contribute to constipation.[76,77]

Patient Evaluations

Clinical history is important in the assessment of constipation. Important questions include the frequency of defecation, time spent defecating, the degree of difficulty, and if there is straining or vomiting associated with defecation, as this information may not be volunteered by the owner. Fecal pellets left around the house may also indicate trouble with defecation. Assessment of hydration status is crucial in these patients and should be recorded in the medical record. Physical examination may find small, hard feces in the descending colon with a buildup of fecal material before the pelvic inlet or, in more severe cases, a large amount of hard fecal material in the colon. Assessment of stifle osteoarthritis may also be helpful, as significant arthritis may affect posturing and make defecation more difficult. A rectal examination should be performed to rule out abnormalities, and the anal glands should be assessed to ensure they are not interfering with fecal evacuation. Appropriate minimum database laboratory tests and imaging to rule out concurrent concerns that could be causing constipation should be performed. Radiographs are helpful in the assessment of the constipated patient to allow assessment the fecal load, ruling out other differentials (masses) and assessing the degree of lumbosacral osteoarthritis that may affect posturing to defecate (**Fig. 3**). Serum biochemistry should include electrolyte assessment so that hypokalemia can be identified and addressed.

Treatment Recommendations

It is not uncommon for constipation in CKD patients to be a contributor to or a concurrent condition associated with a uremic crisis. In this instance, hospitalization with intravenous fluids, including intravenous potassium supplementation when appropriate, should be instituted before enemas are performed. Radiographic assessment of the fecal load helps the clinician determine if the degree of constipation is potentially amenable to enema therapy or if manual deobstipation under anesthesia will be required (the latter of which is suboptimal in a uremic crisis). Regardless, correction of hydration and hypokalemia is necessary before any action is taken and assists with breakdown of fecal material and colonic motility. A common enema formula is warm water, sterile lubricant, and dioctyl sodium sulfosuccinate (Pet-enema) administered slowly through a 10F to 12F red rubber feeding tube at a volume of 5 to 10 mL/kg and repeated intermittently (typically every 8–12 hours). Between enemas, abdominal palpation and manual massage of the colon, physical activity, and food ingestion (to simulate the gastro-colic reflex) can help encourage colonic motility. Some patients will tolerate manual assistance of a fecal mass caught within the rectum without sedation or anesthesia. After relieving an episode of constipation, it should be determined through careful history and assessment if it is a chronic problem that requires medical management to prevent future crises.

In patients experiencing chronic intermittent constipation the following considerations apply. Because the primary inciting cause of constipation secondary to CKD is considered to be chronic dehydration, hydration should be addressed before

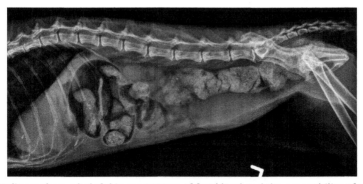

Fig. 3. Radiographs are helpful in assessment of fecal load and the amenability of constipation to therapy. Presence of osteoarthritis can also be assessed.

other medical therapies. Recommendations such as canned diet, adding water to the diet, and providing multiple sources of fresh water should be discussed. Ultimately CKD patients with repeated bouts of constipation are more likely to be prescribed subcutaneous fluids earlier in the course of the disease than others who do not present with this clinical manifestation. Hypokalemia should be identified and addressed (see earlier section on potassium supplementation). Although the efficacy of prophylactic potassium supplementation has not been evaluated, patients with constipation seem an appropriate patient group in whom to prescribe it.

After correction of hydration imbalance and hypokalemia, oral laxatives are often a major part of management of constipation. Polyethylene glycol 3350 (Miralax) is an osmotic laxative that has been assessed in normal cats and found to be effective for softening stool.[78] Although its efficacy in CKD patients has not been evaluated, it is commonly prescribed and is thought by some to be more effective than lactulose (0.5 mL/kg orally every 8–12 hours as needed), which is processed by intestinal microflora and may lead to bloating.[78] Another important consideration is that polyethylene glycol comes as a powder that appears to be well tolerated as opposed to the sticky lactulose syrup.

Bulk-forming laxatives such as pumpkin or psyllium as fiber sources may also be useful in the management of constipation associated with CKD. A psyllium-enriched diet was found to be helpful in management of feline constipation (not associated with CKD) in a previous open field trial and led to a decrease in the concurrent use of laxatives and promotility agents.[79] However, in CKD patients, the renal diet is the preferred therapeutic diet of choice; therefore, fiber sources (pumpkin or psyllium, 1–4 tsp daily) are most commonly added to canned food. The efficacy of these types of fiber on the management of constipation has not been assessed in patients with CKD.

Promotility agents are perhaps a second tier of medical management for constipation associated with CKD as the degree to which inherent colonic motility is affected has not been assessed in veterinary CKD patients. Typically, efforts are first centered on hydration and electrolyte imbalance. Cisapride (1 mg/kg every 8 hours) is the most common promotility medication used, and not only have pharmacokinetics been performed in cats, but it is found to affect contractility in normal and abnormal feline colonic smooth muscle in vitro.[80,81]

Medical management of osteoarthritis may be an important adjunctive treatment for constipation in CKD patients to facilitate appropriate posturing during defecation. Joint supplements such as glucosamine/chondroitin sulfate and medications such as gabapentin (5–10 mg/kg every 8 hours) are potential first-line choices in patients for whom the safety of nonsteroidal anti-inflammatory drugs is somewhat controversial.[82] The effect of the concurrent treatment of osteoarthritis on constipation has not been assessed in CKD patients.

Evaluation of Outcome/Complications

A common recommendation is to have the owner keep a log of defecation events and any associated difficulties. Tracking frequency of bowel movements can help determine response to therapy but can be understandably tricky if multiple pets or dog doors are present in the household. When rechecking the patient, assessment of the character of feces within the descending colon during abdominal palpation and rectal examination can help guide titration of therapies.

Patients refractory to management are typically on multiple therapies and may need repeated enemas, deobstipation, or eventually subtotal colectomy, which may be a difficult choice given the age and poor anesthetic risk of most CKD patients. The syndrome of feline megacolon has not typically been associated with CKD.

BALANCING MEDICAL MANAGEMENT AND QUALITY OF LIFE

Because of the number of medical complications that a patient with CKD could have throughout the course of the disease, a staggering number of medications could potentially be prescribed. If a feeding tube is not present so that medications, food, and water can be administered to the patient in a relatively nonstressful manner, the administration of multiple medications and treatments such as subcutaneous fluids can become an onerous task for the owner. Patient resistance to medication administration has the ability to greatly stress the human-animal bond and call into question quality of life. Discussion should be had with owners regarding quality versus quantity of life for the CKD patient and the importance of balancing the potential benefit of therapies with the stress of administering them. The treatment plan should be individualized to each patient based on the appropriateness of the medication for their condition, the ability of the owner to afford and administer the medication, and the likelihood the medication will benefit the patient based on available evidence. Treatments may need to be ranked in order of importance based on these factors so that the owner has a clear understanding of what order medications should be administered on any given day. Compliance can also be increased by ensuring that owners understand why a medication is being administered and the potential clinical outcome associated with it. Follow-up telephone interaction and recheck visits are also an important component of determining response to therapy and troubleshooting and adjusting treatments. Fostering a good relationship between veterinary care staff and the pet owner will only serve to enhance the outcome for the patient as they progress through the stages of their disease.

REFERENCES

1. Jepson RE. Feline systemic hypertension: classification and pathogenesis. J Feline Med Surg 2011;13:25–34.
2. Jacob F, Polzin DJ, Osborne CA, et al. Association between initial systolic blood pressure and risk of developing a uremic crisis or of dying in dogs with chronic renal failure. J Am Vet Med Assoc 2003;222:322–9.
3. Wehner A, Hartmann K, Hirschberger J. Associations between proteinuria, systemic hypertension and glomerular filtration rate in dogs with renal and non-renal diseases. Vet Rec 2008;162:141–7.
4. Brown S, Atkins C, Bagley R, et al. Guidelines for the identification, evaluation, and management of systemic hypertension in dogs and cats. J Vet Intern Med 2007;21:542–58.
5. Maggio F, DeFrancesco TC, Atkins CE, et al. Ocular lesions associated with systemic hypertension in cats: 69 cases (1985-1998). J Am Vet Med Assoc 2000; 217:695–702.
6. Bartges JW. Chronic kidney disease in dogs and cats. Vet Clin North Am Small Anim Pract 2012;42:669–92, vi.
7. Henik RA, Stepien RL, Bortnowski HB. Spectrum of M-mode echocardiographic abnormalities in 75 cats with systemic hypertension. J Am Anim Hosp Assoc 2004;40:359–63.
8. Bijsmans ES, Jepson RE, Chang YM, et al. Changes in systolic blood pressure over time in healthy cats and cats with chronic kidney disease. J Vet Intern Med 2015;29(3):855–61.

9. Bragg RF, Bennett JS, Cummings A, et al. Evaluation of the effects of hospital visit stress on physiologic variables in dogs. J Am Vet Med Assoc 2015;246:212–5.

10. Quimby JM, Smith ML, Lunn KF. Evaluation of the effects of hospital visit stress on physiologic parameters in the cat. J Feline Med Surg 2011;13:733–7.

11. Polzin DJ. Evidence-based step-wise approach to managing chronic kidney disease in dogs and cats. J Vet Emerg Crit Care 2013;23:205–15.

12. Huhtinen M, Derre G, Renoldi HJ, et al. Randomized placebo-controlled clinical trial of a chewable formulation of amlodipine for the treatment of hypertension in client-owned cats. J Vet Intern Med 2015;29:786–93.

13. Polzin DJ. Chronic kidney disease in small animals. Vet Clin North Am Small Anim Pract 2011;41:15–30.

14. Jepson RE, Elliott J, Brodbelt D, et al. Effect of control of systolic blood pressure on survival in cats with systemic hypertension. J Vet Intern Med 2007;21:402–9.

15. Jepson RE, Syme HM, Elliott J. Plasma renin activity and aldosterone concentrations in hypertensive cats with and without azotemia and in response to treatment with amlodipine besylate. J Vet Intern Med 2014;28:144–53.

16. Syme H. Hypertension in small animal kidney disease. Vet Clin North Am Small Anim Pract 2011;41:63–89.

17. Helms SR. Treatment of feline hypertension with transdermal amlodipine: a pilot study. J Am Anim Hosp Assoc 2007;43:149–56.

18. Brown S, Elliott J, Francey T, et al. Consensus recommendations for standard therapy of glomerular disease in dogs. J Vet Intern Med 2013;27(Suppl 1): S27–43.

19. DiBartola SP, Rutgers HC, Zack PM, et al. Clinicopathologic findings associated with chronic renal disease in cats: 74 cases (1973-1984). J Am Vet Med Assoc 1987;190:1196–202.

20. Elliott J, Barber PJ. Feline chronic renal failure: clinical findings in 80 cases diagnosed between 1992 and 1995. J Small Anim Pract 1998;39:78–85.

21. Nakhoul GN, Huang H, Arrigain S, et al. Serum Potassium, End-Stage Renal Disease and Mortality in Chronic Kidney Disease. Am J Nephrol 2015;41:456–63.

22. Korgaonkar S, Tilea A, Gillespie BW, et al. Serum potassium and outcomes in CKD: insights from the RRI-CKD cohort study. Clin J Am Soc Nephrol 2010;5: 762–9.

23. Reungjui S, Roncal CA, Sato W, et al. Hypokalemic nephropathy is associated with impaired angiogenesis. J Am Soc Nephrol 2008;19:125–34.

24. Buffington CA, DiBartola SP, Chew DJ. Effect of low potassium commercial non-purified diet on renal function of adult cats. J Nutr 1991;121:S91–2.

25. Adams LG, Polzin DJ, Osborne CA, et al. Effects of dietary protein and calorie restriction in clinically normal cats and in cats with surgically induced chronic renal failure. Am J Vet Res 1993;54:1653–62.

26. Chakrabarti S, Syme HM, Elliott J. Clinicopathological variables predicting progression of azotemia in cats with chronic kidney disease. J Vet Intern Med 2012;26:275–81.

27. King JN, Tasker S, Gunn-Moore DA, et al. Prognostic factors in cats with chronic kidney disease. J Vet Intern Med 2007;21:906–16.

28. Forrester SD, Adams LG, Allen TA. Chronic kidney disease. In: Thatcher CD, Remillard RL, editors. Small animal clinical nutrition. 5th edition. Topeka (KS): Mark Morris Institute; 2010. p. 765–810.

29. Theisen SK, DiBartola SP, Radin MJ, et al. Muscle potassium content and potassium gluconate supplementation in normokalemic cats with naturally occurring chronic renal failure. J Vet Intern Med 1997;11:212–7.

30. Sparkes AH, Caney SM, Chalhoub S, et al. ISFM consensus guidelines on the diagnosis and management of feline chronic kidney disease. J Feline Med Surg 2016;18:219–39.

31. Dow SW, LeCouteur RA, Fettman MJ, et al. Potassium depletion in cats: hypokalemic polymyopathy. J Am Vet Med Assoc 1987;191:1563–8.

32. Chalhoub S, Langston C, Eatroff A. Anemia of renal disease: what it is, what to do and what's new. J Feline Med Surg 2011;13:629–40.

33. McLeland SM, Lunn KF, Duncan CG, et al. Relationship among serum creatinine, serum gastrin, calcium-phosphorus product, and uremic gastropathy in cats with chronic kidney disease. J Vet Intern Med 2014;28(3):827–37.

34. Gest J, Langston C, Eatroff A. Iron status of cats with chronic kidney disease. J Vet Intern Med 2015;29:1488–93.

35. Nangaku M. Chronic hypoxia and tubulointerstitial injury: a final common pathway to end-stage renal failure. J Am Soc Nephrol 2006;17:17–25.

36. Chalhoub S, Langston CE, Farrelly J. The use of darbepoetin to stimulate erythropoiesis in anemia of chronic kidney disease in cats: 25 cases. J Vet Intern Med 2012;26:363–9.

37. Markovich JE, Freeman LM, Labato MA, et al. Survey of dietary and medication practices of owners of cats with chronic kidney disease. J Feline Med Surg 2015; 17:979–83.

38. Neyra R, Chen KY, Sun M, et al. Increased resting energy expenditure in patients with end-stage renal disease. JPEN J Parenter Enteral Nutr 2003;27:36–42.

39. Carrero JJ, Stenvinkel P, Cuppari L, et al. Etiology of the protein-energy wasting syndrome in chronic kidney disease: a consensus statement from the International Society of Renal Nutrition and Metabolism (ISRNM). J Ren Nutr 2013;23: 77–90.

40. Parker VJ, Freeman LM. Association between body condition and survival in dogs with acquired chronic kidney disease. J Vet Intern Med 2011;25:1306–11.

41. Freeman L, Lachaud MP, Matthews S, et al. Evaluation of weight loss over time in cats with chronic kidney disease. J Vet Intern Med 2015;29:1272.

42. Bijsmans ES, Jepson RE, Syme HM, et al. Psychometric Validation of a General Health Quality of Life Tool for Cats Used to Compare Healthy Cats and Cats with Chronic Kidney Disease. J Vet Intern Med 2016;30:183–91.

43. Reynolds CA, Oyama MA, Rush JE, et al. Perceptions of quality of life and priorities of owners of cats with heart disease. J Vet Intern Med 2010;24:1421–6.

44. Borison HL, Hebertson LM. Role of medullary emetic chemoreceptor trigger zone (CT zone) in postnephrectomy vomiting in dogs. Am J Physiol 1959;197:850–2.

45. Goldstein RE, Marks SL, Kass PH, et al. Gastrin concentrations in plasma of cats with chronic renal failure. J Am Vet Med Assoc 1998;213:826–8.

46. Liptak JM, Hunt GB, Barrs VR, et al. Gastroduodenal ulceration in cats: eight cases and a review of the literature. J Feline Med Surg 2002;4:27–42.

47. El Ghonaimy E, Barsoum R, Soliman M, et al. Serum gastrin in chronic renal failure: morphological and physiological correlations. Nephron 1985;39:86–94.

48. Gunta SS, Mak RH. Ghrelin and leptin pathophysiology in chronic kidney disease. Pediatr Nephrol 2013;28:611–6.

49. Freeman L, Becvarova I, Cave N, et al. WSAVA nutritional assessment guidelines. Compend Contin Educ Vet 2011;33:E1–9.

50. Michel KE, Anderson W, Cupp C, et al. Correlation of a feline muscle mass score with body composition determined by dual-energy X-ray absorptiometry. Br J Nutr 2011;106(Suppl 1):S57–9.

51. Hutchinson D, Sutherland-Smith J, Watson AL, et al. Assessment of methods of evaluating sarcopenia in old dogs. Am J Vet Res 2012;73:1794–800.

52. Hickman MA, Cox SR, Mahabir S, et al. Safety, pharmacokinetics and use of the novel NK-1 receptor antagonist maropitant (Cerenia) for the prevention of emesis and motion sickness in cats. J Vet Pharmacol Ther 2008;31:220–9.

53. Quimby JM, Brock WT, Moses K, et al. Chronic use of maropitant for the management of vomiting and inappetence in cats with chronic kidney disease: a blinded placebo-controlled clinical trial. J Feline Med Surg 2014;17(8):692–7.

54. Quimby JM, Lake RC, Hansen RJ, et al. Oral, subcutaneous, and intravenous pharmacokinetics of ondansetron in healthy cats. J Vet Pharmacol Ther 2014; 37:348–53.

55. Saynor DA, Dixon CM. The metabolism of ondansetron. Eur J Cancer Clin Oncol 1989;25(Suppl 1):S75–7.

56. Zajic LB, Herndon A, Sieberg L, et al. Investigation of the pharmacokinetics of transdermal ondansetron in normal purpose-bred cats. J Vet Intern Med 2016; 30:TBD.

57. Herndon A, Sieberg L, Davis L, et al. Pharmacokinetics of intravenous and subcutaneous dolasetron and pharmacodynamics of subcutaneous dolasetron in purpose-bred cats. J Vet Intern Med 2016;30:TBD.

58. Timmer CJ, Sitsen JM, Delbressine LP. Clinical pharmacokinetics of mirtazapine. Clin Pharmacokinet 2000;38:461–74.

59. Kast RE, Foley KF. Cancer chemotherapy and cachexia: mirtazapine and olanzapine are 5-HT3 antagonists with good antinausea effects. Eur J Cancer Care (Engl) 2007;16:351–4.

60. Pae CU. Low-dose mirtazapine may be successful treatment option for severe nausea and vomiting. Prog Neuropsychopharmacol Biol Psychiatry 2006;30: 1143–5.

61. Quimby JM, Lunn KF. Mirtazapine as an appetite stimulant and anti-emetic in cats with chronic kidney disease: A masked placebo-controlled crossover clinical trial. Vet J 2013;197:651–5.

62. Giorgi M, Yun H. Pharmacokinetics of mirtazapine and its main metabolites in Beagle dogs: a pilot study. Vet J 2012;192:239–41.

63. Quimby JM, Gustafson DL, Lunn KF. The pharmacokinetics of mirtazapine in cats with chronic kidney disease and in age-matched control cats. J Vet Intern Med 2011;25:985–9.

64. Quimby JM, Gustafson DL, Samber BJ, et al. Studies on the pharmacokinetics and pharmacodynamics of mirtazapine in healthy young cats. J Vet Pharmacol Ther 2011;34:388–96.

65. Ferguson LE, McLean MK, Bates JA, et al. Mirtazapine toxicity in cats: retrospective study of 84 cases (2006-2011). J Feline Med Surg 2015. [Epub ahead of print].

66. Benson KK, Zajic LB, Lunghofer PJ, et al. Pharmacodynamics of transdermal mirtazapine in healthy client-owned cats. J Vet Int Med 2015;29:1225.

67. Zollers B, Allen J, Kennedy C, et al. Capromorelin, an orally active ghrelin agonist, caused sustained increases in IGF-1, increased food intake and body weight in cats. J Vet Intern Med 2015;29:1219.

68. Zollers B, Rhodes L. Capromorelin, an orally active ghrelin agonist, stimulates appetite and weight gain in inappetent dogs in a multi-site field study. J Vet Intern Med 2014;28:1032.

69. Zollers B, Rhodes L. Capromorelin, an orally active ghrelin agonist, stimulates growth hormone, sustained increases in IGF-1, increased food intake and weight gain in beagle dogs. J Vet Intern Med 2014;28:1034.
70. Parkinson S, Tolbert K, Messenger K, et al. Evaluation of the Effect of Orally Administered Acid Suppressants On Intragastric pH in Cats. J Vet Intern Med 2015;29:104–12.
71. Sutalo S, Ruetten M, Hartnack S, et al. The effect of orally administered ranitidine and once-daily or twice-daily orally administered omeprazole on intragastric pH in cats. J Vet Intern Med 2015;29:840–6.
72. Lazarus B, Chen Y, Wilson FP, et al. Proton Pump Inhibitor Use and the Risk of Chronic Kidney Disease. JAMA Intern Med 2016;176:238–46.
73. Michel KE. Management of anorexia in the cat. J Feline Med Surg 2001;3:3–8.
74. Chan DL. The Inappetent Hospitalised Cat: clinical approach to maximising nutritional support. J Feline Med Surg 2009;11:925–33.
75. Chen JZ, Deng AW, Xu JF. Electroenterogram manifestations and significance in hypokalemia. Di Yi Jun Yi Da Xue Xue Bao 2005;25:7–9.
76. Kidder AC, Chew D. Treatment options for hyperphosphatemia in feline CKD: what's out there? J Feline Med Surg 2009;11:913–24.
77. Quimby JM, Lappin MR. Evaluating sucralfate as a phosphate binder in normal cats and cats with chronic kidney disease. J Am Anim Hosp Assoc 2016;52:8–12.
78. Tam FM, Carr AP, Myers SL. Safety and palatability of polyethylene glycol 3350 as an oral laxative in cats. J Feline Med Surg 2011;13:694–7.
79. Freiche V, Houston D, Weese H, et al. Uncontrolled study assessing the impact of a psyllium-enriched extruded dry diet on faecal consistency in cats with constipation. J Feline Med Surg 2011;13:903–11.
80. LeGrange SN, Boothe DM, Herndon S, et al. Pharmacokinetics and suggested oral dosing regimen of cisapride: a study in healthy cats. J Am Anim Hosp Assoc 1997;33:517–23.
81. Washabau RJ, Sammarco J. Effects of cisapride on feline colonic smooth muscle function. Am J Vet Res 1996;57:541–6.
82. KuKanich B. Outpatient oral analgesics in dogs and cats beyond nonsteroidal antiinflammatory drugs: an evidence-based approach. Vet Clin North Am Small Anim Pract 2013;43:1109–25.

Nephroureteral Obstructions
The Use of Stents and Ureteral Bypass Systems for Renal Decompression

Carrie A. Palm, DVM[a], William T.N. Culp, VMD[b],*

KEYWORDS

- Interventional radiology • Interventional urology • Stent
- Subcutaneous ureteral bypass • Nephroureterolithiasis • Ureteral obstruction

KEY POINTS

- The treatment of benign nephroureteral obstructions is challenging and often involves a combination of medical and surgical/interventional therapeutic options.
- Historical surgical treatments of nephroureteral obstructions have demonstrated varying results; however, newer interventional radiology therapies, such as stent and subcutaneous ureteral bypass system placement, are being used more commonly.
- The indications for the placement of stents and subcutaneous ureteral bypass systems still need to be fully elucidated, but early results are showing promise.

INTRODUCTION

Canine and feline nephroureteral obstruction is a complex disease process that can be challenging to treat. Although the availability of various imaging modalities allows for a straightforward diagnosis to be made in most cases, the decision-making process for when a case should be taken to surgery, as well as the optimal treatment modality that should be used for renal decompression, remains controversial. In the following discussion, an overview of the perioperative management of cases with nephroureterolithiasis and nephroureteral obstruction is reviewed, with a focus on the use of renal decompressive procedures, such as ureteral stenting and subcutaneous ureteral bypass (SUB) system placement.

The authors teach laboratories where some of the instrumentation discussed in this article are utilized.

[a] Department of Medicine and Epidemiology, School of Veterinary Medicine, University of California-Davis, One Garrod Drive, Davis, CA 95616, USA; [b] Department of Surgical and Radiological Sciences, School of Veterinary Medicine, University of California-Davis, One Garrod Drive, Davis, CA 95616, USA

* Corresponding author. Veterinary Medical Teaching Hospital, University of California-Davis, One Garrod Drive, Davis, CA 95616.

E-mail address: wculp@ucdavis.edu

http://dx.doi.org/10.1016/j.cvsm.2016.06.008
0195-5616/16/$ – see front matter

Diagnosis

To effectively diagnose, treat, and manage patients with benign upper urinary tract obstructions, it is important to try and identify the underlying causes for these obstructions. The diagnosis of nephroliths and ureteroliths has increased over the last few decades because of advancements in diagnostic imaging and client and clinician education. In cats, nephroliths and ureteroliths are most commonly composed of calcium oxalate[1–3]; however, other stone types, including dried solidified blood calculi and struvite stones,[1,4] are also found. It is also important to note that in many cases of feline ureteral obstruction discrete calculi may not be identified. In these cases, it is likely that ureteritis, scarring from previous inflammation, and/or cellular or crystalline debris may be the cause of obstruction. Identifying the underlying cause for ureteral obstruction will help to guide the optimal treatment plan as well as long-term medical management after renal decompression has been performed.

A serum biochemistry profile should be performed in any dog or cat suspected of having an upper urinary tract obstruction. Most cats with ureteroliths have been shown to be azotemic,[3,5] even when unilateral ureteral obstruction is present. This finding emphasizes the fact that a large percentage of cats have preexisting chronic kidney disease (often times from a previous obstruction of the contralateral kidney) before diagnosis of obstruction. Evaluating the severity of azotemia, in addition to electrolytes, such as potassium, can help to guide whether patients should be taken to surgery on an emergency basis. The severity of azotemia (in conjunction with diagnostic imaging) also provides information regarding the degree of underlying chronic kidney disease that is present, a variable that may guide an owner's decision to pursue surgical intervention. The decision to pursue surgical intervention is not always straightforward, especially in nonazotemic patients that may appear clinically healthy. With the discovery of newer biomarkers of early kidney injury and dysfunction that are much more sensitive than creatinine, earlier diagnosis of and intervention for ureteral obstruction may become possible.[6,7]

The complete blood count often demonstrates anemia in cats with ureteral obstruction; in some cases, this may indicate the presence of longer-standing chronic kidney disease.[3,5] Additionally, the presence of an inflammatory leukogram may suggest an underlying infection associated with the presence of a stone or as the sole cause for the obstruction (ie, ureteritis).

Urinalysis and urine culture should be performed in all patients affected with nephroureterolithiasis. Assessment of urine pH may be useful in differentiating between stone types. Sediment evaluation can help to identify the presence of bacteria and pyuria. In dogs, struvite stones are most commonly associated with urease-producing bacteria (ie, Staphylococcus, Proteus, Klebsiella). The presence of these bacteria should raise the clinician's suspicion for the presence of a struvite stone. If a partial ureteral obstruction is present (and the ureteral stone is, therefore, bathed in urine), it is possible that medical management could be used as the sole treatment; however, concurrent ureteral stent placement may be necessary (see later discussion). In the authors' experience, sterile pyuria is found commonly in patients with ureteral obstruction, likely due to the inflammatory processes that are initiated soon after development of ureteral obstruction. Nonetheless, a urine culture should be performed in all patients with ureteral obstruction. In patients with complete ureteral obstruction, or in anuric patients, a sample of renal pelvic urine can be taken for culture if patients are undergoing surgical decompression.

Abdominal ultrasound should be performed in all cases of suspected nephroureteral obstruction. Ultrasound is the primary imaging method used for diagnosis of ureteral obstruction; however, it is important to note that ureteral obstruction can be missed in early obstruction, partial obstruction, and in patients that are dehydrated or hypovolemic at the time of evaluation. As discussed earlier, ultrasound can be used to evaluate for chronic changes in the kidneys and can also be used as a monitoring tool for changes in renal pelvic and ureteral diameters that can either indicate spontaneous renal decompression (without surgical intervention) or progressive dilation, indicating a need for surgical intervention. Ultrasound can also be used to visualize stones and other obstructing debris in the kidney and ureter.[3] In the authors' practice, ultrasound is commonly used to monitor response to therapy by evaluating renal pelvic and ureteral size after intervention.

In patients with ureteral obstruction, plain abdominal radiographs can be used to complement ultrasound. The sensitivity of radiographs in the identification of ureteral calculi has been shown to be 81%.[3] Additionally, in severe cases, hydroureter can also be diagnosed on survey abdominal radiographs. Many surgeons value the use of abdominal radiographs before surgery, as the number and location of stones can often be identified.

Fluoroscopy is often used during renal decompression surgery. During these procedures, nephrocentesis is performed to allow for contrast medium injection. During and after contrast medium administration, fluoroscopy is performed to evaluate the degree of hydronephrosis, the location and course of the ureter, and the location of ureteral obstruction. Although performed uncommonly at the authors' institution, preoperative antegrade nephropyelograms can also be performed with the use of fluoroscopy in cases where diagnosis of obstruction is not straightforward.

In veterinary medicine, advanced cross-sectional imaging, including computed tomography (CT) and MRI, is not commonly used in the assessment of patients with nephroureteral obstruction. These imaging modalities provide high-quality, detailed images of the upper urinary tract, including identification of kidney and ureteral size, and the presence of calculi. When more traditional surgeries, such as ureterotomy without stent placement, are performed, CT can be useful for identification of multiple ureteral stones, so that all stones can be addressed at the time of surgery; however, results of these advanced imaging techniques do not typically impact the clinical decision-making when newer minimally invasive techniques (eg, stents and SUBS) are used. In addition, increases in intra-renal pressures secondary to nephroureteral obstruction can prevent contrast uptake by the kidneys and obscure diagnostic results.

Decision-making

The decision-making process for optimal treatment timing and modality for cases affected with nephroureteral obstruction is impacted by several factors. Nephroliths that are not causing clinical signs and have been found incidentally are generally monitored without intervention. If patients are experiencing chronic urinary tract infections or the nephrolith has grown large enough to obstruct urine outflow from the renal pelvis, removal can be considered. If a stent or SUB system can be placed to allow urine to flow from the renal pelvis to the bladder in these cases, surgical removal of the nephroliths may not be required.

In cases whereby patients are oliguric or anuric secondary to a ureteral obstruction, intervention is mandatory. Historically, treatment options for these cats included stabilization with hemodialysis (if indicated and available), followed by ureterotomy or other traditional ureteral surgery. In the authors' practice, when a ureteral obstruction is highly suspected or confirmed with imaging, surgery is performed as the first-line therapy in nearly every case. As hemodialysis only provides temporary stabilization in this scenario and requires patients to be anticoagulated, performing this procedure before surgery is generally not indicated and may lead to the need for postponement of surgery. The need for systemic anticoagulation can be avoided with the use of extracorporeal citrate anticoagulation. With immediate and aggressive medical management, however, it is the authors' experience that almost every patient can be stabilized for surgery without instituting hemodialysis.

In patients with ureteral calculi that are nonobstructive (ie, no evidence of ureteral dilation or hydronephrosis), intervention to remove or bypass the calculi is generally not indicated, especially given the potential morbidity. However, serial monitoring of these patients with blood work and abdominal ultrasound is recommended, as unilateral obstruction can occur with minimal to no clinical signs present. Serial creatinine trending for each individual patient and the use of newer biomarkers may allow for earlier diagnosis in patients with unilateral ureteral obstruction. In stable patients (ie, no electrolyte derangements and no overhydration) with ultrasonographic evidence of ureteral obstruction, medical management can be considered, although, in the authors' hands, this is often unsuccessful. The decision to pursue surgical intervention is not always straightforward, especially in nonazotemic patients that may appear clinically healthy. Significant renal injury develops within hours after ureteral obstruction and prolonged obstruction leads to progressive inflammation and fibrosis, which will ultimately develop into chronic kidney disease that will remain after renal decompression. Given this, along with the risk for contralateral obstruction to develop over time and the high incidence of chronic kidney disease (especially in feline patients), preservation of as much renal function via early surgical intervention is likely indicated in many cases.

Once the decision to pursue renal decompression is made, there are several factors that play a role in selecting the optimal surgery type for each case. These factors include surgeon expertise and comfort with each procedure as well as availability of equipment (eg, stents, SUBs, fluoroscopy, surgical microscope). The focus of this article is on the use of stents and SUBs for renal decompression, but it is important to note that some clinicians still prefer to manage patients with ureteral obstruction with traditional surgery techniques. The authors prefer ureteral stenting in dogs experiencing ureteral obstruction secondary to urolithiasis, as these stents can be placed minimally invasively (percutaneous or endoscopic guided) and removed minimally invasively and are generally well tolerated. Stents can be exchanged when partial migration or blockage occurs, and often this can be performed without performing a celiotomy. The placement of a SUB system is considered in cases with known ureteral strictures, circumcaval ureters (**Fig. 1**), when stents cannot be placed successfully, and when stents have not been tolerated by patients.[8]

Treatment

As stated earlier, this discussion focuses on the use of stents and SUB systems in the treatment of ureteral obstructions in dogs and cats. Different considerations need to be made for dogs as compared with cats, and these are discussed later. In addition, the limited amount of available literature is discussed later, but it is important to note that continued scientific evaluation of outcomes with the different surgery types is warranted so that the best treatment decisions can be made for veterinary patients.

Ureteral stenting

Ureteral stents (also called ureteric stents) are tubes placed into the ureter to allow for urine to flow from the kidney (renal pelvis) to the bladder. Additionally, stents can be

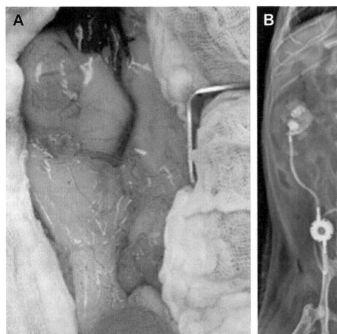
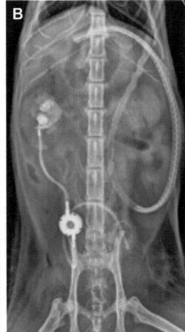

Fig. 1. (*A*) Intraoperative image of a 12-year-old female spayed domestic longhair. A right circumcaval ureter is seen here. (*B*) To treat a ureteral obstruction in this case, an SUB system has been placed.

placed as a means of splinting a ureter that has been anastomosed after a surgical incision or trauma.[9,10] Ureteral stents have been shown to stimulate ureteral dilation.[11]

Ureteral stents can be made of various materials; but currently, there are 3 major categories: polymeric compounds, metal, and biodegradable.[12–14] Although each stent type has its own advantages, no single ureteral stent is perfect. In human patients undergoing stent placement, morbidity is reported in up to 80% of cases[15,16]; therefore, an emphasis has been placed on the development of new stents.[13] Although complications can occur in dogs and cats with ureteral stents, the tolerance of stents tends to be better than in humans.

The use of ureteral stents for treatment of both benign and malignant ureteral obstructions has been described in several veterinary studies.[5,17–24] The most commonly reported indications for ureteral stenting in dogs and cats have been for treatment of benign obstructions with calculi or strictures.[18,19,21,23]

Ureteral stents can be placed in dogs and cats using several different techniques. A percutaneous technique has been described in the treatment of malignant ureteral obstructions in dogs[24]; but a description of this technique for benign obstructions is lacking in veterinary patients, except for an isolated report in a tiger.[25] To perform this technique, ultrasound guidance is used to visualize the renal pelvis and percutaneous nephrocentesis is performed. A guidewire is then passed through the renal access needle and manipulated through the ureter and into the bladder and urethra with fluoroscopic guidance. This technique allows for retrograde placement (from the urethra and into the kidney) of the stent over the guidewire. Antegrade placement can also be performed with use of a sheath placed percutaneously through the nephrocentesis puncture site into the renal pelvis. In the authors' practice, percutaneous stent placement is generally considered only in canine patients, as it has not been successful in cats.

Both antegrade and retrograde placement of stents can be performed in dogs and cats after a celiotomy. The authors prefer antegrade placement of ureteral stents, as this allows for through-and-through guidewire access (ie, the guidewire can be grasped outside of the entry point into the kidney and at the exit point from the bladder). This technique has been described in veterinary studies.[17–19] After performing a ventral midline celiotomy, the affected kidney is isolated by draping the other abdominal organs away and dissecting perirenal fat as necessary. A 22-gauge over-the-needle catheter is introduced into the greater curvature of the kidney aiming toward the ureteral-pelvic junction; generally, this is a location that is equidistant dorsal-ventral and cranial-caudal on the greater curvature. When urine is obtained from the over-the-needle catheter, the needle is removed and the catheter is left in the renal pelvis. A T-port that had been primed with a 50%/50% mixture of saline/iodinated contrast is attached to the catheter and the renal pelvis is filled under fluoroscopic guidance. Fluoroscopy confirms the presence of the catheter within the renal pelvis. A 0.018-in hydrophilic guidewire is then introduced into the catheter and passed antegrade down the ureter and into the bladder. A cystotomy is performed, and the wire is grasped from the bladder and passed externally (out of the bladder). The catheter is removed over the guidewire. A ureteral dilator is then passed normograde over the guidewire through the renal parenchyma into the renal pelvis and through the ureter until it is exits through the ureterovesicular junction (UVJ). The dilator is then removed, and a ureteral stent is passed over the guidewire. The cranial pigtail of the stent is positioned within the renal pelvis using fluoroscopic guidance. When placement is confirmed, the guidewire is removed normograde from the stent allowing a pigtail to form in the bladder.

One study evaluated 12 cats that underwent antegrade placement of ureteral stents. Nine cats underwent unilateral stent placement, and 3 cats received bilateral stents.[19] A ureterotomy was required in 3 cats, and 4 cats required ureteral resection and anastomosis to allow for stent placement. Of the 12 cats treated in that study, 11 were discharged and all cats demonstrated improvement in azotemia. Postoperatively, serum creatinine and renal pelvic size improved significantly when compared with preoperative values.[19] In the largest study to date, the antegrade technique was the preferred approach by the authors, although other techniques were also described.[18] In that study, ureteral stent placement, using a newer stent device specifically designed for cats, was successful in 52 of 53 (98%) cats.[18] Complications occurring during the procedure, immediately postoperative, and in the short-term occurred in less than 10% of cases; long-term complications occurred in 33% of cats, although most were considered minor.[18]

Retrograde stent placement can also be performed with the use of endoscopy or during an open abdominal approach after cystotomy.[18,22,26] Endoscopic ureteral stent placement is the preferred technique by the authors for treating benign ureteral obstructions in dogs (**Fig. 2**). In one study, retrograde ureteral stenting was attempted in the treatment of obstructive ureterolithiasis with secondary pyonephrosis in 13 dogs.[26] The procedure was successfully performed with cystoscopic and fluoroscopic guidance in 11 of 13 dogs. Long-term complications were uncommon and included stent encrustation, stent migration, and tissue proliferation at the UVJ. Overall, the procedure was determined to be effective.[26] Retrograde ureteral stents placed with endoscopy has also been reported in feline cases, although this is rarely performed.[17,18]

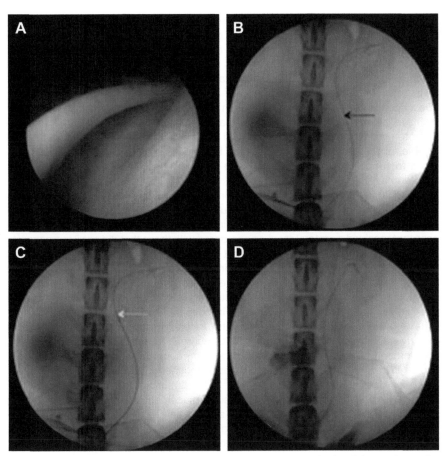

Fig. 2. (*A*) Cystourethroscopic view of the left ureteral orifice. A hydrophilic guidewire has been introduced into the left ureter using cystoscopy. (*B*) Ventrodorsal fluoroscopic image. The guidewire (*black arrow*) has been passed into the renal pelvis. (*C*) Ventrodorsal fluoroscopic image. A ureteral stent (tip marked by *yellow arrow*) is being passed retrograde into the ureter over the guidewire. (*D*) Ventrodorsal fluoroscopic image: after placement of the ureteral stent, the guidewire has been removed; the pigtails of the stent can be seen in the renal pelvis and bladder.

For retrograde ureteral stenting performed with cystoscopic and fluoroscopic guidance, patients are placed in dorsal recumbency and cystourethroscopy is performed. Once the UVJ has been identified, a hydrophilic guidewire is introduced through the working channel of the cystoscope and passed into the ureter and past the obstruction into the renal pelvis. Once in the renal pelvis, the guidewire is formed into a curl to prevent backing out. An open-ended ureteral catheter is introduced over the guidewire to allow for nephropyelography and stent sizing. Once a nephropyelogram has been performed, the guidewire is reintroduced into the ureteral catheter and the catheter is removed. A ureteral stent is then introduced over the guidewire (through the working channel of the scope) and into the ureter until the cranial pigtail can be visualized over the leading end of the guidewire. The guidewire is withdrawn while the cystoscope is positioned within the bladder to direct the caudal aspect of the stent (still in the working channel) into the bladder with a ureteral pusher catheter.

The retrograde placement of ureteral stents has also been described in cats after performance of a celiotomy.[17,18] This procedure is performed similar to the endoscopic technique after a cystotomy has been performed to expose the UVJ. With this technique, a cystoscope is not used and the caudal pigtail of the stent is manually placed in the bladder after placement of the cranial pigtail in the renal pelvis.

Descriptions of stent placement through ureterotomy sites or after ureteral resection have been reported.[17,21] In these cases, a guidewire is introduced into the ureterotomy site or up the open end of the ureter. Dilation is performed when possible, and stents are generally placed in retrograde fashion. Stents can also be placed to support anastomoses that have been performed during stone removal or after trauma.[5,17]

Traditional ureteral surgery has been compared with ureteral stenting in the treatment of ureteral obstruction in 2 recent studies.[5,27] In one study,[5] the occurrence of lower urinary tract signs and urinary tract infections was significantly higher in those cases that received a ureteral stent as compared with those that did not.[5] In a separate study, cats that underwent ureteral stent placement had significantly greater decreases in blood urea nitrogen and creatinine 1-day postoperatively and at discharge as compared with cats that underwent ureterotomy without stent placement. Additionally, in that study, cats that underwent ureteral stent placement were significantly more likely to have resolution of azotemia in-hospital.[27]

The short-term outcome associated with ureteral stents is considered good, as most treated dogs and cats survive to discharge from the hospital; in addition, improvement in azotemia and ultrasonographic findings occurs regularly.[17,18,20,23,26,27] Long-term complications associated with ureteral stent placement have been described in several studies.[5,17–21,23] Dysuria, hematuria, and stranguria have been noted to occur in cats after stent placement[5,18]; in one study, dysuria was noted in 37% of cats.[18] Additionally, stents need to be exchanged or replaced in up to 27% of cases because of stent migration, fracture, encrustation, obstruction, or lower urinary tract signs that are refractory to medical management.[5,17,18]

Ureteral bypass

The placement of ureteral bypass systems (in particular the SUB) has become more commonplace in companion animals over the last several years. The concept of the SUB system is that a nephrostomy tube and cystostomy tube are placed permanently and connected via a shunting port. Urine can then flow through the attached catheters and is delivered into the bladder.

The veterinary literature on the topic is currently limited to 2 case series[8,20] and 1 case report.[28] Early results associated with the SUB system placement are promising. In a study evaluating both stents and SUBs for the treatment of benign ureteral obstructions in cats, all cases had successful decompression of the renal pelvis postoperatively and survival was considered good.[20] In a separate study, a SUB system was used in the treatment of cats with both circumcaval and noncircumcaval ureters, of which most cases had ureterolithiasis.[8] In that groups of cats, the SUB system was shown to reobstruct less commonly than ureteral stents.[8]

The placement of the SUB system is performed after a ventral midline celiotomy. An 18-gauge over-the-needle catheter is inserted into the caudal pole of the kidney equidistant ventral-dorsal and directed to the renal pelvis. Similar to ureteral stent placement, nephropyelography is performed. A 0.035-in guidewire is then placed into the 18-gauge catheter and coiled in the renal pelvis. The 18-gauge catheter is removed over the guidewire. A 6.5F pigtail locking-loop nephrostomy tube is placed over the guidewire into the renal pelvis and secured to the renal capsule with tissue glue. A 7F cystostomy tube is then inserted into the bladder and secured to the bladder with sutures. The tube ends of both the nephrostomy and cystostomy tubes are tunneled through the body wall and attached to a titanium shunting port that is secured to the body wall.

Proposed benefits of SUB system placement include the fact that ureteral surgery is not required, the cystostomy tube enters at the bladder apex (and not through the UVJ as is the case with stents), and flushing of the SUB system can be done, to possibly prevent obstruction of the tubing.

REFERENCES

1. Cannon AB, Westropp JL, Ruby AL, et al. Evaluation of trends in urolith composition in cats: 5,230 cases (1985-2004). J Am Vet Med Assoc 2007;231:570–6.
2. Low WW, Uhl JM, Kass PH, et al. Evaluation of trends in urolith composition and characteristics of dogs with urolithiasis: 25,499 cases (1985-2006). J Am Vet Med Assoc 2010;236:193–200.
3. Kyles AE, Hardie EM, Wooden BG, et al. Clinical, clinicopathologic, radiographic, and ultrasonographic abnormalities in cats with ureteral calculi: 163 cases (1984-2002). J Am Vet Med Assoc 2005;226:932–6.
4. Westropp JL, Ruby AL, Bailiff NL, et al. Dried solidified blood calculi in the urinary tract of cats. J Vet Intern Med 2006;20:828–34.
5. Wormser C, Clarke DL, Aronson LR. Outcomes of ureteral surgery and ureteral stenting in cats: 117 cases (2006-2014). J Am Vet Med Assoc 2016; 248:518–25.
6. Palm CA, Segev G, Cowgill LD, et al. Urinary neutrophil gelatinase-associated lipocalin as a marker for identification of acute kidney injury and recovery in dogs with gentamicin-induced nephrotoxicity. J Vet Intern Med 2016;30:200–5.
7. Hokamp JA, Nabity MB. Renal biomarkers in domestic species. Vet Clin Pathol 2016;45:28–56.
8. Steinhaus J, Berent AC, Weisse C, et al. Clinical presentation and outcome of cats with circumcaval ureters associated with a ureteral obstruction. J Vet Intern Med 2015;29:63–70.
9. Chew BH, Lange D. Advances in ureteral stent development. Curr Opin Urol 2016;26:277–82.
10. Wormser C, Clarke DL, Aronson LR. End-to-end ureteral anastomosis and double-pigtail ureteral stent placement for treatment of iatrogenic ureteral trauma in two dogs. J Am Vet Med Assoc 2015;247:92–7.
11. Lennon GM, Thornhill JA, Grainger R, et al. Double pigtail ureteric stent versus percutaneous nephrostomy: effects on stone transit and ureteric motility. Eur Urol 1997;31:24–9.
12. Fiuk J, Bao Y, Calleary JG, et al. The use of internal stents in chronic ureteral obstruction. J Urol 2015;193:1092–100.
13. Brotherhood H, Lange D, Chew BH. Advances in ureteral stents. Transl Androl Urol 2014;3:314–9.
14. Auge BK, Preminger GM. Ureteral stents and their use in endourology. Curr Opin Urol 2002;12:217–22.
15. Joshi HB, Stainthorpe A, MacDonagh RP, et al. Indwelling ureteral stents: evaluation of symptoms, quality of life and utility. J Urol 2003;169:1065–9.

16. Joshi HB, Newns N, Stainthorpe A, et al. Ureteral stent symptom questionnaire: development and validation of a multidimensional quality of life measure. J Urol 2003;169:1060–4.

17. Kulendra NJ, Syme H, Benigni L, et al. Feline double pigtail ureteric stents for management of ureteric obstruction: short- and long-term follow-up of 26 cats. J Feline Med Surg 2014;16:985–91.

18. Berent AC, Weisse CW, Todd K, et al. Technical and clinical outcomes of ureteral stenting in cats with benign ureteral obstruction: 69 cases (2006-2010). J Am Vet Med Assoc 2014;244:559–76.

19. Manassero M, Decambron A, Viateau V, et al. Indwelling double pigtail ureteral stent combined or not with surgery for feline ureterolithiasis: complications and outcome in 15 cases. J Feline Med Surg 2013;16:623–30.

20. Horowitz C, Berent A, Weisse C, et al. Predictors of outcome for cats with ureteral obstructions after interventional management using ureteral stents or a subcutaneous ureteral bypass device. J Feline Med Surg 2013;15:1052–62.

21. Nicoli S, Morello E, Martano M, et al. Double-J ureteral stenting in nine cats with ureteral obstruction. Vet J 2012;194:60–5.

22. Lam NK, Berent AC, Weisse CW, et al. Endoscopic placement of ureteral stents for treatment of congenital bilateral ureteral stenosis in a dog. J Am Vet Med Assoc 2012;240:983–90.

23. Zaid MS, Berent AC, Weisse C, et al. Feline ureteral strictures: 10 cases (2007-2009). J Vet Intern Med 2011;25:222–9.

24. Berent AC, Weisse C, Beal MW, et al. Use of indwelling, double-pigtail stents for treatment of malignant ureteral obstruction in dogs: 12 cases (2006-2009). J Am Vet Med Assoc 2011;238:1017–25.

25. Delk KW, Wack RF, Burgdorf-Moisuk A, et al. Percutaneous ureteral stent placement for the treatment of a benign ureteral obstruction in a Sumatran tiger (Panthera tigris sumatrae). Zoo Biol 2015;34:193–7.

26. Kuntz JA, Berent AC, Weisse CW, et al. Double pigtail ureteral stenting and renal pelvic lavage for renal-sparing treatment of obstructive pyonephrosis in dogs: 13 cases (2008-2012). J Am Vet Med Assoc 2015;246:216–25.

27. Culp WTN, Palm C, Hsueh C, et al. A comparison of perioperative outcome in cats undergoing ureterotomy or ureteral stenting for the treatment of benign ureteral obstructions. J Vet Intern Med 2015;29:1213.

28. Johnson CM, Culp WT, Palm CA, et al. Subcutaneous ureteral bypass device for treatment of iatrogenic ureteral ligation in a kitten. J Am Vet Med Assoc 2015;247:924–31.

Update on the Current Status of Kidney Transplantation for Chronic Kidney Disease in Animals

Lillian R. Aronson, VMD

KEYWORDS

- Transplantation • Immunosuppressive therapy • Cyclosporine • Allograft rejection
- Retroperitoneal fibrosis • Lymphoma

KEY POINTS

- Renal transplantation is a viable treatment option for cats in chronic renal failure or those that have suffered irreversible acute kidney injury.
- Extensive screening of a potential recipient is critical to prevent both short- and long-term complications.
- Renal donation was not found to affect normal life expectancy in cats.
- Lifelong immunosuppression, consisting of a combination of cyclosporine and prednisolone are necessary to prevent allograft rejection.
- Treatment of complications directly related to the allograft or those secondary to chronic immunosuppressive therapy still remain a significant challenge for the clinician.

INTRODUCTION

Chronic kidney disease (CKD) is a progressive and debilitating disease in cats and dogs with no known cure. Although medical management may be effective initially in stabilizing a patient and improving his or her quality of life, it is not sufficient to maintain a patient with end-stage renal failure. Kidney transplantation was first introduced in 1984 as a novel therapy for cats suffering from CKD and continues to remain an accepted treatment option for this population of patients. Although some question the justification for the technique, in a report comparing survival time of cats that had undergone transplantation to a population of cats treated medically, renal transplantation improved patient quality of life and prolonged survival times compared with the medical management of the disease.[1] The majority of this article focuses on cats, because historically they have been the most predominant species to undergo renal transplantation in veterinary therapeutics.

The author has nothing to disclose.
Department of Clinical Studies, School of Veterinary Medicine, University of Pennsylvania, 3900 Delancey Street, Philadelphia, PA 19104-6010, USA
E-mail address: laronson@vet.upenn.edu

Vet Clin Small Anim 46 (2016) 1193–1218
http://dx.doi.org/10.1016/j.cvsm.2016.06.013
0195-5616/16/© 2016 Elsevier Inc. All rights reserved.

CANDIDATE PRESENTATION

Transplantation is often performed in patients when evidence of kidney decompensation is identified in the face of appropriate medical therapy or in patients with acute irreversible kidney injury. Clinical signs indicative of decompensation include worsening of the anemia and azotemia and continued weight loss. Although objective data are lacking with regard to the optimal time for intervention, based on studies investigating prognostic factors and survival in cats with naturally occurring CKD, conversation with owners regarding transplantation should occur proactively when a cat is in International Renal Insufficiency Society CKD stage 3.[2–5] At 1 facility, a serum creatinine of greater than 4.0 mg/dL or significant aberrations in calcium and phosphorus levels are indications for transplantation.[6] In a review of 156 cases performed at the author's facility from 1998 to 2015, 15% of the cats were in International Renal Insufficiency Society CKD stage 3 and 85% were in International Renal Insufficiency Society CKD stage 4 at presentation. Limited information regarding the degree of azotemia as a risk factor for postoperative morbidity and mortality exists. In 1 study, cats with a serum creatinine greater than 10 mg/dL and increased blood urea nitrogen (specific value not given) were more likely to die before discharge.[1] In a second study, the severity of azotemia significantly increased the risk of neurologic complications in the perioperative period, but was not related to long-term survival.[7]

Both congenital and acquired disorders have been treated successfully with renal transplantation (**Box 1**). It is unclear whether patients in chronic renal failure secondary to amyloidosis are appropriate candidates because of the potential effects on the transplanted kidney. Patients with a history of pyelonephritis or recent infection have been treated successfully with transplantation if the infection is confined to one kidney and that kidney is removed before immunosuppression and transplantation. Cats with renal failure secondary to ethylene glycol toxicity should only be considered for transplantation after the elimination of the ethylene glycol and its metabolites from the body.

RECIPIENT EVALUATION

Extensive screening (**Box 2**) is performed before transplantation to identify any contraindications to moving forward with the procedure. At our facility, findings that preclude transplantation include severe cardiac disease, underlying neoplastic disease,

---

Box 1
Conditions successfully treated with transplantation

Acquired conditions
- Chronic interstitial nephritis (cat, dog); most common
- Oxalate nephrosis (cat)
- Membranous glomerulonephropathy (cat, dog)
- Toxic nephropathy; ethylene glycol, Lily (cat)
- Pyelonephritis (cat)

Congenital disorders
- Polycystic kidney disease (cat)
- Renal dysplasia (cat, dog)

Box 2
Preoperative screening for a potential feline renal transplant recipient
Complete blood cell count
Serum chemistry profile
Blood type and major and minor cross-match to donor (cat, dog)
Dog erythrocyte antigen matching and mixed lymphocyte response testing (dog)
Coagulation profile (dog)
Thyroid hormone level (T4)
Urinalysis, urine culture, urine protein: creatinine ratio
Abdominal radiography
Abdominal ultrasonography
Thoracic radiography
Electrocardiography, echocardiography, arterial blood pressure
Feline leukemia virus and feline immunodeficiency virus testing
Toxoplasmosis titer (IgG and IgM)
Heartworm testing (dog)

positive feline leukemia or feline immunodeficiency virus status, heartworm-positive status, recurrent or existing urinary tract infections that fail medical therapy or a cyclosporine challenge, uncontrolled hyperthyroidism, and a fractious temperament. Although cats with inflammatory bowel disease historically were not considered candidates because of the assumption that they may be at increased risk for allograft rejection, 6 cats with confirmed inflammatory bowel disease and 8 cats with suspected inflammatory bowel disease based on biopsy or ultrasonographic findings have been transplanted successfully at our facility with no episodes of allograft rejection reported (LR Aronson, personal communication, 2014). Recipient age has been identified as a factor associated with survival after discharge in both cats and dogs. In 1 feline study, median survival times decreased with advancing age, and in a second study, cats older than 10 years of age had higher mortality rates, particularly during the first 6 months after surgery. However, if no complications developed during the first 6 months, these patients did similarly to the younger population in the long term.[1,7] A third study found cats older than 12 years of age had a lower overall survival rate than younger cats.[8] In a study of 26 dogs that had undergone renal transplantation, for every 1-year increase in age, the odds of death by 6 months after surgery increased by 42%.[9] In cats, preoperative blood pressure and weight have also been shown to influence overall survival.[1]

Thoracic radiography performed preoperatively has identified significant soft tissue mineralization in 9 of 156 cats that have undergone renal transplantation at the author's facility (**Fig. 1**). All 9 cats had an elevated calcium × phosphate product that was significantly greater than cats that did not have evidence of soft tissue mineralization at the time of presentation. This finding was not associated with any complications preoperatively, during the surgical procedure, or in the long term.

Typing and Cross-Matching Incompatibilities

Because an owner may live a significant distance from a transplant facility, blood typing as well as determination of red blood cell crossmatch compatibility between

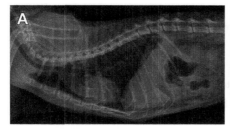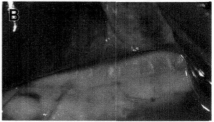

Fig. 1. Lateral thoracic radiograph of a cat in chronic renal failure. Note the significant soft tissue mineralization present involving the thoracic and abdominal aorta and the brachiocephalic trunk (A). Necropsy of a 4-year-old male castrated domestic short hair cat that died of complications after renal transplantation surgery (B). Note the striations of soft tissue mineralization within the thoracic aorta.

the recipient and potential feline kidney donors and blood donors should be performed before travel to the transplantation facility. Although uncommon, incompatible cross-match tests between AB-compatible donor and recipient pairs have been identified. Absence of a novel red blood cell antigen, identified as Mik, has resulted in naturally occurring anti-Mik alloantibodies after an AB-matched blood transfusion.[10] Additionally in dogs, dog erythrocyte antigen matching as well as mixed lymphocyte response testing is performed between recipients and potential donors.

Cardiovascular Disease and Hypertension

Systolic murmurs are common on presentation and most are thought to be physiologic and associated with anemia of chronic renal failure.[11] Structural cardiac abnormalities are also common in patients presenting for transplantation and most changes are no longer seen as a contraindication to surgery. In 1 study evaluating 84 potential recipients, 78% of patients had abnormalities including papillary muscle and septal muscle hypertrophy. It was suggested that these changes may be related to age, hypertension, chronic uremia, or early changes of hypertrophic cardiomyopathy.[12] No preoperative echocardiographic changes in that study were significant predictors of 1-month survival. In a second study evaluating 127 feline renal transplant recipients, preoperative echocardiographic changes including the presence of an arrhythmia, mitral and tricuspid regurgitation, systolic anterior motion of the mitral valve, septal muscle and left ventricular free wall hypertrophy, and increased aortic peak flow velocity, as well as radiographic evidence of heart failure at presentation were not associated with survival to discharge or long-term survival.[13] One study, however, did find increased left ventricular wall thickness as a risk factor for perioperative mortality.[1]

Preoperative hypertension is common in human transplant recipients and hypertension persisting in the postoperative period has been associated with graft damage and suboptimal outcomes.[14–17] The effect of preoperative and postoperative hypertension in cats is unclear. In 1 study, preoperative hypertension negatively influenced overall survival[1]; however, in our experience evaluating 127 transplant recipients, 38% were diagnosed with preoperative hypertension yet this factor was not associated with survival to discharge or decreased survival time.[13] In another study, preoperative hypertension did not predict episodes of postoperative hypertension and treatment with antihypertensive medication preoperatively did not decrease significantly the postoperative incidence of the condition.[7] Antihypertensive therapy should be initiated before transplantation if indicated. Intraoperative hypotension was a risk factor for perioperative mortality and decreased long-term survival in 1 report.[7] Cats with severe hypertrophic cardiomyopathy and atrial dilatation are rejected as candidates for renal transplantation. For cats with less severe disease, a decision regarding candidacy is made on a case-by-case basis.

Urinary Tract Evaluation

A thorough evaluation of the urinary tract is essential to identify underlying infection, obstruction, or neoplastic disease. A cyclosporine (Neoral, Sandoz Pharmaceuticals) challenge is required for patients with a history of urinary tract infections. Cyclosporine is administered for approximately 2 weeks at a recommended dose necessary to obtain therapeutic blood levels. Once appropriate levels are obtained, urine is subsequently evaluated at that time and at the end of the 2-week trial for the presence of an infection. Although negative urine culture results will not guarantee a patient will remain free from infection after transplantation, positive urine culture results will eliminate cats and dogs with occult infections as candidates for transplantation. It has been the author's experience that patients harboring an infection will often show clinical signs (lethargy, depression, anorexia) and have a positive urine culture within 48 to 72 hours after initiation of the cyclosporine trial.

Renal transplantation is a treatment option for cats whose underlying cause of renal failure is associated with calcium oxalate urolithiasis in conjunction with chronic interstitial nephritis.[18] For patients presenting with hydronephrosis secondary to obstructive calcium oxalate urolithiasis or another cause, pyelocentesis and culture are recommended. Immunosuppression in a patient harboring an infection can not only potentiate the rejection process but also lead to increased morbidity and mortality. If neoplasia or feline infectious peritonitis is suspected, a fine-needle aspirate or biopsy should be performed.

Evaluation for Infectious Disease

Significant morbidity and mortality has occurred secondary to the reactivation of latent *Toxoplasma gondii* infections, and for this reason serologic testing (IgG and IgM) for toxoplasmosis is now performed on all potential transplant recipients. Seropositive recipients are placed on lifelong prophylactic clindamycin (25 mg orally [PO] every 12 hours) in conjunction with their immunosuppressive therapy. Trimethoprim-sulfa (15 mg/kg PO every 12 hours) has also been used in cats that did not tolerate clindamycin therapy. Although seropositive donors are no longer used for seronegative recipients, successful transplantation has been performed between a seropositive donor and a seropositive recipient. Three patients at the author's facility that tested negative for *T gondii* before immunosuppression and transplantation, subsequently tested positive for the parasite within 3 months after surgery, and the infection was fatal in 2 of the 3 patients. For this reason, the author now recommends serologic testing (IgG and IgM) during the first 3 months after transplantation in patients that were seronegative before transplantation, and depending on the findings, subsequent evaluation should be performed regularly in the future.

Successful transplantation has been performed in cats with a history of upper respiratory tract infection. Cats with a history of an upper respiratory tract infection or those that have developed clinical signs of an upper respiratory tract infection during the perioperative period have been treated successfully with L-lysine, oral antibiotics, topical antibiotics, antiviral medication, and an appetite stimulant used alone or in combination (LR Aronson, personal communication, 2014).

KIDNEY DONORS

Standard screening of kidney donors includes a serum chemistry profile, complete blood count, blood typing, urinalysis and culture, and serologic testing for toxoplasmosis (IgG and IgM). Feline leukemia and feline immunodeficiency virus testing is performed additionally in cats and heartworm testing is performed in dogs. Computed tomographic angiography is performed to characterize the renal vasculature and to evaluate the renal parenchyma for any abnormalities such as infarcts that might exclude an animal from being a donor (**Fig. 2**).[19,20] In a study of 114 potential feline donors, 45 had multiplicity of the right renal vein, and 8 had multiple left renal arteries.[19] A suitable home is found for any donor candidate that fails the screening process. Perioperative morbidity and long-term outcome of unilateral nephrectomy has been evaluated recently in 99 feline kidney donors with a median interval between nephrectomy and follow-up of 10 years. Three cats developed stable, chronic renal insufficiency a median of 6.2 years after nephrectomy; 2 cats had episodes of acute kidney injury 4 and 6 years after kidney donation which resolved with medical therapy, and 1 cat was diagnosed with idiopathic cystitis, which resolved spontaneously. Renal-related deaths were identified in 6 cats; 4 died of acute ureteral obstruction secondary to calcium oxalate urolithiasis a median of 7 years after surgery, and 2 cats died of chronic renal failure, 12 and 13 years after kidney donation.[21] Although renal donation was not found to affect normal life expectancy in cats, because of the morbidity and mortality associated with stone formation in cats with 1 functioning kidney, abdominal radiographs are now recommended at yearly wellness visits to identify

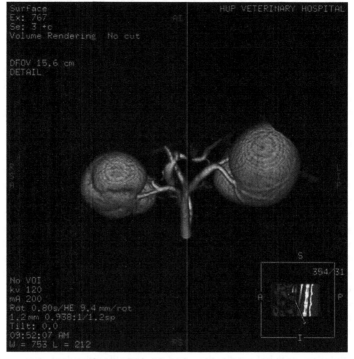

Fig. 2. Computed tomographic angiography of a potential renal donor. Note the multiple infarcts present associated with the right kidney. This cat was excluded as a potential donor.

any early evidence of new stone formation. In a study of 14 canine donors, renal and hematologic variables were normal in dogs evaluated up to 2.5 years after unilateral nephrectomy for kidney donation.[22]

PREOPERATIVE TREATMENT

Hemodialysis is performed before transplantation in anuric patients and those that are severely azotemic and develop pulmonary edema and/or pleural effusion when intravenous (IV) fluid therapy is initiated. After successful transplantation, IV fluid therapy can often be administered without complication in this population of patients. For hypertensive cats, the calcium channel blocker amlodipine (Norvasc) is often indicated before surgery. If a delay in the transplant procedure is expected and the patient is anemic, darbepoetin (6.25 mg/kg once a week for 2–4 weeks until the packed cell volume is approximately 25% and then every other week) can be administered and can reduce greatly the need for blood products during the perioperative period. At the time of surgery, depending on the stability of the patient, anemia is corrected with either packed red blood cells or whole blood transfusions. The first unit administered is preferably one that was collected previously from the crossmatch-compatible donor cat. If the patient is anorectic, an esophagostomy tube may be placed to administer nutritional support before and after surgery. Gastrointestinal protectants and phosphate binders are given if deemed necessary.

Immunosuppressive Therapy

The immunosuppressive protocol currently used for cats at our facility consists of the calcineurin inhibitor cyclosporine in combination with the glucocorticoid prednisolone. This combination also has been an essential component for immunosuppression in canine transplantation between related dogs. The mechanism of action of cyclosporine and glucocorticoids has more recently been elucidated in the cat. In 1 report, cyclosporine inhibited expression of messenger RNA for IL-2, IL-4, interferon-γ, and tumor necrosis factor-α in a dose-dependent manner.[23] In a second report, the use of cyclosporine significantly decreased production of interferon-γ, IL-2, and granulocyte macrophage colony stimulating factor.[24] Dexamethasone alone suppressed production of only granulocyte macrophage colony stimulating factor; when combined with cyclosporine, however, a significant decrease in production of interferon-γ, IL-2, and granulocyte macrophage colony stimulating factor occurred.[24] Inhibition of these cytokines is thought to be critical to graft survival, because they are known to play a role in human graft rejection.[25–27]

In cats, an oral liquid microemulsified formulation of cyclosporine (Neoral, 100 mg/mL) is recommended, so the dose can be titrated for each individual cat. Neoral also is preferred because of its better gastrointestinal absorption and more predictable and sustained blood concentrations.[11] Currently, cyclosporine therapy is initiated 72 hours before transplantation at a dose of 1 to 4 mg/kg PO every 12 hours depending on the patient's appetite. It has been the author's experience cats that are anorectic or hyporexic have a much lower drug requirement to obtain appropriate preoperative drug levels. Because of its bitter taste, cyclosporine is placed into a gelatin capsule before dosing. A 12-hour, whole-blood, trough concentration is obtained the day before surgery to allow adjustment of the preoperative oral dose into a therapeutic range. The ideal 12-hour trough concentration is 300 to 500 ng/mL measured by high-pressure liquid chromatography.[28] This level is maintained for approximately 3 months after surgery and then tapered to approximately 250 ng/mL for maintenance therapy.

Prednisolone therapy is begun the morning of surgery at 0.5 to 1.0 mg/kg every 12 hours PO and continued at that dosage for the first 3 months. The dosage is then tapered to once daily.

Antifungal medications delay the metabolic clearance of cyclosporine and have been used in conjunction with cyclosporine particularly in related dogs to help reduce the cost of posttransplant immunosuppression as well as improve the convenience of dosing for owners. In 1 protocol, after the administration of ketoconazole (10 mg/kg PO every 24 hours), cyclosporine and prednisolone are administered once a day, and cyclosporine doses are adjusted into the therapeutic range by measuring 24-hour whole blood trough levels.[29,30] Ketoconazole inhibits hepatic and intestinal cytochrome P450 oxidase activity, resulting in increased blood cyclosporine concentrations.[30] If signs of hepatotoxicity are identified, ketoconazole administration should be discontinued. Additionally, in dogs, cataract formation has been identified with use of ketoconazole. Itraconazole has been shown to exhibit less toxicity in human renal transplant patients and has recently been investigated in cats.[31] In a separate pharmacokinetic study and case report, the coadministration of the antibiotic clarithromycin with cyclosporine resulted in a significant increase in the bioavailability of cyclosporine in 4 research cats and was used successfully in conjunction with cyclosporine in a once a day protocol for a feline kidney transplant recipient.[32]

Mesenchymal Stem Cell Therapy

An area of growing interest is human transplantation is the use of autogenous mesenchymal stem cells (MSC) to lower the incidence of acute rejection, decrease the risk of opportunistic infections, and improve long-term outcomes. In preclinical models, MSC therapy has been shown to influence renal function and graft survival positively.[33,34] In a randomized controlled study in living-related kidney transplants in humans, the use of autogenous MSCs given at the time of reperfusion improved outcomes at 1 year, including better allograft function and a reduction in adverse events.[35] Recent in vitro work in cats found that feline MSCs and their supernatant reduced the formation of neutrophil reactive oxygen species in a dose-dependent manner when cocultured with feline neutrophils.[36] Although the use of stem cell therapy has the potential to offer great benefits to the feline renal transplant recipient, harvesting autogenous MSC's would require that the recipient undergo an additional surgical procedure performed 7 to 10 days before the transplant procedure. Performing an additional surgery will add to the overall cost of the transplant procedure and, in a debilitated patient, may result in significant morbidity.

ANESTHETIC MANAGEMENT

The anesthetic management for the feline renal transplant recipient has been described previously.[37] A sample anesthetic protocol for both recipient and donor is listed in **Box 3**. There are some practical points to consider with regard to the anesthetic management of these patients. Because both donor and recipient may be under anesthesia for an extended period of time, esophageal temperatures are monitored continuously, and a forced air warmer is used throughout the procedure to prevent hypothermia. A double-lumen indwelling jugular catheter is placed, preferably into the recipient's right jugular vein preserving the left side of the neck in the event esophagostomy tube placement is required. Electrolytes, packed cell volume/total protein, and venous blood gases as well as systemic arterial blood pressure via a noninvasive Doppler technique are monitored throughout the operation. Mannitol is administered to the donor cat at the time of the abdominal incision (0.25 g/kg of

---

Box 3
Sample anesthetic protocol for a renal donor and recipient

Donor

Preoperative
  Butorphanol: 0.5 mg/kg IM
  Telazol: 3-4 mg/kg IM

Epidural
  Bupivacaine: 0.1 mg/kg
  Morphine: 0.15 mg/kg

Induction
  Oxymorphone: 0.1 mg/kg
  Midazolam: 0.5 mg/kg
  Lidocaine: 1 mg/kg
  Etomidate: 0.2 mg/kg ± glycopyrrolate or atropine

Intraoperative
  Mannitol: 0.25 g/kg at the time of incision and 1 g/kg before nephrectomy

Postoperative
  Buprenorphine: 0.02 mg/kg 8 hr postinduction

Recipient

Epidural
  Bupivacaine: 0.1 mg/kg
  Morphine: 0.15 mg/kg

Induction
  Oxymorphone: 0.1 mg/kg
  Midazolam: 0.5 mg/kg
  Lidocaine: 1 mg/kg
  Etomidate: 0.2 mg/kg ± glycopyrrolate or atropine

Intraoperative
  Fentanyl infusion

Postoperative
  Buprenorphine: 0.02 mg/kg 8 hr postinduction
  Hydralazine if needed for hypertension: 2.5 mg/4 kg cat SC

Abbreviations: IM, intramuscularly; SC, subcutaneously.

---

mannitol IV) and 20 minutes before nephrectomy to minimize renal arterial spasms, improve perfusion, and to prevent tubular necrosis that can occur during the warm ischemia period. Mannitol (0.5–0.1 g/kg IV) is occasionally administered to the recipient if there is concern regarding perfusion of the allograft. Recently, the influence of anesthetic variables on both short- and long-term survival in the feline renal transplant recipient has been reported.[8] Prolonged anesthesia (>6 hours), intraoperative hypoxemia, and cats older than 12 years of age were all associated with reduced overall survival.[8] If severe hypertension occurs in the immediate postoperative period, it is treated with the subcutaneous administration of hydralazine (2.5 mg subcutaneously [SC] for a 4-kg cat).

For canine patients, enoxaparin (0.5–1.0 mg/kg SC every 24 hours) is administered the day before surgery and continued for 7 days after transplantation to prevent complications associated with thromboembolic disease. Additionally, because of the potential for an intussusception to occur after surgery, morphine is used as a premedicant to induce ileus, at the time of the initial incision and for pain management after surgery.

SURGERY

Allograft preparation and the surgical technique for feline and canine transplantation have been described previously.[38] Briefly, 3 surgeons participate in each procedure: 2 surgeons work on both the donor and recipient, and a third surgeon closes the donor after nephrectomy. At the time of the abdominal incision and just before nephrectomy, mannitol is administered to the donor. Some surgeons also recommend the alpha-adrenergic agonist, acepromazine (0.1 mg/kg IV).[29]

Preoperative computed tomographic angiography of the donor provides information about the renal vasculature, identifying cats that would be suitable for the surgical procedure. A single renal artery and vein with a minimal length of 0.5 cm are preferable (**Fig. 3**). The left kidney is preferred because it provides a longer vein than the right kidney. If multiple renal veins are present, the smaller vein can be sacrificed. The vasculature is cleared of as much fat and adventitia as possible, and the ureter is isolated for its entire length. Templates are made to accurately measure the width of the artery and vein to determine the sizes of aortotomy and venotomy to be performed in the recipient. At the authors' facility, vascular ligation and nephrectomy are performed when the recipient is prepared to receive the kidney. Alternatively, hypothermic storage to preserve the donor kidney can be performed until the recipient is prepared for surgery.[29,39] This technique minimizes ischemic injury that can occur to the kidney and can reduce personnel and resources needed for the procedure. If multiple arteries are identified in the donor, with the use of hypothermic storage, removing a segment of aorta that includes all arteries (Carrel patch), can be used to harvest the kidney.

An operating microscope with $5\times$ to $22\times$ magnification capabilities is used for the majority of the recipient's surgery. In the current technique, after the placement of vascular occlusion clamps, windows are created in the aorta and vena cava using the previously made templates. The aorta and vena cava are flushed with heparinized saline solution, and sutures of 8-0 nylon are preplaced at the cranial and caudal aspects of the window created in the aorta. The graft is harvested after the second mannitol infusion and then flushed with an ice cold phosphate-buffered sucrose organ preservation solution. The renal artery is anastomosed end-to-side to the caudal aorta using 8-0 nylon, and the renal vein is anastomosed end-to-side to the caudal vena cava using 7-0 silk (**Fig. 4**). The vascular clamps are removed and any hemorrhage

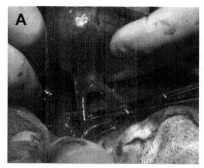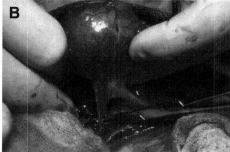

Fig. 3. Vascular dissection of the renal vein (*A*) and renal artery (*B*) in the kidney donor. The vasculature is cleared of as much fat and adventitia as possible down to the vena cava and aorta. The left kidney is preferred because it has a longer vein.

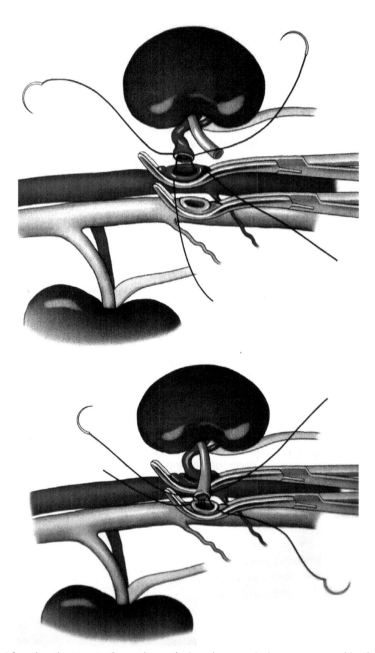

Fig. 4. After the placement of vascular occlusion clamps, windows are created in the aorta and vena cava and the aorta and vena cava are flushed with a heparinized saline solution. The renal artery is anastomosed end-to-side to the caudal aorta using 8-0 nylon and the renal vein is anastomosed end-to-side to the caudal vena cava using 7-0 silk.

along the suture lines are controlled with light pressure (**Fig. 5**). Any significant leaks may need to be repaired with additional sutures. If renal arterial spasm occurs after the release of the vascular clamps the application of topical lidocaine, chlorpromazine, or acepromazine has been effective in some cases to eliminate this problem.[29]

After the vascular anastomosis, a ureteroneocystostomy is performed to appose the ureteral and bladder mucosa. Both intravesicular and extravesicular techniques have been described.[11,40,41] At the authors' facility, an intravesicular mucosal apposition technique is used. After a ventral midline cystotomy, a mosquito hemostat is placed through the apex of the bladder and the end of the ureter grasped and brought into the bladder lumen. The bladder is everted, and the distal end of the ureter removed. The end of the ureter is spatulated, and the mucosa is sutured to the bladder mucosa using 8-0 nylon or Vicryl in a simple interrupted pattern (**Fig. 6**). After completion of the anastomosis, the bladder is inverted and closed routinely.

Two extravesicular techniques have also been described. In the first technique, the entire ureter and ureteral papilla with a 2-mm cuff of bladder are harvested from the donor and anastomosed to a 4-mm defect made at the apex of the recipient's bladder. The ureteral papilla is sutured in a 2-layer pattern—mucosa to mucosa and seromuscular layer to seromuscular layer.[41] (**Fig. 7**) In a second technique, a 1-cm seromuscular incision is made on the ventral surface of the bladder, allowing the bladder mucosa to bulge through the incision. A smaller incision (3–4 mm) is made through the bladder mucosa and the ureteral mucosa is sutured to bladder mucosa using 8-0 nylon (**Fig. 8**A). Once complete, the seromuscular layer is apposed in a simple interrupted pattern over the ureter with 4-0 absorbable suture (**Fig. 8**B).[11,42]

After cystotomy closure, the allograft is pexied to the abdominal wall to prevent torsion (**Fig. 9**). The recipient's native kidneys are typically left in place unless there is an indication for removal. Patients with polycystic kidney disease may require a unilateral nephrectomy to create space in the abdomen for the allograft. Before closure, a biopsy of one of the native kidneys is performed.

The surgical techniques for canine renal transplantation are similar to those described previously for cats, with a few minor differences. Magnification may or may not be necessary in dogs depending on patient size. For the vascular

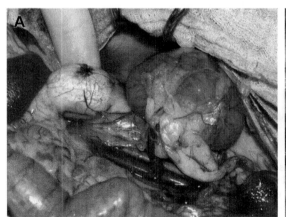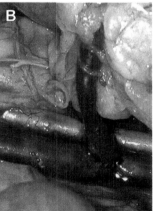

Fig. 5. Allograft after release of vascular clamps (*A*). Any hemorrhage along the suture lines are controlled with light pressure. Significant leaks may need to be repaired with additional sutures. Note a biopsy has been taken of the native kidney. Close up view of the vascular anastomosis (*B*).

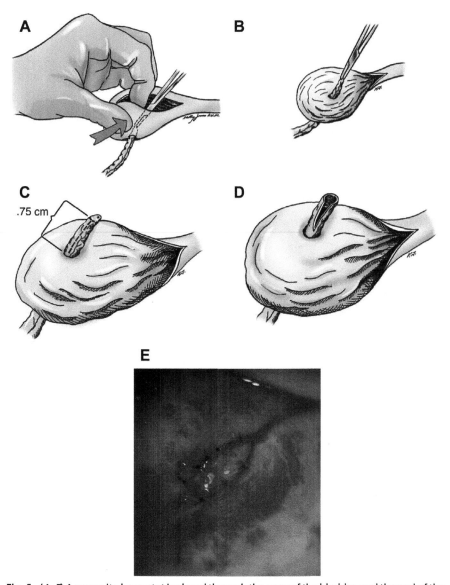

Fig. 6. (*A–E*) A mosquito hemostat is placed through the apex of the bladder, and the end of the ureter grasped and brought into the bladder lumen (*A, B*). The bladder is everted, and the distal end of the ureter removed. The end of the ureter is spatulated (*C, D*), and the mucosa is sutured to the bladder mucosa using 8-0 nylon or Vicryl in a simple interrupted pattern. It is important that no periureteral fat is exposed. ([*A–D*] *From* Aronson LR, Philips H. Renal transplant. In: Tobias KM, Johnston SA, editors. Veterinary surgery: small animal. Philadelphia: Saunders, 2012; with permission; and [*E*] *Courtesy of* Dr Daniel Degner, Animal Surgical Center of Michigan, Burton, MI).

anastomosis, the renal vessels can be anastomosed end to side to either the iliac vessels or to the caudal aorta and vena cava. Intestinal intussusception after renal transplantation and immunosuppression is common. For this reason, enteroplication is performed in all recipients.[43,44]

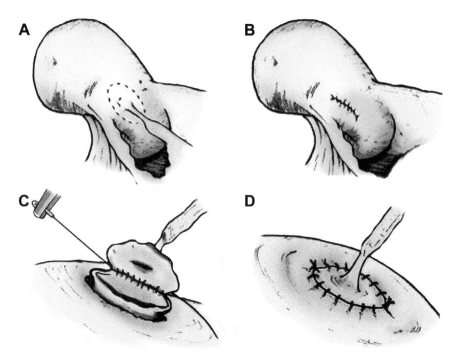

Fig. 7. Extravesicular technique for ureteroneocystostomy. The entire ureter and ureteral papilla are harvested from the donor (*A*, *B*) and anastomosed to a defect made at the apex of the recipient's bladder (*C*). The ureteral papilla is sutured in a 2-layer pattern—mucosa to mucosa and seromuscular layer to seromuscular layer (*C*, *D*). (*From* Renal transplant, in Tobias and Johnston. Veterinary Surgery Small Animal. Saunders; 2012. p. 2019-e407, Figure 119-6; with permission.)

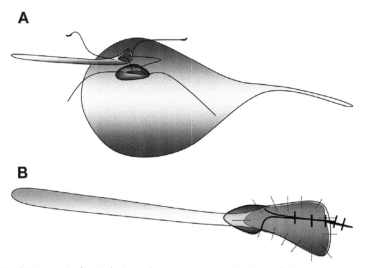

Fig. 8. (*A*, *B*) Extravesicular technique for ureteroneocystostomy. A 1-cm seromuscular incision is made on the ventral surface of the bladder, allowing the bladder mucosa to bulge through the incision. A smaller incision is made through the bladder mucosa, and the ureteral mucosa is sutured to bladder mucosa using 8-0 nylon. The seromuscular layer is apposed in a simple interrupted pattern over the ureter with 4-0 absorbable suture (*B*).

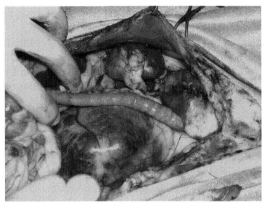

Fig. 9. The allograft is pexied to the left abdominal wall with nonabsorbable Prolene suture in an interrupted pattern to prevent torsion of the allograft. Note that, because of severe polycystic kidney disease, a left nephrectomy was required in this patient to create space in the abdomen for the allograft.

POSTOPERATIVE MONITORING AND TROUBLESHOOTING PERIOPERATIVE COMPLICATIONS

There are a number of aspects that need to be considered with regard to postoperative management that are critical to the success of each case (**Box 4**). Fine suture material is used for the vascular anastomosis and pexy of the allograft, and inappropriate patient handling can lead to catastrophic results and any patient struggling should be avoided. The placement of a double lumen catheter before the surgical procedure allows for minimal stress and handling during blood sampling. Many patients are under anesthesia for approximately 4 to 6 hours and hypothermia is a concern during the recovery period. Prevention or correction of hypothermia if needed in conjunction with prevention of hypotension will help to ensure appropriate allograft perfusion. If hypotension occurs (mean arterial pressure of <100), it needs to be treated aggressively with IV fluid boluses and then adjustments in maintenance fluid therapy and/or the

---

Box 4
Critical aspects to postoperative care

- Minimizing stress and handling
- Prevent hypothermia
- Fluid therapy and treating electrolyte imbalances
- Antibiotic therapy
- Pain management
- Monitor for seizure
- Treatment of hypertension
- Prevent hypotension
- Management of anorexia
- Regulate cyclosporine levels

administration of blood products to prevent acute tubular necrosis and delayed graft function.

Perioperative antibiotic therapy is continued until removal of the double lumen catheter and the patient is then switched to oral antibiotic therapy until the feeding tube is removed. If the cat is positive for *T gondii*, clindamycin (25 mg PO every 12 hours) administration is continued for the lifetime of the cat. Postoperative pain has been controlled successfully at our facility with methadone (0.15–0.3 mg/kg IV every 4–6 hours), buprenorphine (0.005–0.02 mg/kg IV every 4–6 hours), or a constant rate infusion of butorphanol (0.1–0.5 mg/kg/h).

Depending on the stability of the cat, packed cell volume, total protein, electrolytes, blood glucose, and acid–base status are evaluated initially 2 or 3 times daily and then as needed. A renal panel is evaluated every 24 to 48 hours, and voided urine is collected daily for assessment. Resolution of azotemia should occur within 24 to 72 hours after surgery. If improvement is not identified or if clinical status and renal function decline after initial improvement, an ultrasonographic examination of the allograft is recommended. The allograft is examined for appropriate renal blood flow and any signs of hydronephrosis or hydroureter. Emergency surgery may be warranted if evidence of obstruction exists. If graft perfusion is adequate and no evidence of obstruction exists, graft function may be delayed. If the transplanted kidney fails to function, the kidney should be biopsied before a second transplant is undertaken.

Hypophosphatemia in the early postoperative period has been reported to occur in 37% of cats after successful transplantation and may require treatment.[45] The development of hypophosphatemia after transplantation in cats does not affect survival. Blood cyclosporine concentrations are measured every 3 to 4 days, and the oral cyclosporine dose is adjusted as needed into the therapeutic range.

The occurrence of severe hypertension (>200 mm Hg) in the postoperative period has been associated with postoperative seizure activity in the feline renal transplant recipient.[46] The incidence of hypertension and its association with seizures has varied among veterinary transplant centers, and so the exact cause of neurologic complications in cats may be difficult to determine.[29] In cats, the occurrence of seizures was not correlated with intraoperative blood pressure, cholesterol or magnesium concentrations, serum electrolyte or blood glucose concentrations, osmolality, erythropoietin or cyclosporine administration, or the degree of azotemia.[47,48] In 1 study, an increase of 10 mg/dL in blood urea nitrogen or 1 mg/dL in serum creatinine would increase the likelihood of postoperative neurologic complications by 1.6- and 1.8-fold, respectively.[7]

Indirect blood pressure should be monitored every 1 to 2 hours during the first 48 to 72 hours for evidence of hypertension. If systolic blood pressure is equal to or greater that 180 mm Hg and the cat is not painful or anxious, the vascular smooth muscle relaxant hydralazine (Sidmack Laboratories; 2.5 mg/4 kg cat SC) should be administered. The dose can be repeated if systolic blood pressure does not decrease within 15 minutes. If hypertension is refractory to hydralazine, acepromazine (0.005–0.01 mg/kg IV) can be administered. The cause of postoperative hypertension is unclear in the feline renal transplant recipient, but it does not seem to be induced by ischemia–reperfusion injury or elevated plasma renin concentration after reperfusion of the graft.[49,50]

With resolution of azotemia and appropriate pain control, most cats will start eating within 24 to 48 hours after surgery. If continued anorexia is thought to be associated with alterations in gastric motility, the administration of metoclopramide (0.2–0.4 mg/kg SC every 6–8 hours) may improve the cat's appetite. If the cat remains anorexic, esophagostomy tube feeding is initiated.

LONG-TERM MANAGEMENT AND COMPLICATIONS

After discharge, patients are evaluated weekly for the first 6 to 8 weeks, and if stable the frequency of visits is gradually decreased. Eventually, the visits can be decreased to every 3 to 4 months for long-term maintenance. A thorough physical examination is essential in these patients; however, firm abdominal palpation should be avoided. Body temperature and weight are monitored carefully, and steady weight gain often begins within the first month after discharge. If the patient is doing well clinically, a renal panel, packed cell volume, total protein, cyclosporine level as well as evaluation of a free catch urine should be adequate at each visit. Typically, anemia secondary to chronic renal failure resolves within 1 month after surgery.[51] If anemia persists, but graft function remains adequate, iron supplementation should be considered. If concerns exist, a full complete blood count and serum chemistry panel as well as a urine culture should be performed. Regardless, a full complete blood count and chemistry profile should also be performed every 6 to 12 months, even in the stable patient. Toxoplasmosis titers should be performed regularly even in patients that tested negative before transplantation and immunosuppression. Echocardiography should be performed every 6 to 12 months in patients diagnosed with underlying cardiac disease before transplantation and treated accordingly if complications exits. If there are any concerns regarding allograft function, an abdominal ultrasound examination should be performed as an initial investigative step to identify any evidence for a urinary obstruction or thrombosis. The feeding tube is removed once oral intake of food and water is deemed appropriate.

LONG-TERM COMPLICATIONS

Complications can be divided into those causing allograft dysfunction and those secondary to immunosuppressive therapy (**Box 5**). Some of the more common complications are acute rejection, retroperitoneal fibrosis, and calcium oxalate urolithiasis.

Acute Rejection

The incidence of acute allograft rejection in the cat ranges from 13% to 26% and occurs most commonly within the first few months after surgery (**Fig. 10**).[1,52] Common

---

Box 5
Long term complications

Causes of allograft dysfunction

- Acute rejection
- Retroperitoneal fibrosis
- Calcium oxalate nephrosis
- Delayed graft function
- Hemolytic uremic syndrome
- Allograft rupture
- Vascular pedicle complications

Complications associated with immunosuppressive therapy

- Infection (bacterial, viral, fungal, parasitic)
- Diabetes mellitus
- Neoplasia

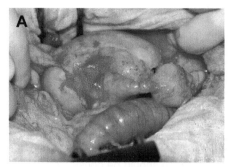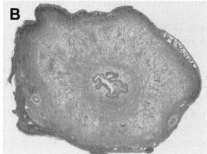

Fig. 10. Acute allograft rejection in an 8-year-old MC domestic long hair cat. The patient developed clinical signs of depression, anorexia, and lethargy with reoccurrence of azotemia within 1 month after surgery. The cat did not respond to the medical treatment for rejection. Ultimately, surgical removal of the graft was performed (*A*). On cross-section of the allograft ureter, severe ureteritis with granulation tissue and hemorrhage was observed (*B*).

causes of rejection include low cyclosporine concentrations, poor owner compliance, and presence of another disease process that potentiates the rejection episode. Clinical signs may include depression, decreased appetite, and polyuria/polydipsia; however, clinical signs in some affected animals may be minimal.[53] For this reason, frequent evaluation of cyclosporine levels is particularly critical during the early postoperative period to maintain the cyclosporine level in a therapeutic range and hopefully prevent changes in serum creatinine. Additionally, temperature should be monitored, because hyperthermia may be associated with allograft rejection.[54] Histopathologic, sonographic, and scintigraphic evidence of allograft rejection in cats has been described previously.[53–59]

The protocol for treatment of acute allograft rejection is listed in **Box 6**. If abdominal ultrasound examination capabilities are available at the clinic, the allograft should be evaluated to rule out a ureteral obstruction, and a urine sediment and culture should be evaluated to rule out an obvious infection. Treatment should not be delayed; therefore, these tests should only be performed before initiating therapy if these diagnostic capabilities are available in-house.

A rare complication of acute allograft rejection that has been identified in 2 cats is allograft rupture. The pathogenesis is thought to be related to an increase in intragraft

---

Box 6
Treatment for acute allograft rejection

Do not delay treatment

1. Place intravenous catheter and submit complete blood count, chemistry panel, packed cell volume, total solids, and cyclosporine level

2. Intravenous cyclosporine (50 mg/mL). Give 6.6 mg/kg of the solution slowly over 6 hours. Each milliliter of the IV solution should be diluted in to 20 to 100 mL 0.9% NaCl or D5W and administered as a constant rate infusion

3. Fluid bag and line should be covered so that the medication is not exposed to light

4. Solu-delta cortef: Give 10 mg/kg IV every 12 hours

5. If azotemia has not resolved, dosing can be repeated the following day

6. After resolution of azotemia, patient is placed back on oral medication

pressure and cortical and capsular ischemia secondary to interstitial/medullary edema and cellular infiltration.[60] A partial ureteral obstruction in conjunction with an infection potentiating a rejection episode was likely the cause of allograft rupture in a 5-year-old domestic shorthair cat.[60]

Retroperitoneal Fibrosis

Although partial and complete ureteral obstructions have occurred secondary to stricture or granuloma formation, the most common cause of ureteral obstruction is retroperitoneal fibrosis.[61,62] **(Fig. 11**A). Twenty-nine of 138 recipients (21%) developed clinically important retroperitoneal fibrosis a median of 62 days (range, 4–730 days) after renal transplantation. Similar to human patients, males were overrepresented (66%). In human transplant patient, the condition has been associated with infection, operative trauma, presence of foreign material such as talc, insufficient immunosuppression, urine leakage, or hemorrhage during the transplant procedure.[61,62] In human surgical patients who have not undergone a transplant, the condition has been identified secondary to a local inflammatory response to atherosclerotic disease and has occurred concurrently in patients with a systemic autoimmune disease. Hydronephrosis often without hydroureter is noted on abdominal ultrasound examination, and occasionally a capsule can be identified surrounding the allograft. Surgical ureterolysis has been successful in relieving the extraluminal compression and restoring normal renal function **(Fig. 11**B). Recurrence of the condition can occur and has been treated successfully with repeating surgical ureterolysis.[62]

Calcium Oxalate Urolithiasis

Previous work in cats has found that renal transplantation is a treatment option for cats whose underlying cause of renal failure is associated with calcium oxalate urolithiasis. No difference in long-term outcome was found in a control group of 49 cats whose underlying cause of renal failure was not related to stone disease and a group of 13 stone formers.[18] Development of calculi within the allograft occurred in 5 of the 13 cats and in 4 of these 5 cats calculi were found attached to the 8-0 nylon suture at the ureteroneocystostomy site **(Fig. 12**). Two cats that formed calculi after surgery were diagnosed with a concurrent urinary tract infection. A change in suture material to the use of absorbable suture material for the ureteroneocystostomy has eliminated the nidus for stone formation. Patients that are known stone formers should be screened more thoroughly for infection.

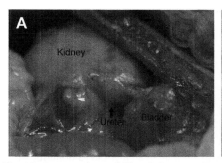 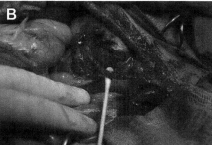

Fig. 11. Retroperitoneal fibrosis in a cat. Note the thick grey-white fibrous tissue surrounding the allograft kidney and ureter (A). Surgical ureterolysis. The ureter has been dissected free from the encasing fibrous tissue (elevated by Q-tip) and the mechanical obstruction of the ureter has been eliminated (B).

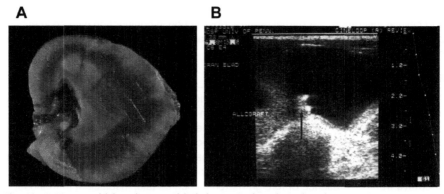

Fig. 12. A 10-year-old female spayed (FS) domestic short hair that developed an acute onset of azotemia 2 years after renal transplantation. Abdominal radiographs and ultrasound examination identified multiple calculi within the renal pelvis causing an obstruction. The owner elected euthanasia. Stone analysis revealed that the stones were 100% calcium oxalate (*A*). Abdominal ultrasound image of a different cat identified a ureteral obstruction secondary to calculi attached to the 8-0 nylon suture at the ureteroneocystostomy site (*arrow*) (*B*). Both cats were diagnosed with calcium oxalate urolithiasis in conjunction with chronic interstitial nephritis at the time of presentation for transplantation.

Immunosuppressive Therapy

Infection

Infectious complications, both acquired and opportunistic, are common in the feline renal transplant recipient and can result in morbidity and mortality and also may activate the rejection process (**Fig. 13**).[63,64] In a retrospective study of 169 feline recipients, 47 infections developed in 43 cats. Bacterial infections were most common followed by viral, fungal, and protozoal.[65] One-half of the infectious complications occurred within the first 3 months after surgery, when higher levels of immunosuppression were maintained. Risk of infection was increased in patients that developed diabetes mellitus.[65] The prevalence of certain types of infections vary depending on

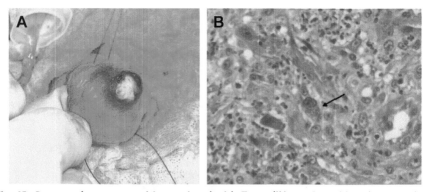

Fig. 13. Pyogranulomatous cystitis associated with *T gondii* in an 8-yr-old FS domestic short hair. A mass was identified on abdominal ultrasound 6 weeks after transplantation, resulting in a ureteral obstruction. Surgery was performed to remove the mass (*A*). Histologic examination of the mass revealed severe necrotizing pyogranulomatous cystitis with numerous intralesional tachyzoites and bradyzoite cysts (*arrow*) (*B*).

the location of the transplant facility. Infection was second only to rejection as the leading cause of death or euthanasia in the feline renal transplant recipient.[65] Treatment protocols and treatment success can vary greatly depending on the pathogen involved.

NEOPLASIA

In 3 separate veterinary studies, lymphoma was the predominant neoplasia identified (**Fig. 14**).[66–68] Similar to posttransplant lymphoproliferative disorders in humans, all lymphomas were mid- to high-grade, diffuse, large B-cell lymphomas.[69] The most likely mechanism for development of neoplasia in humans is the activation of latent oncogenic viruses such as the Epstein- Barr virus. Other potential mechanisms include promotion of DNA mutations from cyclosporine therapy, decreased immune surveillance and neoplastic cell clearance, and chronic antigenic stimulation from the allograft. In 2 recent studies, posttransplant malignant neoplasia occurred in 24% and 22.5% of the cases and cats that underwent transplantation and immunosuppression had a 6.1 and 6.6 times higher odds of developing a malignancy than a group of age-matched controls.[66,67] Additionally, cats undergoing renal transplantation and cyclosporine-based therapy had a 6.7 times higher odds of developing lymphoma compared with controls.[67] The development of neoplasia did not significantly affect overall survival.

DIABETES MELLITUS

The feline renal transplant recipient is 5.45 times as likely to develop diabetes mellitus compared with cats in chronic renal failure that have not undergone transplantation.[70] In a large multicenter study of 187 patients, 13.9% of cats developed posttransplant diabetes at a median of 132 days from the time of surgery.[70] The mortality rate for cats with diabetes mellitus was 2.38 times higher than that of the feline renal transplant recipients that did not develop diabetes and the median time from diagnosis until death was 275 days. Glycemic control can be successfully maintained with a number of management techniques, including dietary management, dose reduction of immunosuppressive therapy, and the use of glipizide or insulin therapy. In some cases, a combination of therapies is necessary.

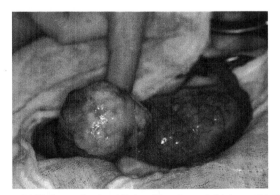

Fig. 14. An 11-year-old FS domestic short hair with a 1-week history of lethargy and vomiting approximately 22 months after renal transplantation. Abdominal ultrasound examination revealed a 10-cm mass involving segments of the small and large intestine. A biopsy of the mass confirmed lymphoma.

COMPLICATIONS IN DOGS

Information regarding the canine renal transplant recipient is limited. Commonly reported complications include thromboembolic disease, allograft rejection, infection (bacterial, fungal, or protozoal) of the respiratory tract, central nervous system, nasal cavity, skin, and upper and lower urinary tracts.[9,71–73] Two canine patients from the author's facility developed skin infections 16 weeks (*Nocardia* spp. and *Staphylococcus aureus*) and 17 weeks (*Mycobacterium* spp.) after transplantation; both responded to appropriate antibiotic therapy. Successful management of pneumonia secondary to a multidrug-resistant *Pseudomonas* has been described.[72]

Multiple types of neoplasia, including transitional cell carcinoma, ceruminous gland adenocarcinoma, and pheochromocytoma, were identified in 1 canine patient that survived 60 months after transplantation surgery.

OUTCOME

Renal transplantation in cats offers a unique method of treatment, improving a patient's quality of life and prolonging life expectancy compared with the medical management of renal failure. Based on published and unpublished reports, 70% to 93% of cats have been discharged after surgery, and median survival times have ranged from 360 to 653 days (LR Aronson, personal communication, 2015).[1,8,52] Currently at the authors' facility, the 6-month and 3-year survivals are 79% and 32%, respectively, and the longest survivor lived for approximately 13 years after his surgery. Continued experience with the management of both short- and long-term complications, as well as the ability to identify specific risk factors during the perioperative and postoperative period, will hopefully continue to improve long-term outcomes in these patients. Median survival was only 24 days (range, 0.5–4014) in a retrospective case series of 26 dogs.[9] One-half of the dogs in this study received a kidney from a related donor and one-half received a kidney from an unrelated donor. The lack of an effective protocol for immunosuppression in unrelated dogs suggests that, at this time, renal transplantation should be reserved only for dogs in which a compatible relative is available as a potential donor.[9]

REFERENCES

1. Schmeidt CW, Holzman G, Schwarz T, et al. Survival, complications and analysis of risk factors after renal transplantation in cats. Vet Surg 2008;37:683–95.
2. Boyd LM, Langston C, Thompson K, et al. Survival in cats with naturally occurring chronic kidney disease (2000-2002). J Vet Intern Med 2008;22(5):1111–7.
3. Kuwahara Y, Ohba K, Kitoh K, et al. Association of laboratory data and death within one month in cats with chronic renal failure. J Small Anim Pract 2006;47: 446–50.
4. King JN, Tasker S, Gunn-Moore DA, et al. Prognostic factors in cats with chronic kidney disease. J Vet Intern Med 2007;21:906–16.
5. Syme HM. Survival of cats with naturally occurring chronic renal failure is related to severity of proteinuria. J Vet Intern Med 2006;20:528–35.
6. Katayama M, McAnulty JF. Renal transplantation in cats: patient selection and preoperative management. Compend Contin Educ Pract Vet 2002;24: 868–72.
7. Adin CA, Gregory CR, Kyles AE, et al. Diagnostic predictors and survival after renal transplantation in cats. Vet Surg 2001;30:515–21.

8. Snell W, Aronson LR, Phillips H, et al. Influence of anesthetic variables on short-term and overall survival rates in cats undergoing renal transplantation surgery. J Am Vet Med Assoc 2015;247:267–77.
9. Hopper K, Mehl ML, Kass PH, et al. Outcome after renal transplantation in 26 dogs. Vet Surg 2012;41:316–27.
10. Weinstein NM, Blais MC, Harris K, et al. A newly recognized blood group in domestic shorthair cats: the Mik red cell antigen. J Vet Intern Med 2007;21:287–92.
11. Gregory CR, Bernsteen L. Organ transplantation in clinical veterinary practice. In: Slatter DH, editor. Textbook of small animal surgery. Philadelphia: WB Saunders; 2000. p. 122–36.
12. Adin DB, Thomas WP, Adin CA, et al. Echocardiographic evaluation of cats with chronic renal failure (abstract). ACVIM Proc 2000;714.
13. Phillips H, Mariano AD, Oyama M, et al. Characterization of preoperative cardiovascular status and association with outcome after feline renal allograft transplantation: 127 cases.
14. Cosio FG, Pelletier RP, Pesaunto TE. Elevated blood pressure predicts the risk of acute rejection in renal allograft recipients. Kidney Int 2001;59:1158–64.
15. Cosio FG, Pelletier RP, Sedmak DD, et al. Renal allograft survival following acute rejection correlates with blood pressure levels and histopathology. Kidney Int 1999;56:1912–9.
16. Opelz G, Wujciak T, Ritz E, et al. Association of chronic kidney graft failure with recipient blood pressure. Kidney Int 1998;53:217–22.
17. Raiss-Jalali GA, Fazelzadeh A, Mehdizadah AR. Effects of hypertension on transplant kidney function:3 years of follow-up. Transplant Proc 2007;39:941–2.
18. Aronson LR, Kyles AE, Preston A, et al. Renal transplantation in cats diagnosed with calcium oxalate urolithiasis:19 cases (1997–2004). J Am Vet Med Assoc 2006;228:743–9.
19. Bouma JL, Aronson LR, Keith DM, et al. Use of computed tomography renal angiography for screening feline renal transplant donors. Vet Radiol Ultrasound 2003; 44:636–41.
20. Caceres AV, Zwingenberger AL, Aronson LR, et al. Characterization of normal feline renal vascular anatomy with dual-phase CT angiography. Vet Radiol Ultrasound 2008;49:350–6.
21. Wormser C, Aronson LR. Peri-operative morbidity and long-term outcome of unilateral nephrectomy in feline kidney donors. J Am Vet Med Assoc 2016;248: 275–81.
22. Urie BK, Tillson DM, Smith CM, et al. Evaluation of clinical status, renal function, and hematopoietic variables after unilateral nephrectomy in canine kidney donors. J Am Vet Med Assoc 2007;230:1653–6.
23. Kuga K, Nishifuji K, Iwasaki T. Cyclosporine A inhibits transcription of cytokine genes and decreases the frequencies of IL-2 producing cells in feline mononuclear cells. J Vet Med Sci 2008;70:1011–6.
24. Aronson LR, Stomhoffer J, Drobatz K, et al. Effect of cyclosporine, dexamethasone and human CTLA4-Ig on production of cytokines in lymphocytes of clinically normal cats and cats undergoing renal transplantation. Am J Vet Res 2011;72: 541–9.
25. Halloran PF, Leung Lui S. Approved immunosuppressants. In: Tobias K, Johnston S, editors. Primer on transplantation. Thorofare (NJ): American Society of Transplant Physicians; 1998. p. 93–102.
26. Kahan BD, Yoshimura N, Pellis NR, et al. Pharmacodynamics of cyclosporine. Transplant Proc 1986;18:238–51.

27. Kim W, Cho ML, Kim SI, et al. Divergent effects of cyclosporine on Th1/Th2 Type cytokines in patients with severe, refractory rheumatoid arthritis. J Rheumatol 2000;27:324–31.
28. Bernsteen L, Gregory CR, Kyles AE, et al. Renal transplantation in cats. Clin Tech Small Anim Pract 2000;15:40–6.
29. Katayama M, McAnulty JF. Renal transplantation in cats: techniques, complications, and immunosuppression. Compend Contin Educ Pract Vet 2002;24:874–82.
30. McAnulty JF, Lensmeyer GL. The effects of ketoconazole on the pharmacokinetics of cyclosporine A in cats. Vet Surg 1999;28:448–55.
31. Katayama M, Katayama R, Kamishina H. Effects of multiple oral dosing of itraconazole on the pharmacokinetics of cyclosporine in cats. J Feline Med Surg 2010;12:512–4.
32. Katayama M, Nishijima N, Okamura Y, et al. Interaction of clarithromycin with cyclosporine in cats: pharmacokinetic study and case report. J Feline Med Surg 2012;14:257–61.
33. Baulier E, Favreau F, Le CA, et al. Amniotic fluid derived mesenchymal stem cells prevent fibrosis and preserve renal function in a preclinical porcine model of kidney transplantation. Stem Cells Transl Med 2014;3:809–20.
34. De Martino M, Zonta S, Rampino T, et al. Mesenchymal stem cells infusion prevents acute cellular rejection in rat kidney transplantation. Transplant Proc 2010;42:1331–5.
35. Tan J, Wu W, Xu X. Induction therapy with autologous mesenchymal stem cells in living-related kidney transplants: a randomized controlled trial. JAMA 2012;307:1169–77.
36. Mumaw JL, Schmiedt CW, Breidling S, et al. Feline mesenchymal stem cells and supernatant inhibit reactive oxygen species production in cultured feline neutrophils. Res Vet Sci 2015;103:60–9.
37. Valverde CR, Gregory CR, Ilkew JE. Anesthetic management in feline renal transplantation. Vet Anes Analgesia 2002;29:117–25.
38. Aronson LR, Phillips H. Renal transplant. In: Tobias K, Johnston S, editors. Textbook veterinary surgery- small animal. St Louis (MO): Elsevier; 2012. p. 2019–32.
39. McAnulty JF. Hypothermic storage of feline kidneys for transplantation: Successful ex vivo storage up to 7 hours. Vet Surg 1998;27:312–9.
40. Gregory CG, Lirtzman R, Kochin EJ, et al. A mucosal apposition technique for ureteroneocystostomy after renal transplantation in cats. Vet Surg 1996;25:13–7.
41. Hardie RJ, Schmiedt C, Phillips L, et al. Ureteral papilla implantation as a technique for neoureterocystotomy in cats. Vet Surg 2005;34:393–8.
42. Mehl ML, Kyles AE, Pollard R, et al. Comparison of 3 techniques for ureteroneocystostomy in cats. Vet Surg 2005;34:114–9.
43. Kelly GE, Drummond JM, Rogers JH, et al. Intussusception in dogs following renal homograft transplantation. Aust Vet J 1971;47:597–600.
44. Kyles AE, Gregory CR, Griffey SM, et al. Modified Noble plication for the prevention of intestinal intussusception after renal transplantation in dogs. J Invest Surg 2003;16:161–6.
45. Paster ER, Mehl ML, Kass PH, et al. Hypophoshatemia in cats after renal transplantation. Vet Surg 2009;38:983–9.
46. Kyles AE, Gregory CR, Wooldridge JD, et al. Management of hypertension controls postoperative neurological disorders after renal transplantation in cats. Vet Surg 1999;28:436–41.

47. Gregory CR, Mathews KG, Aronson LR, et al. Central nervous system disorders following renal transplantation in cats. Vet Surg 1997;26:386–92.
48. Mathews KG. Renal transplantation in the management of chronic renal failure. In: August J, editor. Consultation in feline internal medicine. 4th edition. Philadelphia: WB Saunders; 2001. p. 319.
49. Schmiedt CW, Mercurio A, Vandenplas M, et al. Effects of renal autograft ischemic storage and reperfusion on intraoperative hemodynamic patterns and plasma renin concentrations in clinically normal cats undergoing renal autotransplantation and contralateral nephrectomy. Am J Vet Res 2010;71:1220–7.
50. Schmiedt CW, Mercurio A, Glassman M, et al. Effects of renal autograft ischemic and reperfusion associated with renal transplantation on arterial blood pressure variables in clinically normal cats. Am J Vet Res 2009;70:1426–32.
51. Aronson LR, Preston A, Bhalereo DP, et al. Evaluation of erythropoiesis and changes in serum erythropoietin concentration in cats after renal transplantation. Am J Vet Res 2003;64:1248–54.
52. Mathews KG, Gregory CR. Renal transplants in cats: 66 cases (1987–1996). J Am Vet Med Assoc 1997;211:1432–6.
53. Kyles AE, Gregory CR, Griffey SM, et al. Evaluation of the clinical and histological features of renal allograft rejection in cats. Vet Surg 2002;31:49–56.
54. Halling KB, Ellison GW, Armstrong D, et al. Evaluation of oxidative stress markers for the early diagnosis of allograft rejection in feline renal allotransplant recipients with normal renal function. Can Vet J 2004;45:831–7.
55. Halling KB, Graham JP, Newell SP, et al. Sonographic and scintigraphic evaluation of acute renal allograft rejection in cats. Vet Radiol Ultrasound 2003;44:707–13.
56. Newell SM, Ellison GW, Graham JP, et al. Scintigraphic, sonographic, and histologic evaluation of renal autotransplantation in cats. Am J Vet Res 1999;60:775–9.
57. Kinns J, Aronson L, Hauptman J, et al. Contrast-enhanced ultrasound of the feline kidney. Vet Radiol Ultrasound 2010;31:168–72.
58. Pollard R, Nyland TG, Bernsteen L, et al. Ultrasonographic evaluation of renal autografts in normal cats. Vet Radiol Ultrasound 1999;40:380–5.
59. Schmiedt CW, Delaney FA, McNaulty JF. Ultrasonographic determination of resistive index and graft size for evaluating clinical feline renal allografts. Vet Radiol Ultrasound 2008;49:73–80.
60. Palm CA, Aronson LR, Mayhew PD. Feline renal allograft rupture. J Feline Med Surg 2010;12:330–3.
61. Aronson LR. Retroperitoneal fibrosis in four cats following renal transplantation. J Am Vet Med Assoc 2002;221:984–9.
62. Wormser C, Phillips H, Aronson LR. Retroperitoneal fibrosis in feline renal transplant recipients: 29 cases (1998-2011). J Am Vet Med Assoc 2013;243:1580–5.
63. Bernsteen L, Gregory CR, Aronson LR, et al. Acute toxoplasmosis following renal transplantation in three cats and a dog. J Am Vet Med Assoc 1999;215:1123–6.
64. Lo AJ, Goldschmidt MH, Aronson LR. Osteomyelitis of the coxofemoral joint due to Mycobacterium species in a feline transplant recipient. J Feline Med Surg 2012;14:919–23.
65. Kadar E, Sykes JE, Kass PH, et al. Evaluation of the prevalence of infections in cats after renal transplantation:169 cases (1987–2003). J Am Vet Med Assoc 2005;227:948–53.
66. Schmiedt CW, Grimes JA, Holzman G. Incidence and risk factors for development of malignant neoplasia after feline renal transplantation and cyclosporine-based immunosuppression. Vet Comp Oncol 2009;7:45–53.

67. Wormser C, Mariano A, Holmes E, et al. Post-transplant malignant neoplasia associated with cyclosporine-based immunotherapy: prevalence, risk factors and survival in feline renal transplant recipients. Vet Comp Oncol 2014. [Epub ahead of print].

68. Wooldridge J, Gregory CR, Mathews KG, et al. The prevalence of malignant neoplasia in feline renal transplant recipients. Vet Surg 2002;31:94–7.

69. Durham AC, Mariano AD, Holmes ES, et al. Characterization of post transplantation lymphoma in feline renal transplant recipients. J Comp Pathol 2014;150: 162–8.

70. Case JB, Kyles AE, Nelson RW, et al. Incidence of and risk factors for diabetes mellitus in cats that have undergone renal transplantation: 187 cases (1986–2005). J Am Vet Med Assoc 2007;230:880–4.

71. Gregory CR, Gourley IM, Taylor NJ, et al. Preliminary results of clinical renal allograft transplantation in the dog and cat. J Vet Intern Med 1987;1:53–60.

72. KyungMee P, Hyunsuk N, HeungMyong W. Successful management of multidrug resistant Pseudomonas aeruginosa pneumonia after kidney transplantation in a dog. J Vet Med Sci 2013;75:1529–33.

73. Mathews KA, Holmberg DL, Miller CW. Kidney transplantation in dogs with naturally occurring end stage renal disease. J Am Anim Hosp Assoc 2000;36: 294–301.

Index

Note: Page numbers of article titles are in **boldface** type.

Vet Clin Small Anim 46 (2016) 1219–1230
http://dx.doi.org/10.1016/S0195-5616(16)30083-3
0195-5616/16/$ – see front matter

UNITED STATES POSTAL SERVICE® Statement of Ownership, Management, and Circulation (All Periodicals Publications Except Requester Publications)

1. Publication Title	2. Publication Number	3. Filing Date
VETERINARY CLINICS OF NORTH AMERICA: SMALL ANIMAL PRACTICE	003 – 150	9/18/2016

4. Issue Frequency	5. Number of Issues Published Annually	6. Annual Subscription Price
JAN, MAR, MAY, JUL, SEP, NOV	6	$310.00

7. Complete Mailing Address of Known Office of Publication (Not printer) (Street, city, county, state, and ZIP+4®)

ELSEVIER INC.
360 PARK AVENUE SOUTH
NEW YORK, NY 10010-1710

Contact Person
STEPHEN R. BUSHING

Telephone (Include area code)
215-239-3688

8. Complete Mailing Address of Headquarters or General Business Office of Publisher (Not printer)

ELSEVIER INC.
360 PARK AVENUE SOUTH
NEW YORK, NY 10010-1710

9. Full Names and Complete Mailing Addresses of Publisher, Editor, and Managing Editor (Do not leave blank)

Publisher (Name and complete mailing address)

LINDA BELFUS, ELSEVIER INC.
1600 JOHN F KENNEDY BLVD. SUITE 1800
PHILADELPHIA, PA 19103-2899

Editor (Name and complete mailing address)

PATRICK MANLEY, ELSEVIER INC.
1600 JOHN F KENNEDY BLVD. SUITE 1800
PHILADELPHIA, PA 19103-2899

Managing Editor (Name and complete mailing address)

ADRIANNE BRIGIDO, ELSEVIER INC.
1600 JOHN F KENNEDY BLVD. SUITE 1800
PHILADELPHIA, PA 19103-2899

10. Owner (Do not leave blank. If the publication is owned by a corporation, give the name and address of the corporation immediately followed by the names and addresses of all stockholders owning or holding 1 percent or more of the total amount of stock. If not owned by a corporation, give the names and addresses of the individual owners. If owned by a partnership or other unincorporated firm, give its name and address as well as those of each individual owner. If the publication is published by a nonprofit organization, give its name and address.)

Full Name	Complete Mailing Address
WHOLLY OWNED SUBSIDIARY OF REED/ELSEVIER, US HOLDINGS	1600 JOHN F KENNEDY BLVD. SUITE 1800 PHILADELPHIA, PA 19103-2899

11. Known Bondholders, Mortgagees, and Other Security Holders Owning or Holding 1 Percent or More of Total Amount of Bonds, Mortgages, or Other Securities. If none, check box ▶ ☐ None

Full Name	Complete Mailing Address
N/A	

12. Tax Status (For completion by nonprofit organizations authorized to mail at nonprofit rates) (Check one)
The purpose, function, and nonprofit status of this organization and the exempt status for federal income tax purposes:
☐ Has Not Changed During Preceding 12 Months
☐ Has Changed During Preceding 12 Months (Publisher must submit explanation of change with this statement)

13. Publication Title	14. Issue Date for Circulation Data Below
VETERINARY CLINICS OF NORTH AMERICA: SMALL ANIMAL PRACTICE	JULY 2016

PS Form 3526, July 2014 [Page 1 of 4 (see instructions page 4)]   PSN 7530-01-000-9931   PRIVACY NOTICE: See our privacy policy on www.usps.com.

15. Extent and Nature of Circulation			Average No. Copies Each Issue During Preceding 12 Months	No. Copies of Single Issue Published Nearest to Filing Date
a. Total Number of Copies (Net press run)			919	971
b. Paid Circulation (By Mail and Outside the Mail)	(1)	Mailed Outside-County Paid Subscriptions Stated on PS Form 3541 (include paid distribution above nominal rate, advertiser's proof copies, and exchange copies)	486	591
	(2)	Mailed In-County Paid Subscriptions Stated on PS Form 3541 (include paid distribution above nominal rate, advertiser's proof copies, and exchange copies)	0	0
	(3)	Paid Distribution Outside the Mails Including Sales Through Dealers and Carriers, Street Vendors, Counter Sales, and Other Paid Distribution Outside USPS®	175	225
	(4)	Paid Distribution by Other Classes of Mail Through the USPS (e.g. First-Class Mail®)	0	0
c. Total Paid Distribution (Sum of 15b (1), (2), (3), and (4))		▶	661	816
d. Free or Nominal Rate Distribution (By Mail and Outside the Mail)	(1)	Free or Nominal Rate Outside-County Copies Included on PS Form 3541	70	85
	(2)	Free or Nominal Rate In-County Copies Included on PS Form 3541	0	0
	(3)	Free or Nominal Rate Copies Mailed at Other Classes Through the USPS (e.g. First-Class Mail)	0	0
	(4)	Free or Nominal Rate Distribution Outside the Mail (Carriers or other means)	70	85
e. Total Free or Nominal Rate Distribution (Sum of 15d (1), (2), (3) and (4))		▶	70	85
f. Total Distribution (Sum of 15c and 15e)		▶	731	901
g. Copies not Distributed (See Instructions to Publishers #4 (page 83))		▶	188	70
h. Total (Sum of 15f and g)		▶	919	971
i. Percent Paid (15c divided by 15f times 100)		▶	90%	91%

* If you are claiming electronic copies, go to line 16 on page 3. If you are not claiming electronic copies, skip to line 17 on page 3.

16. Electronic Copy Circulation		Average No. Copies Each Issue During Preceding 12 Months	No. Copies of Single Issue Published Nearest to Filing Date
a. Paid Electronic Copies	▶	0	0
b. Total Paid Print Copies (Line 15c) + Paid Electronic Copies (Line 16a)	▶	661	816
c. Total Print Distribution (Line 15f) + Paid Electronic Copies (Line 16a)	▶	731	901
d. Percent Paid (Both Print & Electronic Copies) (16b divided by 16c × 100)	▶	90%	91%

☒ I certify that 50% of all my distributed copies (electronic and print) are paid above a nominal price.

17. Publication of Statement of Ownership

☒ If the publication is a general publication, publication of this statement is required. Will be printed in the NOVEMBER 2016 issue of this publication. ☐ Publication not required.

18. Signature and Title of Editor, Publisher, Business Manager, or Owner

Stephen R. Bushing   Date 9/18/2016

STEPHEN R. BUSHING - INVENTORY DISTRIBUTION CONTROL MANAGER

I certify that all information furnished on this form is true and complete. I understand that anyone who furnishes false or misleading information on this form or who omits material or information requested on the form may be subject to criminal sanctions (including fines and imprisonment) and/or civil sanctions (including civil penalties).

PS Form 3526, July 2014 (Page 2 of 4)

Moving?

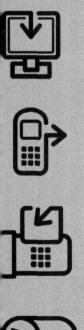

Make sure your subscription moves with you!

To notify us of your new address, find your **Clinics Account Number** (located on your mailing label above your name), and contact customer service at:

Email: journalscustomerservice-usa@elsevier.com

800-654-2452 (subscribers in the U.S. & Canada)
314-447-8871 (subscribers outside of the U.S. & Canada)

Fax number: 314-447-8029

Elsevier Health Sciences Division
Subscription Customer Service
3251 Riverport Lane
Maryland Heights, MO 63043

*To ensure uninterrupted delivery of your subscription, please notify us at least 4 weeks in advance of move.

Edwards Brothers Malloy
Ann Arbor MI. USA
March 13, 2017